THE

ART OF MASSAGE:

ITS

PHYSIOLOGICAL EFFECTS AND THERAPEUTIC APPLICATIONS.

BY J. H. KELLOGG, M. D.,

MEMBER OF THE BRITISH GYNÆCOLOGICAL SOCIETY, THE INTERNATIONAL PERIODICAL CONGRESS
OF GYNÆCOLOGY AND OBSTETRICS, AMERICAN AND BRITISH ASSOCIATIONS FOR THE
ADVANCEMENT OF SCIENCE, THE SOCIÉTÉ D'HYGIÈNE OF FRANCE, AMERICAN
SOCIETY OF MICROSCOPISTS, AMERICAN CLIMATOLOGICAL SOCIETY, AMERI-
CAN ELECTRO-THERAPEUTIC ASSOCIATION, TRI-STATE MEDICAL
SOCIETY, AMERICAN MEDICAL ASSOCIATION, MICHIGAN
STATE MEDICAL SOCIETY, SUPERINTENDENT OF
THE BATTLE CREEK (MICH.) SANITARIUM.

BATTLE CREEK, MICH.

Must Have Books
503 Deerfield Place
Victoria, BC
V9B 6G5
Canada

ISBN: 9781773238395

Copyright 2022 – Must Have Books

PREFACE.

Massage is a subject which to the rational physician is one of greatest interest and importance. Twenty years ago its employment, as well as the use of electricity and hydrotherapy, was generally regarded by the profession as closely allied to quackery. Up to that time, scientific massage was almost unknown in this country, although various rude manipulations were practiced by bonesetters, so-called "magnetic healers;" and a few superannuated nurses who claimed to be specially gifted in "rubbin'." Twenty-two years ago, when the writer first made a study of massage and passive movements as a therapeutic means, even the term "massage" was as unfamiliar to the medical profession of this country as it still is to the majority of the laity. After obtaining such a knowledge of massage as was at that time possible at home, I visited Sweden, Germany, France, and other European countries, with the purpose of becoming acquainted with the methods employed by the most expert manipulators abroad; and from the knowledge thus obtained, as well as that gleaned from the various treatises and papers which have appeared upon the subject within the last twenty years, added to my personal experience in the constant employment of ten to twenty masseurs and masseuses, in the treatment of patients suffering from a great variety of chronic ailments, I have endeavored to summarize and condense in this little work the facts which are essential to a scientific knowledge of the art and science of massage and its rational employment.

It should be mentioned that, since this manual is intended for the use of medical students and student nurses, technical expressions have been omitted, as far as possible, only such anatomical facts and terms having been presented as are essential to a correct understanding of the subject.

One of the most conspicuous faults of a majority of the treatises upon the subject which have heretofore appeared, has been the absence of specific directions for the various procedures recommended. There has also been, in many instances, a failure to present in a sufficiently lucid and concise manner, the indications and contra-indications for the employment of this important therapeutic means. It is not expected that this little work will, in itself, be capable of rendering any one an adept in the art of massage, as personal instruction is absolutely indispensable, to give even to a person possessed of much natural ability, the dexterity necessary for real expertness. Nevertheless, it is believed that the work will be found of very great assistance to all who wish to practice this art, and especially in the training of classes in connection with Training Schools for Nurses.

A special feature of the work to which the writer desires to call attention is the classification of the different procedures of massage, which is believed to be more complete and systematic than any which has heretofore appeared. By a careful study of all the different procedures described by the best authorities and employed by expert manipulators, it was found possible to include all in seven different general classes with subdivisions, each of which has been described with a very considerable degree of painstaking care.

A careful study of the physiological effects of massage and its practical use during many years, based upon a knowledge of its physiological effects, has enabled the writer to develop a number of new procedures which are presented for the first time in this work, and which it is believed will be found to be of great practical value. Among these may be named as especially worthy of mention, Reflex Stroking and Percussion, Inspiratory Lifting, and several procedures in connection with pelvic and abdominal massage, two of the most important forms in which this valuable therapeutic agent is employed.

It is hoped that the numerous illustrations presented with the text will be found a valuable aid in obtaining exact ideas of the mode of applying to the different parts of the body the various procedures described. The half-tone engravings were made directly from photographs prepared with great care, under the author's immediate supervision. The anatomical plates are copies of the famous studies by Bock.

The most important paragraphs in the book, especially those of a practical character, have been numbered, both for handy reference from one part of the book to another, and also for the convenience of the practitioner who may wish to give special directions to the masseur. It should be remembered that it is not expected that the formulæ for either general or local massage will be slavishly followed. The experienced masseur or the physician may modify the typical formulæ given, by omitting certain procedures or giving special prominence to others, as the indications in each case may suggest.

Nearly every patient who requires massage, sooner or later reaches a stage of improvement at which active voluntary exercises should, in part at least, take the place of those of a passive character.

As a means of systematic, graduated exercise the author especially commends the excellent system of medical gymnastics developed by Ling, of Sweden. With the concurrence of Professor Hartelius, for many years director of the Central Institute of Gymnastics at Stockholm, the excellent work published by him has been translated, and is published by the Modern Medicine Co. simultaneously with this volume. It ought to be in the hands of every masseur.

In the first Appendix will be found a few cases illustrative of the benefits to be derived from massage. The number of cases might be increased sufficiently to fill several large volumes, but only a few — those of a typical character — have been selected for the purpose of demonstrating to those not personally familiar with the great benefits to be derived from this rational mode of treatment, the efficiency of skillful manipulations as a therapeutic measure.

Among the various works consulted by the author in the

preparation of this manual, special mention should be made of the excellent treatises by Graham, Reibmayr, Murrell, Dowse, Schreiber, and Tibbitts, together with numerous articles which have appeared in English, French, and German medical literature within the last few years, among which particular mention should be made of papers by Eccles, Poliakow, Vineberg, Rosenblith, Franks, Landerer, Kesch, Oertel, Petit, Gilles, Dujardin-Beaumetz, and Mervy. J. H. K.

Battle Creek, Mich., April, 1895.

PREFACE TO SECOND EDITION.

SCARCELY two years had elapsed after the publication of the first edition of two thousand copies of this work before the author was admonished by the publishers that nearly the entire edition was exhausted, and a new edition was called for.

In carefully looking through the work to prepare it for the new edition, the writer has been able to correct numerous little verbal and typographical errors which are the almost unavoidable defects of a first edition ; and has also been able to add to the text a few items of practical interest, which it is believed will be appreciated. Perhaps chief among these is the description of the so-called Schott method of treatment in cardiac disease, employed so successfully at Nauheim, in connection with the effervescing baths. This method, while more properly belonging to the Swedish system of Manual Swedish Movements than to massage, is in practice so inseparable from the procedures technically known as "massage" that it does not seem improper to make it a part of this work. This important addition to the subject matter of the work will be found in Appendix II, beginning with page 277.

Thanking the medical profession for the cordial welcome accorded the first edition of this work, and the hundreds of nurses who have honored the author by accepting this work as a practical guide and text-book, the author dares to express the hope that in its present revised and improved form his effort to systematize and elucidate the important subject considered in this little work may still be recognized as a useful contribution to the armamentarium of rational therapeutics.

J. H. K.

Battle Creek, Mich., November, 1897.

TABLE OF CONTENTS.

1 *

LIST OF PLATES.

[xi]

THE ART OF MASSAGE.

ITS HISTORY.

MASSAGE, or systematic rubbing and manipulation of the tissues of the body, is probably one of the oldest of all means used for the relief of bodily infirmities. There is evidence that massage was employed by the Chinese as early as 3000 B. C. Their literature contains treatises upon the subject written some thousands of years ago. An ancient Chinese book entitled, "The Cong-Fou of the Tao-Tse," of which a French translation appeared about a century ago, was probably the foundation both of our modern massage and of the manual Swedish movements so admirably elaborated and systematized by Ling. Massage is still very extensively employed by the Chinese, and also by the Japanese, who doubtless learned the art from the Chinese.

Among the Japanese, massage is employed almost exclusively by blind men, who go about the streets soliciting patronage by shouting in a loud voice the words *Amma! amma!* (shampooing, or massage). Fig. 1 represents one of these blind masseurs crying his vocation upon the streets of Mito, Japan. Fig. 2 shows one of them administering massage to a lady patient. These engravings are photo-reproductions from photographs kindly sent to the writer by a friend in Japan. The same friend also sent the following description of his personal experience with Japanese massage, which was administered to him by a first-class manipulator, for the relief of a severe cold accompanied with fever : —

[9]

"The shampooer sat in Japanese fashion at the side of the patient, as the latter lay on a *futon* (thick comforter or quilt) on the floor, and began operations on the arm ; then took the back and the back of the neck, afterward the head (top and forehead), and ended with the legs. On the arms, back, back of the neck, and legs, he used sometimes the tips of his fingers, sometimes the palms or the backs of his hands, sometimes his knuckles, sometimes his fists. The movements consisted of pinching, slapping, stroking, rubbing, knuckling, kneading, thumping, drawing in the hand, and snapping the knuckles. The rubbing in the vicinity of the ribs was slightly ticklish, and the knuckling on the back of the neck, and at the side of the collar bone, a little painful. On the head he used gentle tapping, a little pounding with his knuckles, stroking with both hands, holding the head tight for a moment, grasping it with one hand and stroking with the other. The operator seemed to have a good practical knowledge of physiology and anatomy, and certainly succeeded in driving away the headache and languor, in producing a pleasant tingling throughout the body, and in restoring the normal circulation of the blood. He is to be criticised, however, for one serious fault in his operations,—that of shampooing down, instead of up. A portion of the good done is thus neutralized, one object of scientific massage being to help back toward the center the blood which is lingering in the superficial veins."

I do not agree with my friend's criticism of the mode of manipulation employed by the Japanese masseur, who seems to have been more skilled than most of our own manipulators, since he was apparently aware of the fact that the limbs should be rubbed down, rather than up, for the relief of the condition of feverishness and irritation from which his patient was suffering.

Massage has been employed from the most ancient times by the Hindoos and Persians, who still practice it, some of their native masseurs being possessed of remarkable skill. The ancient Greeks and Romans also employed massage constantly in connection with their famous baths. Hippocrates, the renowned Greek physician, made extensive use of this mode of

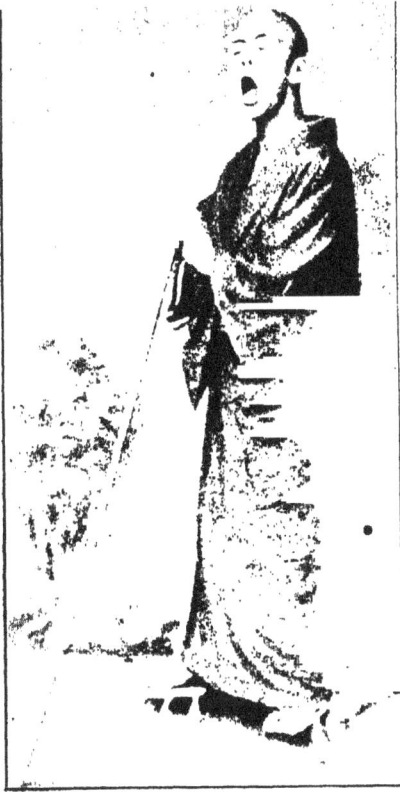

Fig. 1. Blind Japanese Masseur
Soliciting Patronage.

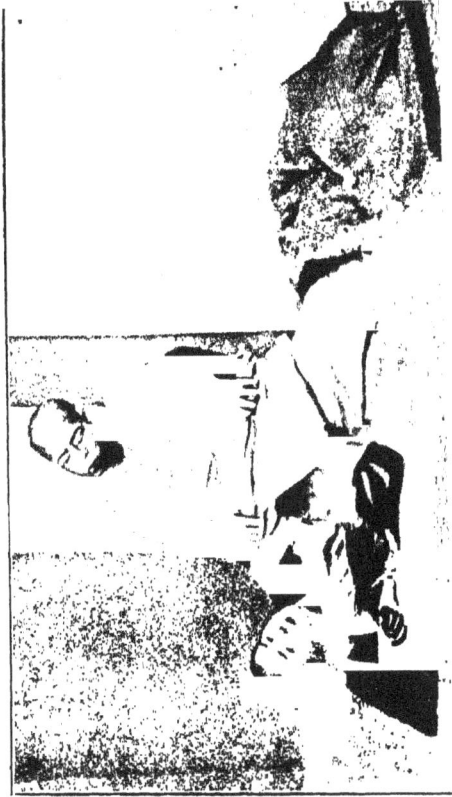

Fig. 2. Blind Japanese Masseur Treating
a Patient.

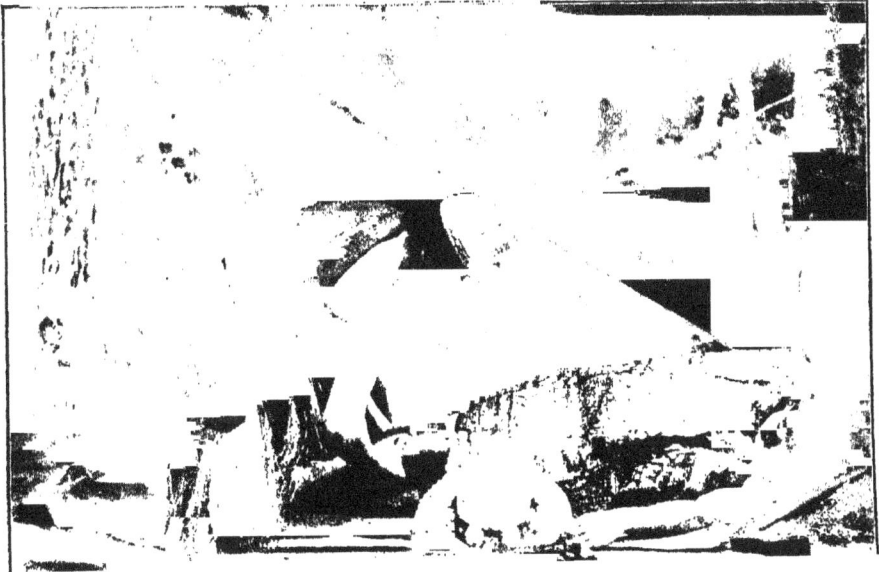

treatment, designating it *anatripsis*. He evidently appreciated the principles of the art very well, as he directed that friction should be applied centripetally, or in the direction of the veins. That he understood the effects of different modes of application is shown by the following quotation from his works: "Friction can relax, brace, incarnate (fleshen), attenuate; hard, braces; soft, relaxes; much, attenuates; and moderate, thickens." [1] Hippocrates learned massage, as well as gymnastics, from his teacher Herodicus, the founder of medical gymnastics. Asclepiades, another eminent Greek physician, held the practice of this art in such esteem that he abandoned the use of medicines of all sorts, relying exclusively upon massage, which he claimed effects a cure by restoring to the nutritive fluids their natural, free movement. It was this physician who made the discovery that sleep might be induced by gentle stroking.

Plutarch tells us that Julius Cæsar, a century before the Christian era, had himself pinched all over daily for neuralgia. It is well known that Julius Cæsar was subject to a severe nervous disorder (epilepsy), and it is more than probable that his prodigious labors were only rendered possible by the aid derived from massage. Pliny, the great Roman naturalist, had himself rubbed for the relief of chronic asthma. Arrian recommended massage for horses and dogs, asserting that it would strengthen the limbs, render the hair soft and glossy, and cleanse the skin. After giving directions for massage of the legs, abdomen, and back, he directed that the treatment should be terminated in the following peculiar manner, which indicates that he understood the value of nerve-stretching, at least for dogs: "Lift her up by the tail, and give her a good stretching; let her go, and she will shake herself and show that she liked the treatment."

Celsus, the most eminent of all Roman physicians, who lived at the beginning of the present era, was very familiar with massage, and used great discretion in its application.

---

[1] Genuine Works of Hippocrates, Vol. II, page 16.

He recommended manipulations of the head for the relief of headache, and general manipulations to restore the surface circulation in fever, making this wise remark: "A patient is in a bad state when the exterior of the body is cold, the interior hot with thirst; but, indeed, also, the only safeguard lies in rubbing." Galen, the greatest physician of his time, in the second century recommended massage in many diseases. He seems to have had a good understanding of the various forms of friction and kneading.

A sort of percussion, called whipping, was employed by the ancient Roman physicians in various diseases, and is still used by the Laplanders and the Finns, who beat the body with bundles of birch twigs.

The natives of the Sandwich Islands have, from the most ancient times, employed massage, which they term *lomi-lomi*. They frequently administer *lomi-lomi* to an exhausted swimmer while in the water, supporting him with their hands until his forces are rallied by the manipulations. The Maoris of New Zealand practice massage under the name of *romi-romi*. The accompanying cut (Fig. 3) shows a Polynesian, a son of a chief, administering the treatment. The natives of Tonga Island employ massage under the name of *toogi-toogi*, the literal meaning of which is "to beat," for the relief of sleeplessness, fatigue, etc. In cases of insomnia, the manipulations are confined to the arms and legs.

Paracelsus, the prince of charlatans, who flourished at Basle, Switzerland, four hundred years ago, made great use of massage, and taught it to his pupils in the medical school of that city. Massage has been used in France for two hundred years. It was much employed in the early part of the present century by eminent English surgeons, especially in the treatment of sprains and other injuries of the joints. Its use in modern times, however, is chiefly due to its systematic development and employment by Mezger, of Amsterdam.

STRUCTURES ESPECIALLY CONCERNED IN MASSAGE.

Massage, in its varied applications, has either direct or indirect relation to every structure and function of the body; but in its ordinary applications, this therapeutic measure directly and immediately affects especially the following : —

1. *The skin*, with its connective tissue network, its sebaceous and sweat glands, hair follicles, and the infinite number of minute blood vessels and sensitive terminal nerve filaments — trophic, vasomotor, and sensory.

2. *The connective tissue* lying just beneath the skin, with its rich supply of veins and lymph vessels and spaces.

3. *The muscles* which chiefly constitute the fleshy portions of the body, and which receive special attention in the various manipulative procedures of massage, both as individual muscles and as functional groups.

4. *The large blood vessels*, both veins and arteries, but principally the veins, the circulation of which may be readily accelerated or impeded according as the manipulations are applied in the direction in which the blood runs in the veins, or in the opposite direction. The large lymph channels which usually accompany the larger veins are also brought directly under the influence of massage through appropriate manipulations. The heart itself may be reached by certain special procedures, and is greatly influenced by nearly all forms of manipulation.

5. *The large nerve trunks*, which, with the terminal nerve filaments, are influenced by all forms of manipulation, but especially so by certain procedures which are particularly efficacious in producing stimulating or sedative effects.

6. *All the large viscera of the abdomen,*— stomach, colon, small intestines, pancreas, spleen, liver, kidneys,—which may be brought more or less directly under the influence of massage by a skilled operator; while less directly, but still effectively, the lungs and heart may also be influenced by certain procedures.

7. *The bones, joints, and ligaments* must also be mentioned as structures which are directly affected by massage.

The student of massage should make a careful study of the muscles, bones, and joints, and, in fact, so far as possible, of the entire anatomy. To facilitate this study, a number of colored plates have been prepared, which are exact reproductions of the famous copper-plate engravings prepared under the direction of the eminent German anatomist, Bock. A careful study of these plates will give the student a very fair idea of the general form of the structures with which he must chiefly deal in administering massage; but it is also important that he should make a careful study of the human body, if possible by attending a course of dissections. If this cannot be done, the dissection of an animal will be helpful. Some valuable knowledge may be gained even by the dissection of so small an animal as a cat or a small dog. If possible, such dissections should be made under the direction of a competent teacher, as their value will thereby be greatly enhanced.

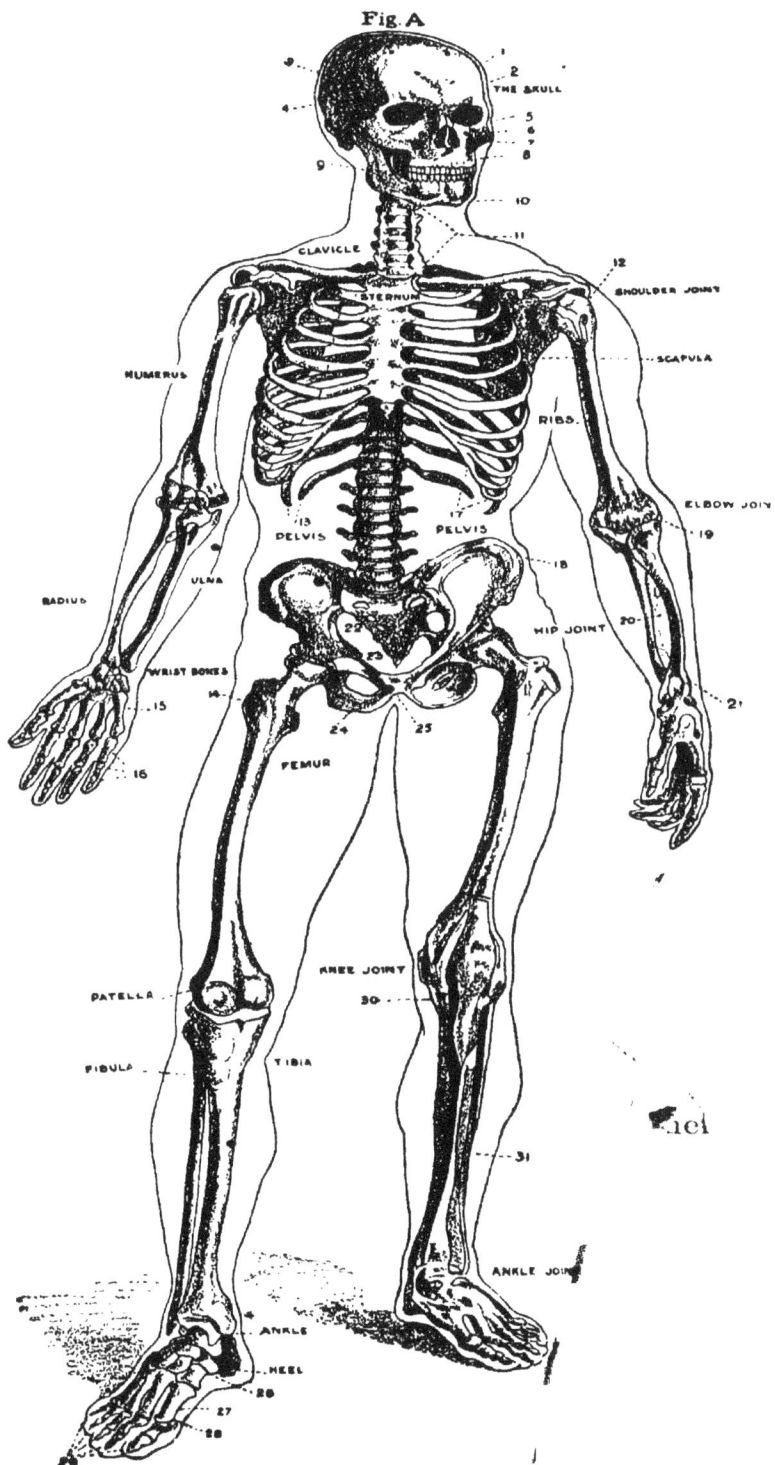

Fig. A

9
1
2
THE SKULL
4
5
6
7
8
9
10
11
CLAVICLE
12
SHOULDER JOINT
STERNUM
SCAPULA
HUMERUS
RIBS
ELBOW JOINT
13
17
19
PELVIS
PELVIS
18
RADIUS
ULNA
20
22
HIP JOINT
23
WRIST BONES
15
14
24
25
21
16
FEMUR
KNEE JOINT
PATELLA
30
FIBULA
TIBIA
31
ANKLE JOINT
ANKLE
HEEL
26
27
28
29

Fig. 4. The Skeleton

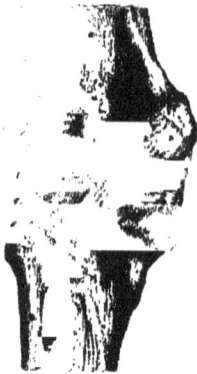

Fig. 10.

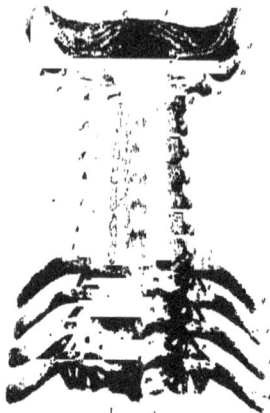

Fig. 6.

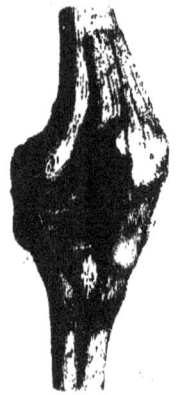

Fig. 8.

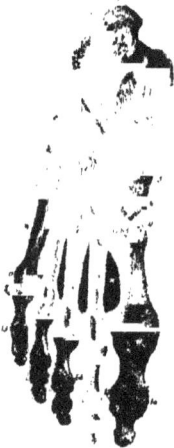

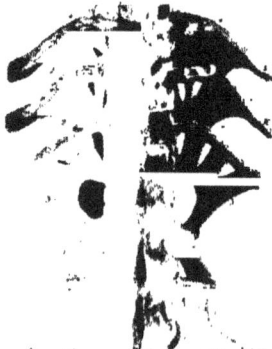

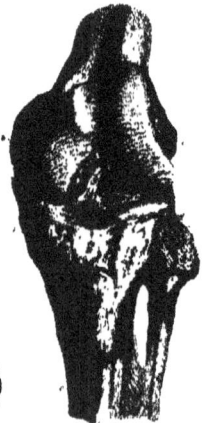

Fig. 11 (a.)

Fig. 11 (b.)

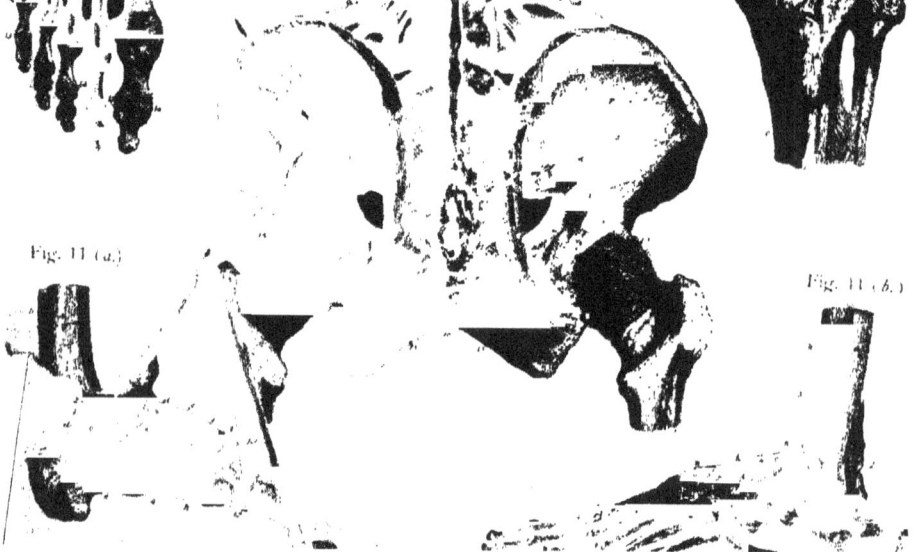

PARTS TO BE ESPECIALLY STUDIED BY THE MASSEUR.

A proper understanding of massage and its skillful application requires a good knowledge of anatomy. Physiology is also of the highest value to the masseur, but a practical study of anatomy is absolutely indispensable. This is not the place for a detailed anatomical consideration of the body, but the learner may perhaps be somewhat assisted by the following brief enumeration of some of the anatomical structures with which he must become familiar : —

The Bones.—First of all, the student of massage should make a serious study of the bones (Fig. 4), as in all the manipulations of massage their conformation must be kept carefully in mind. Every bony prominence, hollow, furrow, ridge, articulating surface, together with the points of origin and insertion of the principal muscles ; in relation to the skull, the points of entrance and exit of nerve trunks, arteries, and veins; also the joints and ligaments (Figs. 5–11b), should be made thoroughly familiar by a minute and careful study of the skeleton. The following points in relation to the skeleton should receive special attention : —

1. *Head :* Vertex, occiput, parietal eminence, mastoid process, zygoma, temporal fossa, orbit, angle of lower jaw.

2. *Neck :* Cervical vertebræ, vertebra prominens, hyoid bone.

3. *Chest :* Dorsal vertebræ ; twenty-four ribs (on each side, seven true ribs, three false ribs, two floating ribs); sternum, cartilages of ribs, xiphoid cartilage.

4. *Arm :* Shoulder bones, consisting of the scapula, or shoulder blade, with its spine, acromion process, coracoid pro-

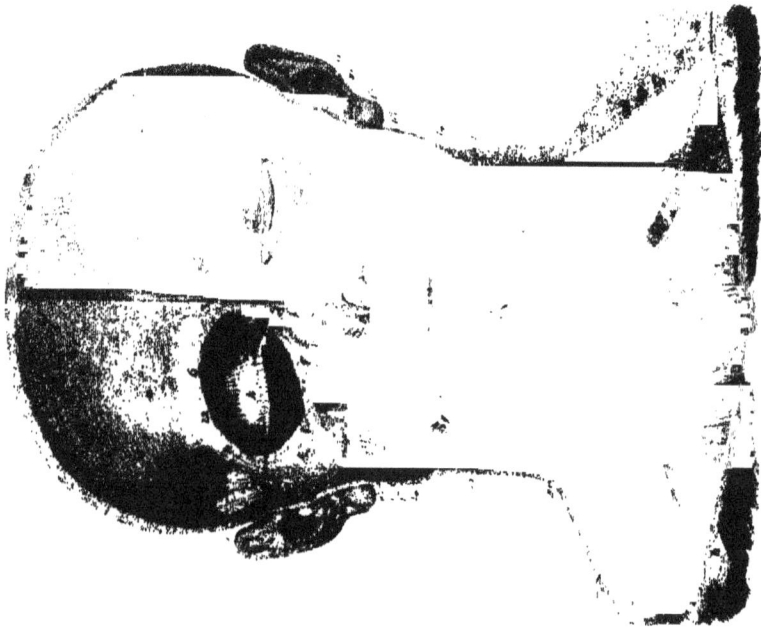

Fig. 13.

Fig. 13. Muscles of Face.

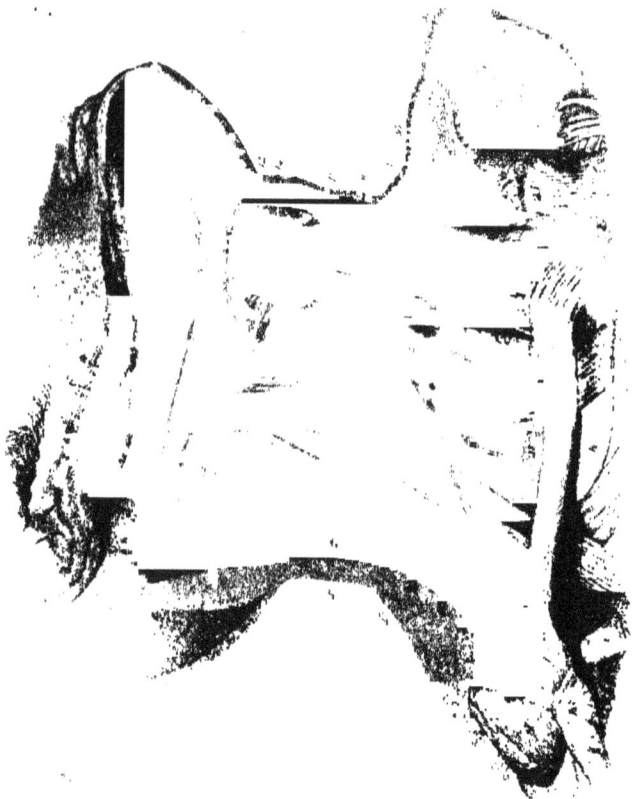

Fig. 14. Muscles of Neck.

7. *Abdomen :* Rectus, external oblique, quadratus lumborum (Fig 15).

8. *Shoulder :* Deltoid and supra-spinatus, which raise the arm ; infra-spinatus and teres minor, which rotate arm outward and hold shoulders back ; teres major and latissimus dorsi, which rotate arm inward and draw arm to side (Fig 16).

9. *Arm :* Anterior, flexors — biceps, coraco-brachialis, and brachialis; posterior, extensor — triceps (Fig. 15).

10. *Forearm :* Radial (thumb) side, supinators, extensors, and thumb flexor; ulnar (little finger) side, flexors, pronator teres (Fig. 15).

11. *Hand:* Palmar surface — short flexors of fingers; dorsal surface — interossei.

12. *Hip:* Glutei, which rotate thigh outward and inward and abduct it; obturators and pyriformis, which tilt pelvis forward, increasing obliquity of the pelvis (important in relation to correct standing). With thighs flexed upon abdomen, nearly all the muscles of the hip except the obturator externus (which rotates femur outward) act as abductors (Figs. 18, 19).

13. *Thigh :* Anterior, extensors, quadriceps (Fig. 17) ; posterior, flexors (Fig. 19) ; internal, adductors (Fig. 20).

14. *Lower Leg:* Inner portion — extensors of foot and flexors of toes, gastrocnemius (Fig. 20) ; anterior, flexors of foot and extensors of leg, tibialis anticus (Fig. 17) ; outer and upper — extensors, peronei (Fig. 18).

15. *Foot :* Plantar surface, flexors of toes; dorsal, interossei.

Veins.— The arteries are not so important in massage as are the veins, as they lie too deep to be influenced to any considerable degree by the manipulations ordinarily employed.

1. *Neck:* Jugular (Fig. 21).

2. *Arm:* Axillary and brachial (upper); cephalic (outer); basilic (inner) (Fig. 21).

3. *Forearm:* Radial (outer) ; anterior ulnar (inner); median anterior, posterior ulnar (posterior) (Fig. 21).

4. *Leg:* Femoral (upper anterior); long saphenous (inner anterior, beginning at arch of foot); short saphenous (posterior

2

outer, beginning behind the outer malleolus); popliteal (Figs. 22, 25).

The Nerves.— So large a proportion of the physiological effects obtained by the employment of massage being the result of reflex action, it is highly important that the masseur or the student of massage should have a good knowledge of the physiology of the nervous system.   The more he knows of anatomy the better, but he must know the names and location of the principal nerve trunks.   The location of those which will be mentioned is so clearly shown upon the colored plates that it will not be necessary to do more than name them here.

1. *Face :* Facial, trifacial (Fig. 27).

2. *Arm :* Median, ulnar, musculo-spiral (Figs. 23 and 24).

3. *Leg :* Crural, sciatic (Fig. 25).

The *sacral nerve* passes across the sacro-iliac synchondrosis, or junction of the sacrum and ilium.

The *pneumogastric*, or *par vagum*, is the large nerve from the brain, which passes down the side of the neck, entering the chest just behind the top of the sternum, near the median line. It is distributed to the heart, lungs, and all the abdominal viscera (Fig. 27).

The *sympathetic nerve* controls the function of the digestive organs, kidneys, liver, and other viscera of the abdomen, all the glands of the body, and the action of the heart and blood vessels.   Its principal divisions of interest to the masseur are the cervical ganglia, the renal plexus, the hepatic plexus, the lumbar or umbilical ganglia (situated at the back of the abdominal cavity and two inches on either side of the umbilicus), and the subumbilical ganglion, or lumbar aortic plexus, located two inches below the umbilicus (Fig. 27).

The Viscera.— Nearly all the contents of the abdomen and pelvis may be brought under the direct influence of massage.   Their general form and normal location should be carefully studied (Figs. 28, 29, 30, 31); viz., the heart, stomach, pancreas, liver and gall bladder, spleen, kidneys (right lower than left), colon, appendix vermiformis, bladder, prostate gland, uterus, Fallopian tubes, and ovaries.

Landmarks and Regions. — While the profound knowledge of surgical landmarks and regions important for the physician is not needed by the masseur, some knowledge of this kind is essential to skillful work. The student is advised to familiarize himself with the following, by the aid of a good anatomy: —

Linea alba, the median line of the body, extending from the sternum to the pubes.

Linea semilunaris, the outer border of the rectus muscle.

Umbilicus, commonly called the navel, located, in symmetrical persons, midway between the end of the sternum and the pubes, normally higher in women than in men.

Poupart's ligament, the fibrous band connecting the anterior superior spine of the ilium with the spine of the pubes.

External inguinal ring, an opening in the abdominal wall just above the spine of the pubes, through which the spermatic cord passes in the male and the round ligament in the female; larger in men than in women.

Femoral ring, an opening below Poupart's ligament, the seat of femoral hernia; larger in women than in men.

Axilla, the armpit, space under the arm bounded by tendons, in front by the pectoral muscles, and behind by the sub-scapular, teres major, and latissimus dorsi muscle. Enlarged glands are often found in the axilla.

Groin, the fold at the junction of the leg with the body, a little below Poupart's ligament. A number of enlarged glands are often felt in this region, even in healthy persons.

Popliteal space, the space underneath the knee. It contains large vessels and nerves, hence too strong pressure in this region should be avoided.

Fold of the buttocks, the furrow just below the buttock, marking the lower border of the large gluteal muscle.

The *regions* of the abdomen may be said to be nine in number, divided by lines drawn upon the surface (Fig. 30), — right hypochondriac, left hypochondriac, epigastric, right lumbar, left lumbar, umbilical, right inguinal, left inguinal, hydrogastric.

THE PHYSIOLOGICAL EFFECTS OF MASSAGE.

1   The interest in the therapeutic applications of massage which has increased so rapidly within the last twenty years has led to numerous investigations by able 'physiologists for the purpose of determining with exactness the physiological effects of the various procedures included under the general term *massage*, and thus obtaining a correct basis for their therapeutic use. Many of these experiments have been repeated and verified by the writer in the physiological laboratory under his charge in connection with the Battle Creek Sanitarium, and some of the results will be recorded in an Appendix, in addition to this brief summary of the conclusions which have thus far been obtained by those who have most carefully studied the subject. These investigations have established beyond all possibility of question, that massage affords one of the most effective means of influencing the functions of the human body.

.   Experiments clearly show that every function of both animal and organic life may be powerfully influenced by some or all of the numerous procedures of massage. The various effects produced may be included under the following heads : —

2   1. *Mechanical*, in which the tissues are wholly passive, being simply acted upon in a mechanical way by the hand of the manipulator, as in the movement of the blood and lymph in the venous and lymph channels, or the restoration of a displaced viscera to its normal positions

3   2. *Reflex*, in which the peripheral and central portions of the nervous system, both cerebro-spinal and sympathetic, are chiefly active, an impression made upon the nerve ends of

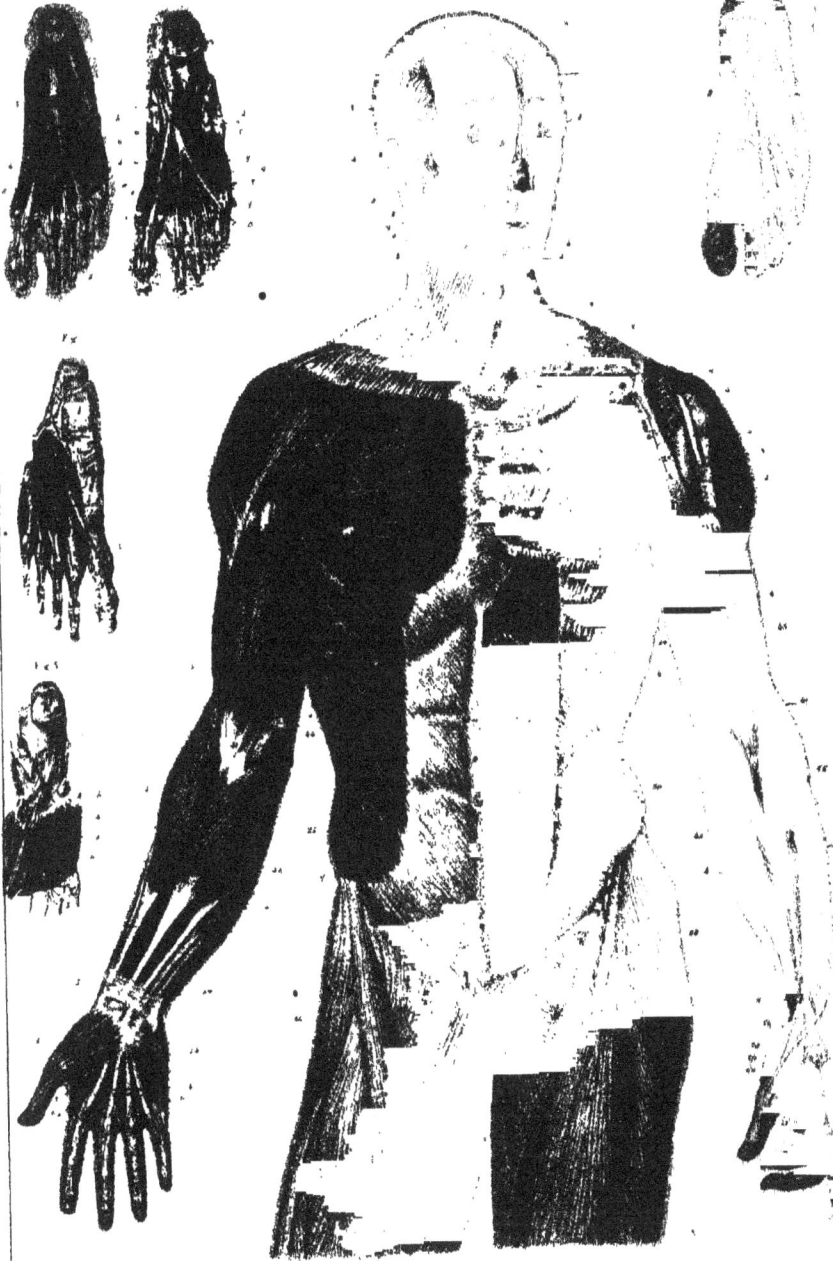

Fig. 16

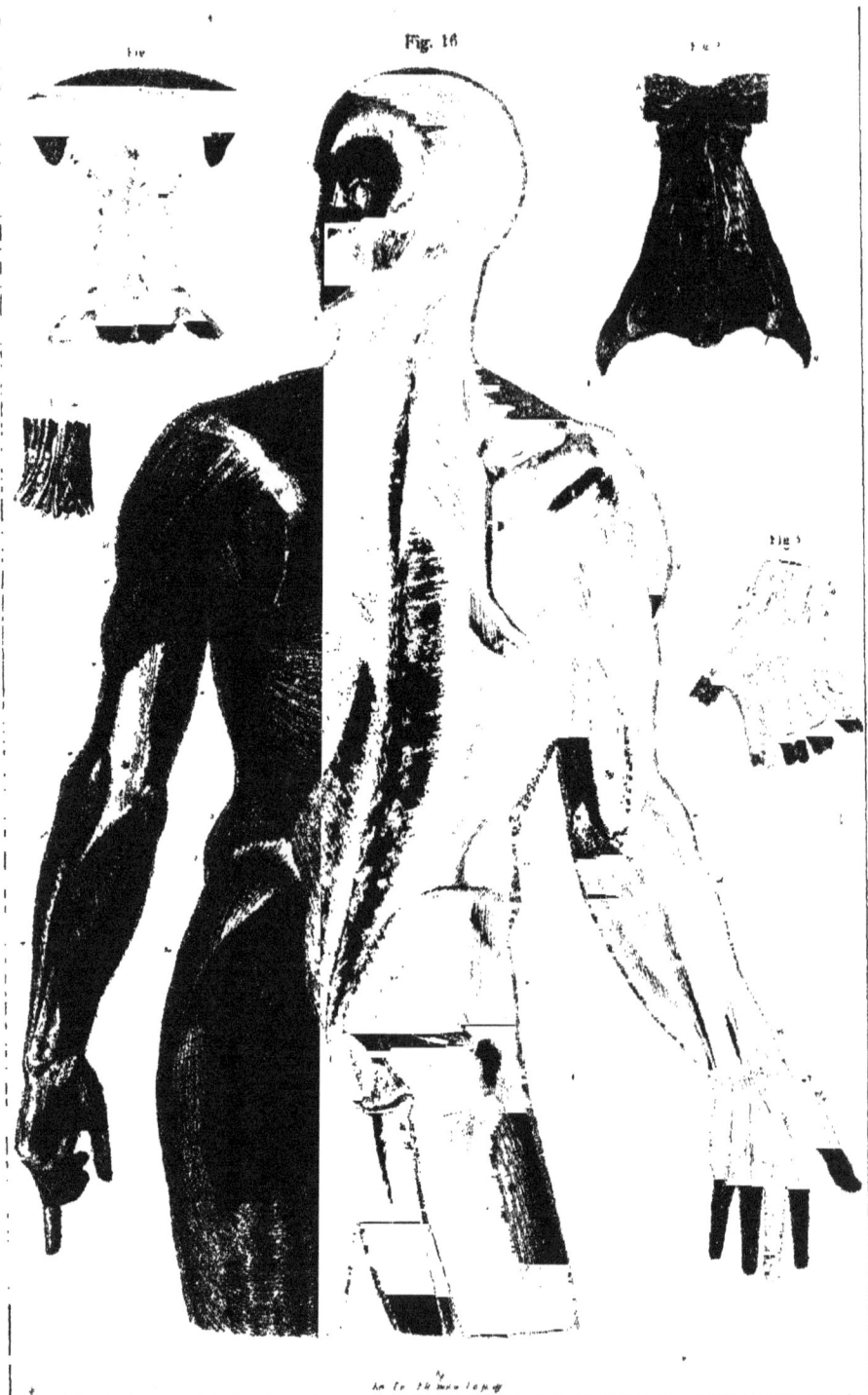

Fig. 16. Muscles of Trunk and Arms — Posterior View.

the sensory or afferent fibers connected with the nerve centers of the cerebro-spinal and sympathetic systems being transmitted to the related centers, where new activities are set up, resulting in the sending out of nerve impulses by which vital changes are effected, not only in the parts directly acted upon, but in related parts.

3. *Metabolic*, in which important modifications occur in the 4 tissue activities both of the parts directly operated upon and of the body as a whole, as the result in part of the direct mechanical effects of massage upon the tissues, and in part of the reflex activities set up by it.

In a brief manual like this there is not space to consider in detail the *modus operandi* of all the different effects of massage. We must be content with a simple enumeration of the specific effects upon the principal systems and functions of the body.

Effects of Massage upon the Nervous System.— 5 All the different procedures of massage produce a decided effect upon the nervous system through the influence of the manipulations upon the nerve endings of both the cerebrospinal and the sympathetic nerves, which are found in so great abundance in the skin and muscles—the former in connection with the special senses of locality, temperature, pressure, and weight; the latter more especially in connection with the glands, blood vessels, and thermic mechanism located in the skin and muscles.

1. *Direct Stimulating Effects.*—Vibration and nerve com- 6 pression may be made to act directly upon nerve trunks, thereby causing powerful stimulation not only of the peripheral nerves but of all the nerve centers with which a nerve trunk is connected.

Friction is an effective means of exciting languid nerves. 7

Light percussion simply increases nervous irritability, while 8 strong percussion may cause so great a degree of nervous irritability as to exhaust the nerves, and thus produce a benumbing effect.

9   Tapping, slapping, clapping, and hacking are the most effective means of exciting nerve trunks.

Beating and vigorous hacking are especially useful for exciting the nerve centers, and hence are especially applicable to the spine. The nerve centers may also be directly excited by deep vibration and by strong percussion.

10   2. *Reflex Effects.*—The reflex effects of massage are very remarkable and exceedingly interesting. All the procedures of massage produce powerful reflex effects. Some of the most striking effects are produced by very light stroking, especially when applied to certain reflex areas. (See Reflex Stroking.)

11   Percussion and vibration are also powerful means of producing reflex effects, which include not simply muscular action, but increase or decrease of vascular and glandular activity, and general tissue change.

12   3. *Sedative Effects.*—The sedative effects of massage are equally as marked as the stimulating effects. Strong percussion relieves pain in the same manner as does strong faradization, by tiring out and thus obtunding nerve sensibility. Pinching produces an anæsthetic effect in essentially the same way. The physician always pinches the skin before introducing the hypodermic needle.

13   Sedative effects are also produced by gentle stroking — the so-called hypnotic effect, doubtless, through reflex influence upon the nerve centers.

14   Very marked sedative effects are produced by derivative friction and kneading. Centrifugal friction (rubbing down) diminishes the blood supply of the brain, and hence lessens cerebral activity.

15   Light friction over a deep-lying organ diminishes its blood supply by increasing the activity of the overlying vessels, thus causing the blood to go around instead of through it.

16   Massage of the soft parts above a joint, and movements of the next joint above, relieve pain by emptying the lymph and blood vessels of the part.

4. *Restorative or Reconstructive Effects.*— Mental fatigue is **17** relieved by massage, through its effect upon the circulation and the eliminative organs. The toxic substances produced by mental activity are more rapidly oxidized and removed from the body, while the hastened blood current more thoroughly repairs and cleanses the wearied nerve tissues.

General reconstructive effects are experienced by the entire **18** nervous system through the improved nutrition induced by massage.

Effects of Massage upon the Muscular System.— **19** Massage, when skillfully administered, has to do chiefly with the muscles. That form of manipulation which consists simply of skin pinching excites the nervous system and the surface circulation, but has little influence upon the muscles. When we reflect that the muscles constitute one half of the bulk of the body, and receive one fourth of all the blood of the body, it is at once apparent that any procedure which acts directly upon them must have a decided influence upon the whole body.

Although the muscles constantly receive a certain blood **20** supply, this supply is comparatively small except during activity; consequently, it may be said that "*the muscles are well fed only when exercising.*" When the muscle is inactive, the blood goes around it rather than through it; but the moment activity of the muscle begins, there is a great increase in its blood supply, even before any acceleration in heart activity has occurred.

Massage may serve to a considerable extent as a substitute **21** for exercise by increasing the blood supply of a muscle, just as exercise may be considered a sort of massage, through the pressing and rubbing of the muscles against each other. When properly administered, the manipulations of massage act upon the muscles in such a way as to produce a suction, or pumping effect, pressing onward the contents of the veins and lymph channels, and thus creating a vacuum to be filled by a fresh supply of fluid derived from the capillaries and the tissues.

22   *Specific Effects of Massage upon the Muscles.*— Massage in its specific effects upon the muscles, may be said to accomplish the following results : —

1. *To Encourage Nutrition and Development of the Muscles.* —The increased blood supply of the muscle induced by massage naturally improves its nutrition. Experience shows that, when systematically and regularly employed, massage produces an actual increase in the size of the muscular structures. The muscle is also found to become firmer and more elastic under its influence.

23   Massage feeds a muscle without exhausting it, in which respect it differs from exercise ; nevertheless, it is not a complete substitute for exercise, for the reason that exercise brings into active play the whole motor mechanism — nerve center, nerve, and muscle — while massage affects chiefly the muscle.

24   The improvement in the nutrition of the muscle, as regards increase in size or firmness, is seldom noticeable for the first three or four weeks, and the most marked effects should not be expected until after two or three months.

25   2. *To Excite Muscular Contraction.*— A smart blow upon a muscle is one of the ways by which contraction may be excited. By a succession of blows, one following another with sufficient rapidity, tetanic contraction of a muscle may be induced.

26   Strong vibration will also cause tetanic contraction of a muscle ; but very rapid and strong vibrations are required to produce tetanus. In voluntary tetanus (ordinary muscular contraction) the number of impulses received by the muscle per second is ten to twenty. It is evident that the rate of vibration required for producing tetanus must be as great or greater, and consequently mechanical means of some sort must be applied, as the highest rate of movement which can be communicated by the hand directly is ten to twelve double movements per second. A vibratory apparatus which I have

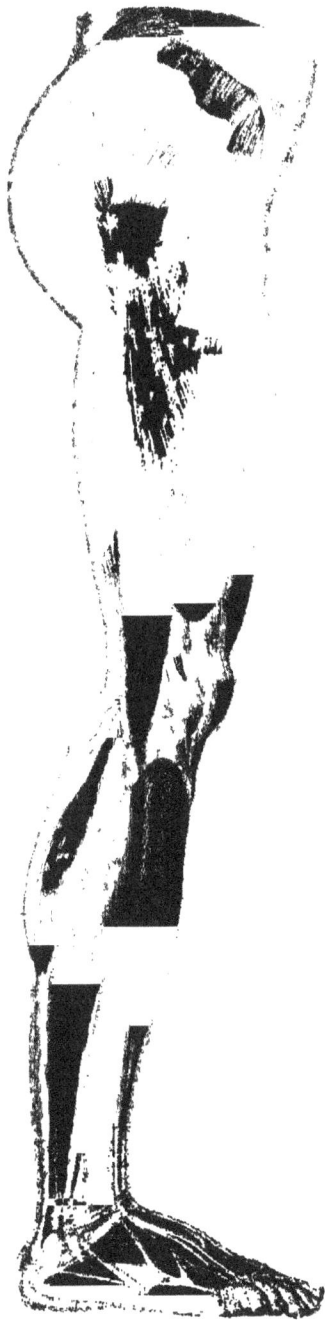

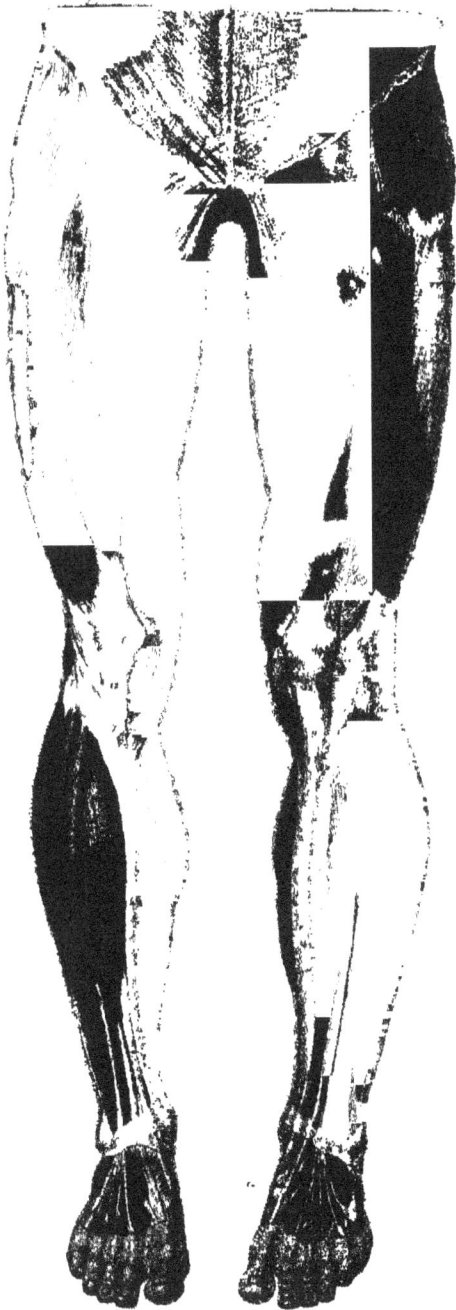

Fig. 18. Outer Side.   Fig. 17. Anterior View.

PLATE VIII.— Muscles of the Leg.

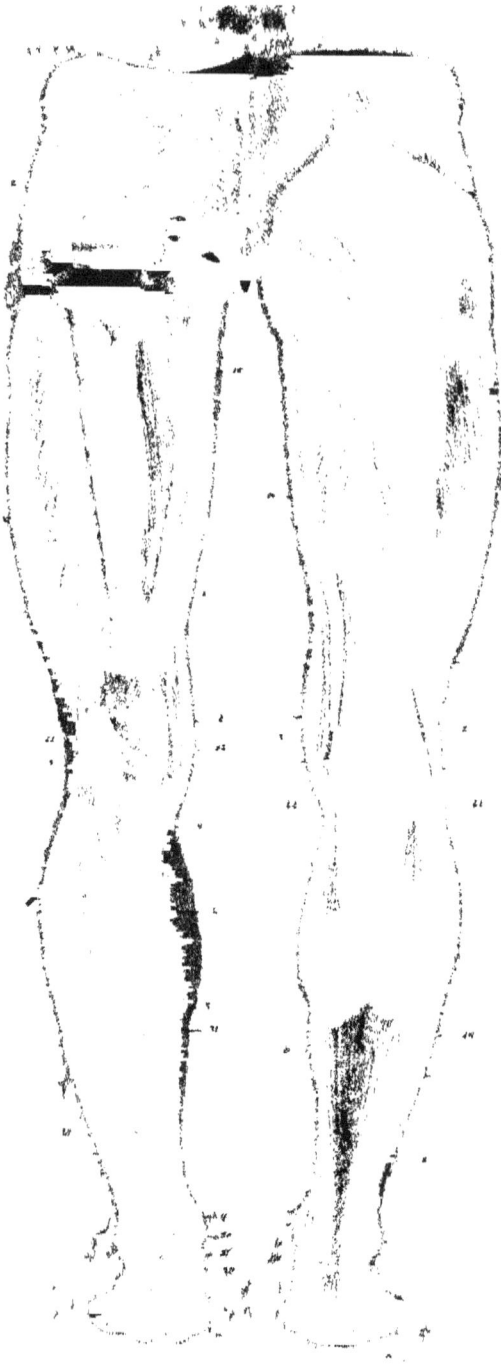

Fig. 19. Posterior View.   Fig. 20. Inner Side.

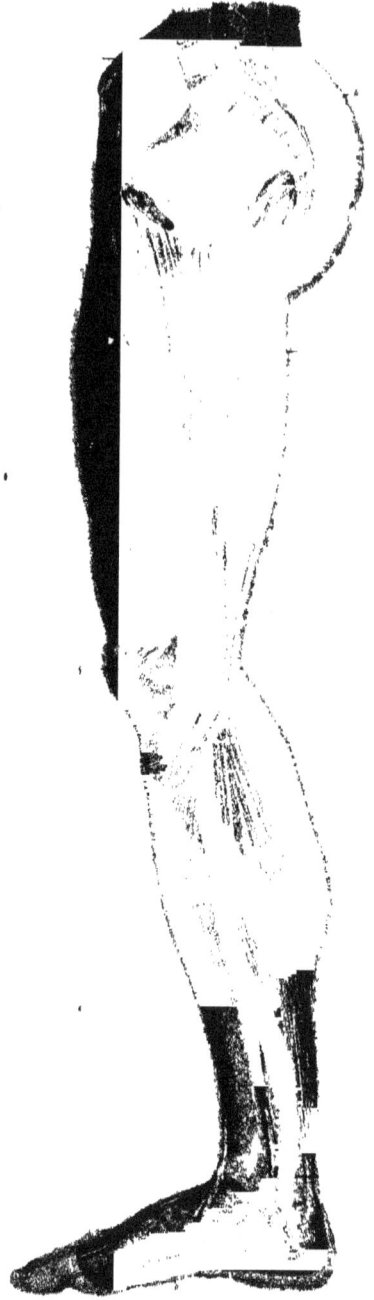

PLATE IX. — Muscles of the Leg.

had in use for many years, and which produces decided muscular contractions, has a movement of thirty per second.

In certain cases, muscular contraction may be induced more 27 readily by the application of percussion than by the faradic current.

3. *To Increase Electro-excitability of the Muscle.*—Numerous 28 experiments have shown that massage increases the electro-excitability of a muscle, as indicated by the fact that a smaller number of milliamperes of current is required to cause contraction of the muscle after massage than before.

According to Kröncker, however, a muscle is less easily 29 tetanized after massage than before, but its power of action is greatly increased. An abnormal degree of muscular irritability is certainly relieved by massage.

This effect of massage may be advantageously utilized as a 30 preparation for applications of electricity in cases in which the electro-excitability of a muscle is diminished by trophic changes, as in infantile paralysis.

4. *To Remove the Effects of Muscular Fatigue.*— Ranke, 31 • Helmholtz, Du Bois-Raymond, Mosso, and more recently, Abelous, have conclusively shown that special toxic substances are produced as the result of muscle work, and that the phenomena of fatigue are due to the influence of these substances upon the nervous and muscular systems.

Abelous has shown that the first effect is a sort of auto-cu- 32 rarization, or paralysis, of the terminal motor plates of the nerves which actuate the muscles, while in advanced fatigue the muscle itself is exhausted by the consumption of the material (glycogen) necessary for work.

The fact that a fatigued muscle can be restored to full vigor 33 at once by simply rinsing its vessels with a normal saline solution, as shown by Ranke, demonstrates the toxic character of the phenomena of fatigue. Bowditch, Bernstein, and others have shown that the nerve itself is indefatigable.

Zabloudowski has shown that frogs completely exhausted 34 by faradization of the muscles, although not restored by fifteen minutes' rest, were revived at once by massage, and were even able to do twice as much work as before.

35   In another experiment, a man lifted with his little finger, one kilo (2 1-5 lbs.) 840 times, lifting the weight once a second. The muscles of his finger were then completely exhausted. After five minutes' massage he was able to lift the same weight 1100 times, and his muscles were even then not greatly fatigued.   •

36   The Sandwich Islanders employ massage under the name of *lomi-lomi* as a means of resting fatigued persons, and sometimes even apply it to restore an exhausted companion when swimming long distances in company. An intelligent native Maori informed the writer that the same method is used by the natives of New Zealand to relieve cramp resulting from cold when swimming in the sea. The term used for massage among the Maoris is *romi-romi*, the literal meaning of which is the same as *petrissage* in the French.

37   The stiffness and soreness of muscles which occur from so-called consecutive or secondary fatigue resulting from over-exercise, is also relieved by massage. It should be remembered, however, that secondary fatigue may be produced by too vigorous an application of massage in a person not accustomed to it, especially in those who are very fleshy.

38   *Muscular Electricity.* — Physiological experiments have demonstrated that with each muscular contraction an electrical discharge takes place, and Mervy has shown that a muscle is a sort of electrical accumulator, electricity doubtless being generated by the muscular and thermic activities which are constantly present in the muscle. As an accumulator it is auto-excitant, and may also be excited by induction or by contact. In this way the muscles of the person masséed may be favorably influenced through induction from the more highly charged muscles of the masseur. This influence, however, must be very slight, and its therapeutic value can scarcely be said to be established.

Effects of Massage upon the Bones, Skeleton, and 39 Ligaments.—That massage is capable of influencing such hard structures as the bones, ligaments, and cartilages, is clearly demonstrated by numerous facts and observations. A bone has essentially the same blood supply as its overlying muscles. It is for this reason that the same exercise which causes increase in the size of a muscle, at the same time induces growth in the bone to which the muscle is attached. The bones and joints of persons who are much addicted to exercise are decidedly larger than those of persons who have made little use of their muscles. This is especially noticeable in comparing the large, strong hand and knotty knuckles of the laboring man with the puny hand and straight, slender fingers of the man of sedentary pursuits.

The blood vessels and lymphatics are largest in the vicinity 40 of the joints, and the change of fluids effected by joint movements, resulting from the action of the muscles upon the bones, necessarily produces increase in the nutrition of the parts, and consequently an increased growth in the cartilages, ligaments, and other structures of the joint.

It is said that among the South Sea Islanders, the chiefs, 41 who have themselves masséed daily, are very much larger than the average of the people. The well-known fact that "cracking" or "snapping" the fingers will cause enlargement of the joints is another evidence of the effects of joint movements in producing change in the growth of the hard structures of the body.

Effects of Massage upon the Circulation.— Mas- 42 sage profoundly affects the circulation, both general and local, its effects differing, however, according to the mode of application and the part acted upon. General massage increases the rate and the force of the heart beat, as does exercise, with the difference that it does not raise the arterial tension as does exercise, and does not accelerate the heart to the same degree, though producing a full, strong pulse. This is due to the fact that the influence of massage is chiefly upon the peripheral circulation.

43   The vigor of the circulatory activity is increased not only in answer to the greater demand for the removal of the poisons resulting from oxidation as in exercise, but through the mechanical assistance afforded by massage, in moving the blood forward in the venous and lymph channels, and in setting up reflex activities whereby the small vessels are dilated and their activities quickened. The reflex influence of massage acts as a tonic for the heart, while the dilatation of the vessels decreases the resistance so that the heart acts more freely and efficiently in performing its functions. Recent experiments by Brunton, verified by the author, show that general massage produces at first, but briefly, a rise in arterial pressure.

44   Locally, the effect of massage is to produce an active hyperæmia of the part. Under the influence of massage the blood vessels become more active, pumping forward the blood into the veins, through which its flow is assisted materially by the manipulations. The increase of blood is usually accompanied by reddening of the surface and an increase of warmth, sensibility, and general vital activity.

45   Light percussion of the surface causes contraction of the blood vessels of that portion of the skin acted upon. Strong percussion very quickly produces dilatation of the blood vessels which may even amount to paralysis. Light percussion, if sufficiently prolonged, also produces dilatation.

46   When applied to a reflex area, percussion doubtless also excites the circulation in the vessels of the related nerve centers. This is the explanation of the influence of percussion of the soles of the feet, the inner portion of the thighs, and the gluteal region, upon the genito-urinary organs (**328, 329**).

47   Massage of the abdomen retards the pulse by causing portal congestion, and thus withdrawing a large quantity of blood from the general circulation. The pulse movements are also somewhat fuller, the result of the influence of abdominal massage upon the great sympathetic centers.

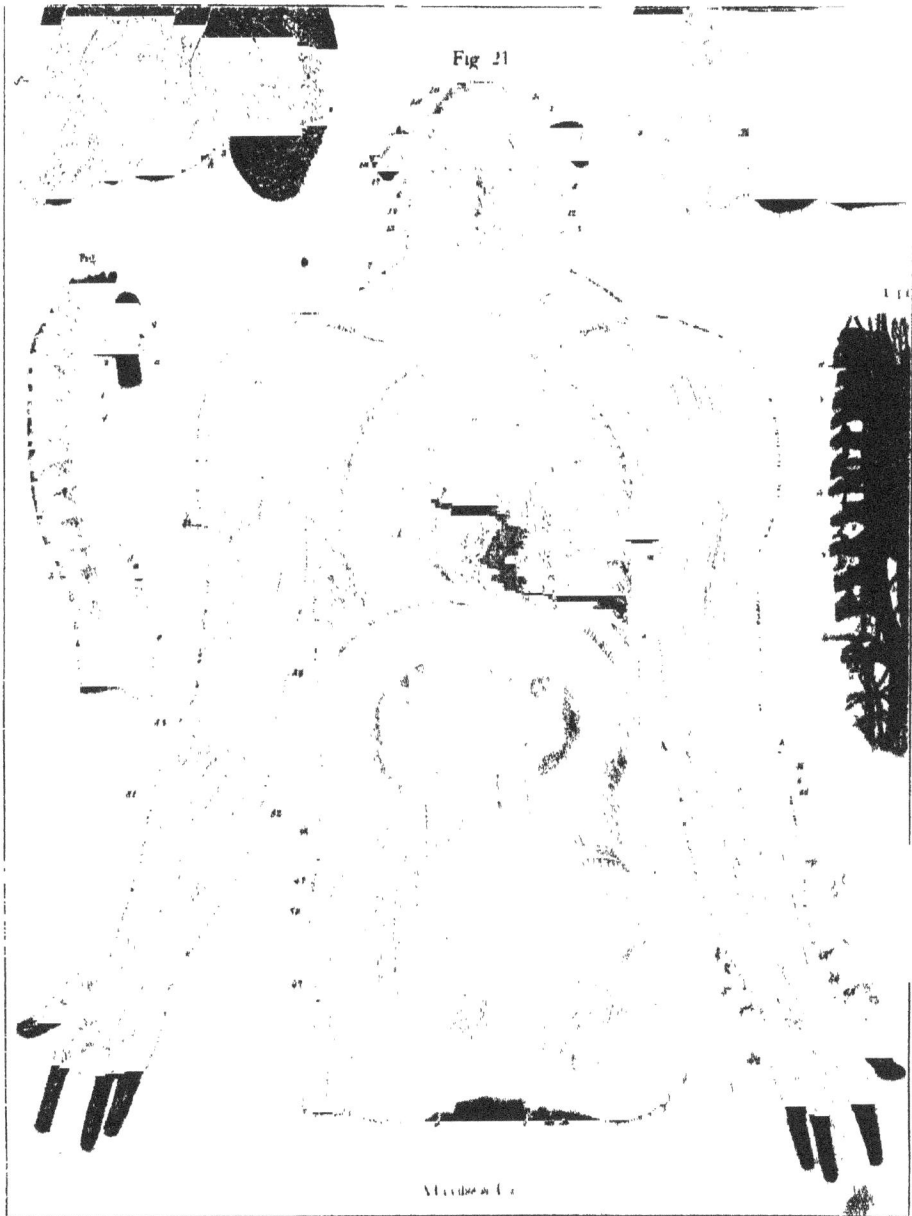

Fig. 21. Blood Vessels of Arms, Neck, and Trunk.

PLATE X.

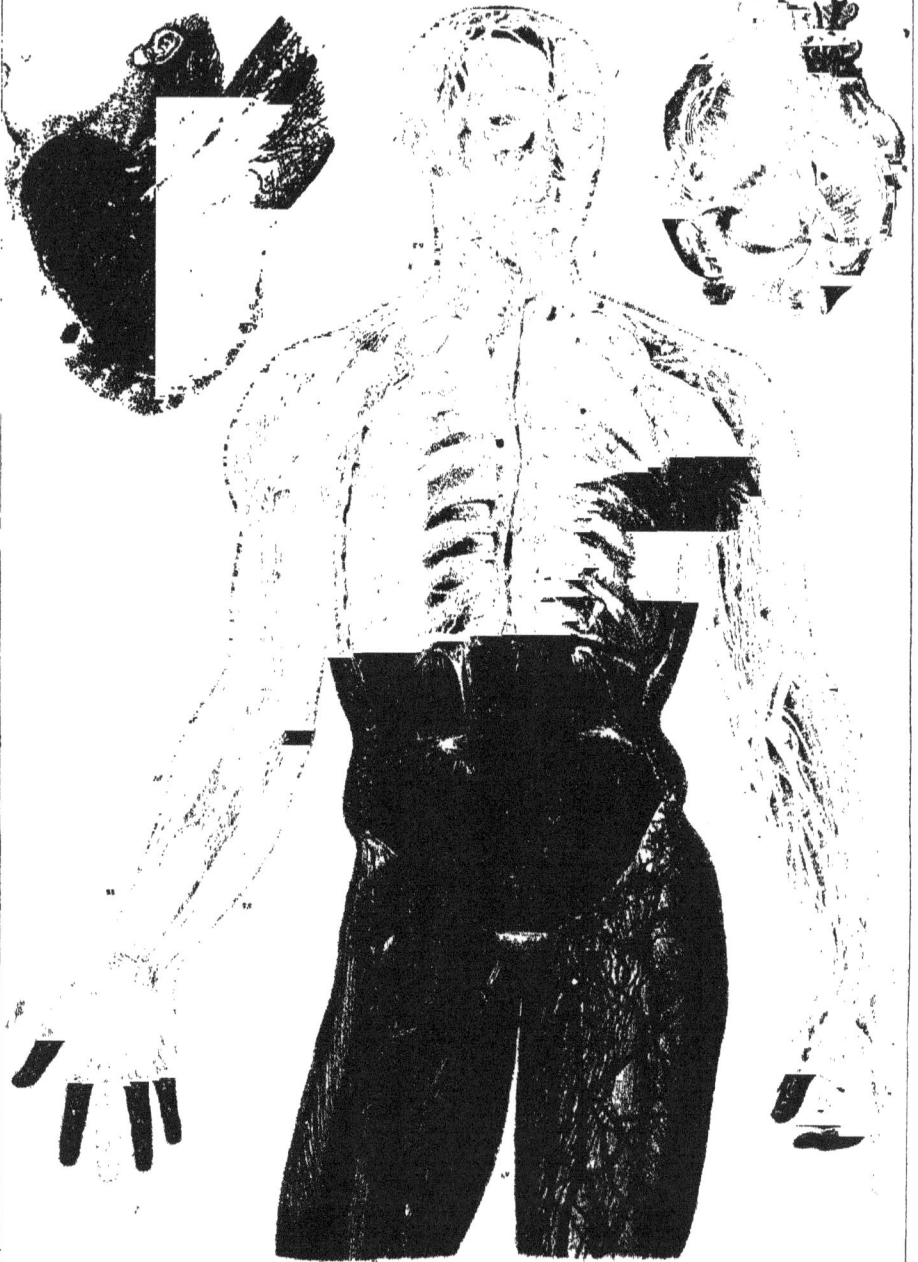

Fig 22

Fig. 22. The Lymphatic System

PLATE XI.

Massage has chiefly to do with the circulation of fluid in the **48** veins and the lymph channels, since these are more readily accessible from the surface than the arteries.

Friction acts chiefly upon the superficial veins, while petris- **49** sage and other forms of deep kneading act upon the deeper vessels as well.

Indirectly, the portal and pulmonary circulations are also **50** influenced by massage. Massage of the extremities, for example, especially if concluded with centrifugal friction, may relieve congestion of both the portal and the pulmonary systems.

Massage of the legs acts more directly upon the portal **51** system, while massage of both extremities favorably influences the pulmonary circulation in case of congestion of the lungs. Massage of the arms and legs also acts derivatively upon the brain and spine. For derivative effects upon the brain, however, care should be taken to avoid such exciting procedures as percussion and reflex stroking.

Massage also has a powerful effect upon the circulation by **52** promoting the action of the diaphragm, which serves efficiently as a pump in assisting the circulation, as well as in carrying on the process of respiration. M. Camus has shown by experiments upon dogs that the increase either of the rate or the depth of respiratory movement increases the flow of lymph in the thoracic duct. The same has been shown in regard to the blood circulation by numerous investigators.

The influence of massage upon the lymph circulation is **53** especially worthy of attention. The lymph vessels drain the tissues of waste and toxic substances, and prevent clogging from wandering cells. Lymph channels are most abundant in the subcutaneous tissue and in the fascia which cover and lie between the muscles, so that these vessels are mechanically acted upon in massage, especially by friction and kneading movements.

That massage and exercise of muscles greatly increase the **54** flow of lymph has been repeatedly demonstrated by experi-

ments upon animals, as, for example, it was found that the flow
in the lymph vessels of a dog's leg nearly ceased when the animal was quiet, but as soon as the limb was exercised or masséed, the flow of lymph began again (Reibmayr).

55   It has also been shown that the flow of lymph from a limb
in a state of inflammation was very easily induced, and was
seven or eight times greater than from a sound limb. A swollen limb was found to diminish during the flow of lymph
(Lessar).

56   The same author has shown that massage of a lymph gland
increases the outflow of the fluid. Deep massage applied to a
limb diminishes its size. The central tendon of the diaphragm
contains a large number of lymph channels. The diaphragm
may be regarded as a great lymph pump, since by its rhythmical movement, the lymph channels are alternately dilated and
contracted.

57   Höffinger has shown that the absorptive power of the peritoneum is greatly increased by massage. In experiments upon
rabbits, the peritoneum was found to absorb under the influence of massage twice as much water in an hour as without
massage.

58   An experiment made by Mosengeil, an eminent German
physiologist, graphically demonstrates the influence of massage
in promoting absorption. The joints of rabbits were injected
with ink. Massage was applied to some of the rabbits and not
to others. In the cases subjected to massage, the swelling
which was produced by the injection rapidly passed away.
When the rabbits were killed, some months afterward, it was
found that the ink had entirely disappeared from the joints
which had been masséed, and was found in streaks between
the muscles, and accumulated in the lymphatic glands, indicating the course of the lymphatic channels. In cases in
which the joints were not masséed, ink was found in the joints,
but none in either the muscles or lymphatic glands. This result affords a striking illustration of the value of massage in
affections of the joints accompanied by exudate.

It is through its power to promote absorption that massage **59** is of great value in the treatment of local œdemas, general dropsy, and ascites.

Effects of Massage upon Respiration.—These effects may be thus enumerated :—

1. *Increase of Respiratory Activity.*—Massage, as does exer- **60** cise, increases the depth of the respiratory movements. This is doubtless in some measure due to the reflex influence of massage, but must also be attributed in part to its effect in bringing into the circulation waste products requiring elimination through the lungs, and in increasing oxidation, or CO_2 production, which necessarily accompanies the increased heat production resulting from the effect of massage upon the muscles.

2. *Increase of Tissue Respiration.*—It should be borne in **61** mind that the function of respiration is not confined to the lungs. Respiration begins and ends in the lungs, but the most important part of the process is effected in the intimate recesses of the tissues themselves.

Massage is certainly a most efficient means of increasing **62** tissue metabolism, by which oxygen is absorbed by the tissues and CO_2 taken up by the blood. This process takes place chiefly in the muscles, through the oxidation of the glycogen, of which they contain one half the total bodily store. Hence it is that massage, by acting directly upon the muscles, increases the tissue respiration by promoting circulation and general tissue activity.

In thus promoting the depth of respiratory movement and **63** the intensity of tissue respiration, massage profoundly affects all the bodily functions. Through the increased lung activity there is also increased circulation, as the lungs materially aid the heart in the circulation of the blood. Increased activity of the diaphragm serves to pump both blood and lymph toward the heart with greater vigor. Digestion, liver action, and other of the vital functions come in for their share of benefit in the increased vigor and efficiency of the respiratory process. The functions of the brain are more easily performed on account of the more perfect movement of venous blood and the better supply of oxygen received.

54   Influence of Massage upon the Heat Functions of the Body.— The heat functions of the body being so intimately connected with the circulation and general tissue activity, it is clear that any agent which profoundly affects the latter must also affect the former proportionately. The heat functions consist of three distinct processes,— heat production, heat elimination, or dissipation, and heat regulation. Massage materially influences all three of these processes.

65   The muscles are the chief seat of heat production in the body, containing a great store of glycogen and a special mechanism which, under the influence of the nervous system, gives rise to increase or decrease of oxidation, or combustion of the glycogen. The muscles may be considered as the furnace of the body. During activity, heat production is very active ; while during rest, it is considerably diminished. In fever there may be either a great increase of heat production or simply a loss of heat regulation, or both conditions may exist. It is thus evident that those procedures of massage which especially concern the muscles, such as different forms of deep kneading and strong percussion, must exert a powerful influence upon heat production.

66   By actual observation it has been shown that massage of a muscle, as well as exercise, may cause a rise of temperature amounting to several tenths of a degree Fahrenheit. The importance of this fact will be recognized when it is recalled that four fifths of all the food eaten goes to the production of heat, only one fifth of the force represented in the food reappearing as work or energy. This explains the enormous increase of CO_2 in connection with muscular exercise. The quantity of CO_2 eliminated during vigorous muscular effort sometimes rises to nearly five times the usual amount. Muscular waste and weakness in fever is chiefly due to the consumption of the glycogen, which occurs under the influence of the toxic substances present in the tissues during febrile states.

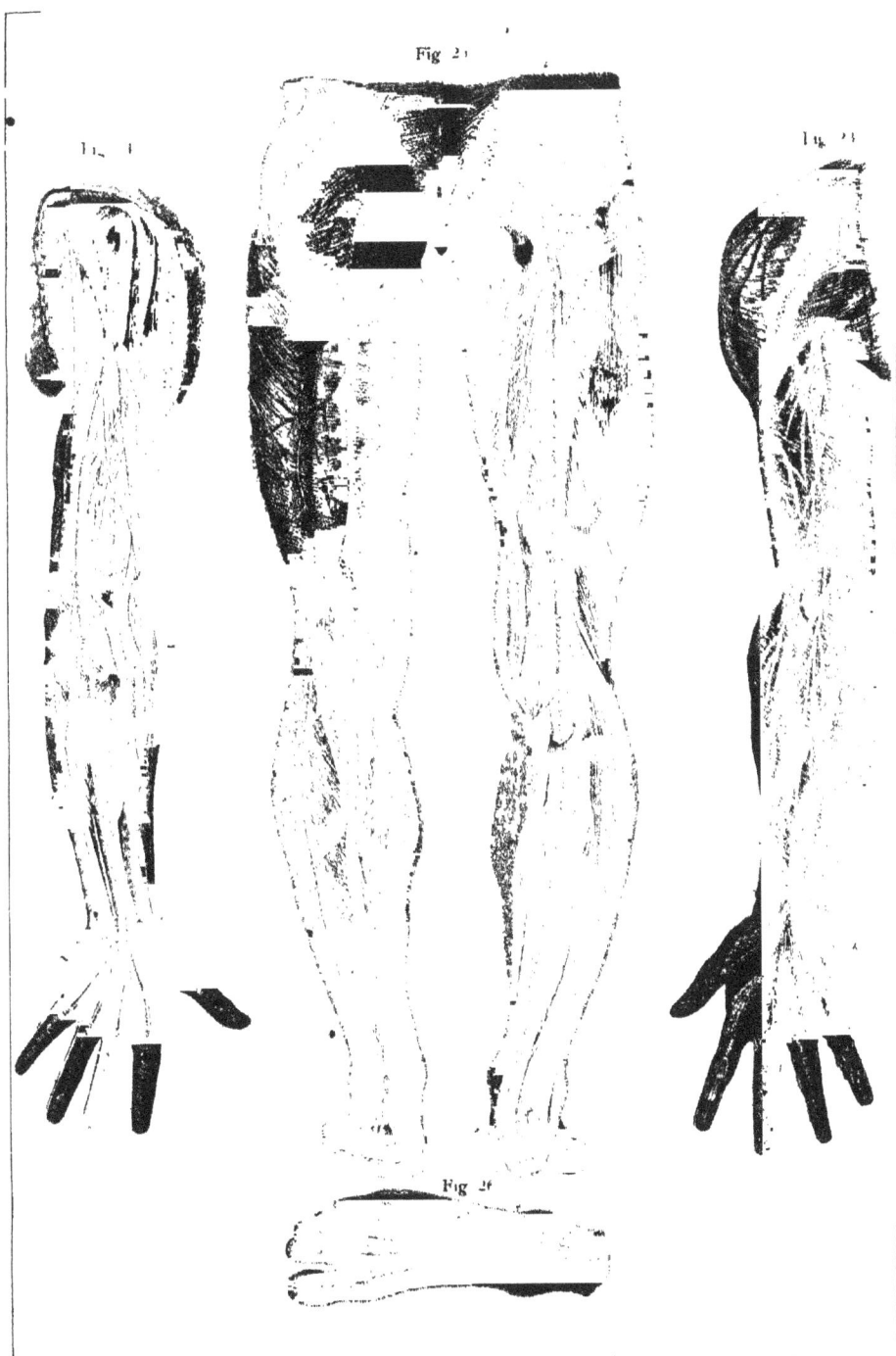

Fig. 23. Superficial Nerves of Arm.
Fig. 24. Deep Nerve Trunks of Arm

Fig. 25. Nerves of Leg.
Fig. 26. Nerves of Foot.

PLATE XII. — The Nervous System.

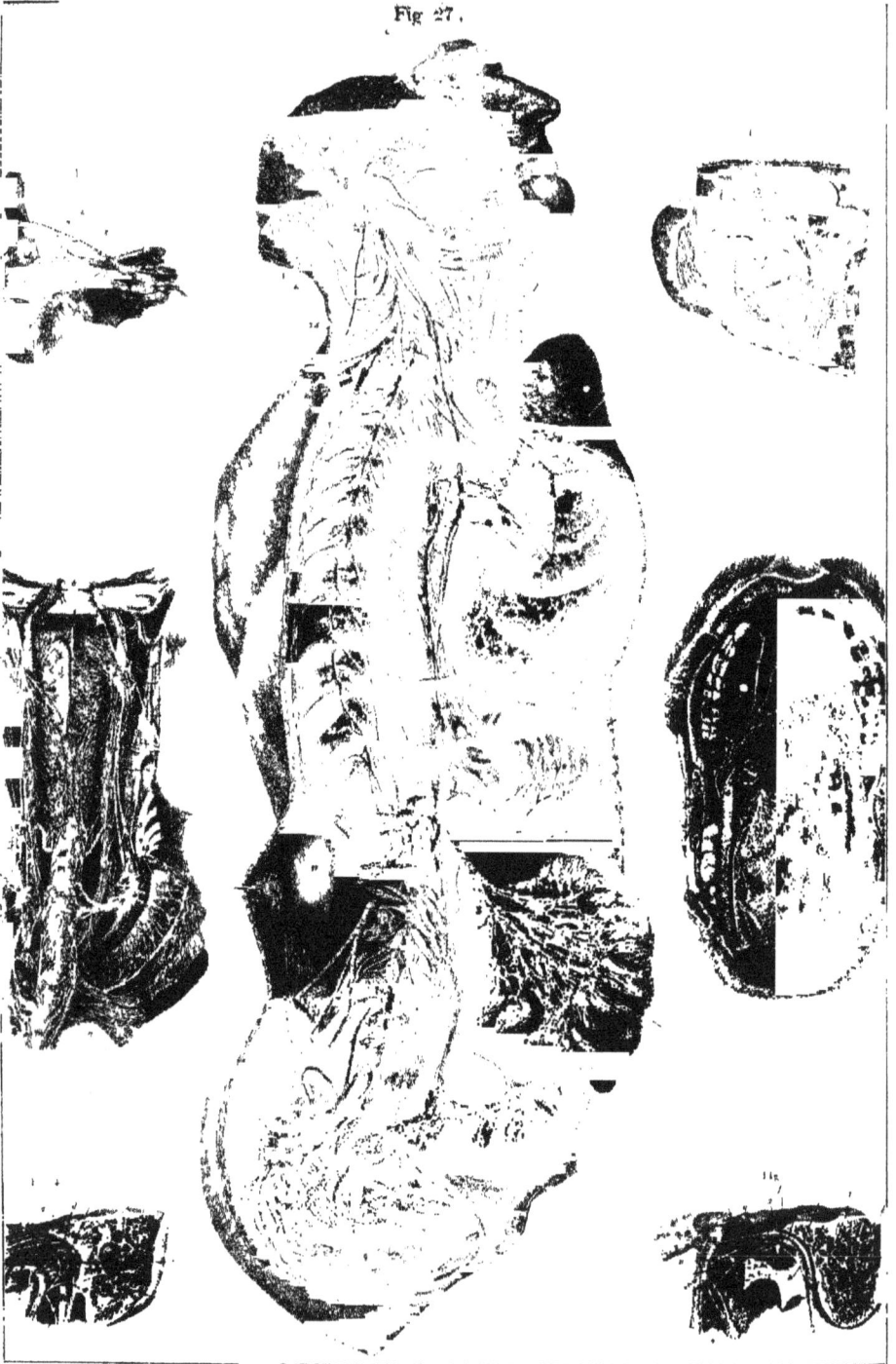

Fig. 27. The Sympathetic Nerves.

PLATE XIII.

The continued activity of the muscles in heat production, 67 even when the body is at rest, is doubtless due to the slight muscular activity constantly present as so-called muscular tone.

Winternitz has shown that under some circumstances heat 68 elimination by the skin may be nearly doubled (increased ninety-five per cent) by friction. He accordingly recommends friction, in connection with the cold bath, for reducing temperature in fevers.

Celsus, the famous old Roman physician, recommended rub- 69 bing in fevers when the surface was cold, although he carefully interdicted rubbing in fevers at other times. The increased heat dissipation resulting from massage is directly due to the increased circulation of blood in the skin. The higher the temperature of the skin the more rapid will be the dissipation of heat from the body. The skin is the principal means by which the blood is cooled, the heat brought from the interior to the surface being dissipated by radiation, conduction, and especially by the evaporation of water poured out of the skin by the sweat glands.

Massage, by dilatation of the blood vessels and accelera- 70 tion of the peripheral circulation, brings an increased quantity of heat to the surface, and at the same time, through increasing the blood supply and by reflex influence upon the sympathetic nerves, it induces increased activity of the sweat glands, which leads them to pour out an increased amount of perspiration. Thus heat dissipation is increased both by radiation and by evaporation as the result of the application of superficial massage.

It thus appears that bodily temperature may be either in- 71 creased or diminished by massage, since by kneading the muscles we may increase heat production, while by friction we may increase heat elimination. It is particularly important to remember that when massage is applied for the purpose of increasing heat dissipation, only such procedures should be adopted as will act upon the surface alone, since any manipulation of the muscles will increase heat production.

3

72   A small amount of heat is communicated to the surface by the hand of the manipulator, and a further small quantity is generated by the friction of the hand upon the surface ; but these sources of heat are too small to deserve more than mere mention.

73   Another point worthy of notice is the fact that while general massage increases heat production, it does not necessarily increase the bodily temperature, for the reason that the increase in heat production may be more than balanced by the increased dissipation of heat. For example, in a case in which general massage increased the surface temperature 1.4° F., the rectal temperature fell .8° F.

74   Abdominal massage, however, exercises an effect the opposite of that of general massage. Massage of the abdomen may cause a fall of surface temperature of .2° F., while the rectal temperature rises 2.2° F.

75   **Effect of Massage upon Digestion.**—There is no single function which may be more clearly demonstrated to be directly encouraged by massage than digestion. By its judicious application, the digestive process is promoted in several ways : —

76   1. *By Improving the Appetite.*— The general improvement in nutrition occasioned by the removal of waste and the acceleration of the blood and lymph circulations, creates a demand for an increased supply of nutriment which nature manifests by an improvement in appetite.

77   2. *By Promoting Secretion of the Digestive Fluids.*—Massage, especially abdominal massage, through its reflex influence upon the glands and circulation of the stomach and intestines, promotes the production of the digestive fluids in sufficient quantity and quality.

78   3. *By Promoting Absorption of the Products of Digestion.*— Hopadzë has shown that massage of the abdomen, for even so short a time as ten minutes, applied at once after eating, diminishes by fifteen to seventy-five minutes the length of time the food is retained in the stomach.

Hirschberg declares that massage of the abdomen hastens the passage of food from the stomach even more efficiently than does either exercise or electricity. This fact the writer has frequently demonstrated.

4. *By Aiding Peristalsis.*—Massage not only aids the **79** absorption of food from the stomach, and its passage from the stomach into the intestine, but also excites the reflexes by which the alimentary mass is moved along in the small intestine to the colon, and finally discharged from the body. Indeed, massage has no rival in its efficiency as a means of promoting intestinal activity.

Influence of Massage upon Nutrition, Hæmato- **80** **genesis, and Phagocytosis.**—That massage encourages the blood-making process is demonstrated by the rapidity with which the number of red blood corpuscles and the amount of hæmoglobin increase in the blood under the influence of this therapeutic means in cases of anæmia. The value of this fact can scarcely be over-estimated. The blood is one of the most important of all the tissues of the body. The total amount of blood contained in the body is about ten pounds, each cubic millimeter of which contains from four and a half to five million corpuscles, making in all 32,500,000,000,000 — more than twenty thousand times the entire population of the globe. These little bodies have a combined area of nearly 2900 square meters, or more than 3100 square yards — equal to a square nearly 175 yards on each side. When we consider that this enormous area of blood must pass through the lungs every twenty-two seconds in order to secure the proper amount of oxygen for the tissues, it is readily apparent how great a loss must be suffered when the quantity of blood is diminished ten to twenty or even seventy-five per cent, as in cases of anæmia, and also the great gain effected by a like increase in the number of corpuscles, or oxygen carriers.

Another important influence of massage upon the blood **81** which has recently been noted is the immediate increase in the number of corpuscles produced by a general application of massage. Winternitz pointed out, a year or two ago, the interesting fact that by the application of cold water to the surface in such a way as to secure vigorous reaction, the number of corpuscles could be immediately increased from twenty-five to fifty per cent. In one case an increase of more than 1,800,000 corpuscles was noted within half an hour after the administration of the cold bath.

82   Winternitz also showed that exercise has a like effect, and Mitchell, of Philadelphia, has proven the same for massage.

83   It is not to be supposed, as is remarked by Winternitz, that this sudden increase of blood corpuscles is due to a new production of blood cells; the apparent increase in numbers is due to the sudden bringing into the circulation of a great number of corpuscles which had previously been retained in the large vascular viscera of the interior of the body, especially the spleen and liver.

84   Quincke has noticed that the corpuscles accumulate in the capillaries of the liver and spleen in great numbers just before they are disintegrated, which naturally leads to the suggestion that the corpuscles set free by massage, and restored to usefulness by being brought into circulation, are at the same time rescued from destruction by the organs devoted to this work in the body, so that we have in massage not only a means of bringing useless cells into activity, but also of combating the anæmia which in certain cases results from the excessive destruction of blood cells rather than from deficient production. The sudden bringing into the circulation of the blood of many extra square yards of blood corpuscles destined to pass through the lungs for the discharge of CO_2 and the absorption of oxygen every twenty-two seconds, very clearly explains the wonderfully rejuvenating effects of massage and its powerful influence in aiding nutrition.

85   *Phagocytosis.*—This interesting phenomenon, the complete demonstration of which was worked out by Metchnikoff in Pasteur's laboratory, is influenced by massage to a remark-

able degree. In the case of exudates in parts which have suffered from inflammatory processes, the removal of the exudate depends first upon its solution. This is effected by the white blood corpuscles, which actually digest the inflammatory products, thus setting them free so they can be carried off by the venous and lymph currents. It is thus apparent that the first thing essential for the removal of chronic exudates is an increased blood supply. Through the influence of massage directly applied, not only is an increased supply of blood made to circulate through the vessels which have remained intact, but old blood and lymph channels which have been obliterated are reopened, and thus the vital streams are made to flow through and about the affected part with greatly increased activity.

Phagocytosis is also the principal means by which the body antagonizes an invasion of foreign microbes which always takes place in connection with infectious disease. Microbes of various sorts, and even animal parasites, such as the plasmodia of malaria, are captured and destroyed by the white blood corpuscles. It is, indeed, through the action of these blood cells that the vital current is kept free from foreign matters of various kinds. They seem to be, in fact, a sort of vital patrol which march up and down the highways of the body, resisting and destroying intruders of various sorts.

It is evident that massage, as already pointed out (**81-83**), by bringing into circulation an increased number of blood cells, must greatly increase the resisting powers of the body. It is especially worthy of notice that while both the red and the white corpuscles are greatly increased by massage, the white corpuscles are increased in much greater proportion than the red ones.

Massage is also valuable as a regulator of the nutritive **86** processes. Hopadze has proven that massage increases the assimilation of nitrogenous food substances, while Zabloudowski has shown that massage both diminishes the weight of very fleshy persons and increases the weight of badly nourished persons, giving increased appetite and sleep. He showed that these effects continue not only during the treatment but for some time afterward.

87   Influence of Massage upon Elimination.— The chief effects of massage upon elimination are : —

1. *To Improve Elimination.*— In general it sets waste matters free, by encouraging oxidation, by encouraging cell exchanges by which the waste matters are poured into the blood and the lymph currents from the tissues, and by stimulating the flow of the venous blood and the lymph, as well as by promoting general activity of the circulation, thus bringing the waste matters in contact with the organs devoted to their elimination.

88   2. *To Encourage Activity of the Liver.*— The liver requiring oxygen in the various branches of its work as an eliminative organ, its action is greatly encouraged by the increased amount of oxygen brought into the blood by massage. The increased activity of the portal circulation produced by abdominal massage especially aids the liver.

89   Hepatic activity may also be directly stimulated by the application of massage to the liver — especially by vibratory movements and percussion applied over the organ. The fact is worthy of notice that not only hepatic activity but renal efficiency depend upon the integrity and activity of the hepatic cell, which, when stored with glycogen, is capable of transforming leucomaines and various other toxic substances normally produced in the body, into less toxic forms, preparing them for elimination by the kidneys, and also actually destroying ptomaines and other alkaloids which may be taken in with the food or generated in the alimentary canal. Massage, by promoting these important activities in the liver, not only aids elimination through both liver and kidneys, but contributes to purity of blood by the destruction of poisons.

90   3. *To Encourage Renal Activity.*— That massage aids renal activity has been actually demonstrated by experiments upon both dogs and human beings. Abdominal massage frequently gives rise to a copious discharge of newly formed urine,

although massage of the back or loins does not produce the same effect. Abdominal massage doubtless promotes kidney activity through its influence upon the lumbar ganglia of the abdominal sympathetic and the solar plexus.

In experiments made upon a dog, it was observed that massage of the legs also promoted renal activity. The increased secretion of urine was, however, observed to be but temporary, probably because the, quantity of fatigue-poisons in the body, the removal of which was especially aided by massage, was soon exhausted. It was found that the same effect was again noticeable after tetanizing the leg, whereby a new quantity of fatigue-poisons was produced, **91**

4. *To Promote Activity of the Skin.*—The activity of the skin is promoted by massage, both in the direct stimulus of the sweat and sebaceous glands and the hair follicles, and also in the reflex influence upon the vasomotor nerves whereby an increased supply of blood is brought to the skin, thus promoting and continuing the glandular activity directly excited. An evidence of this stimulation of the skin as the result of massage is to be seen in the reddening of the surface; the increased perspiration, which may be so great as to interfere with the manipulations; the increased production of oil, which is particularly noticeable in cases in which the skin is abnormally dry at the beginning of a course of treatment; and the increased growth of hair, especially upon the legs and arms. Winternitz has shown that friction of the skin increases the elimination of water sixty per cent. **92**

When it is remembered that the skin is an organ of respiration as well as perspiration, its increased activity must be regarded as one of the most valuable effects of massage. **93**

It is also noticeable that massage of the skin increases its reactive power and so gives it increased ability to defend itself against changes in temperature, weather changes, etc. **94**

Local Effects of Massage.— The local effects of massage may be briefly stated to be : — **95**

1. Increase of blood and lymph circulation.

2. Increase in both constructive and destructive tissue change.

3. Absorption of waste or effused products.

4. Development of the muscles, ligaments, and other structures acted upon.

5. Increased heat production and tissue respiration.

6. Reflex or sympathetic effects upon the vasomotor centers, and through them upon the large internal organs,—the liver, spleen, stomach, intestines, kidneys, and the general glandular system of the whole body.

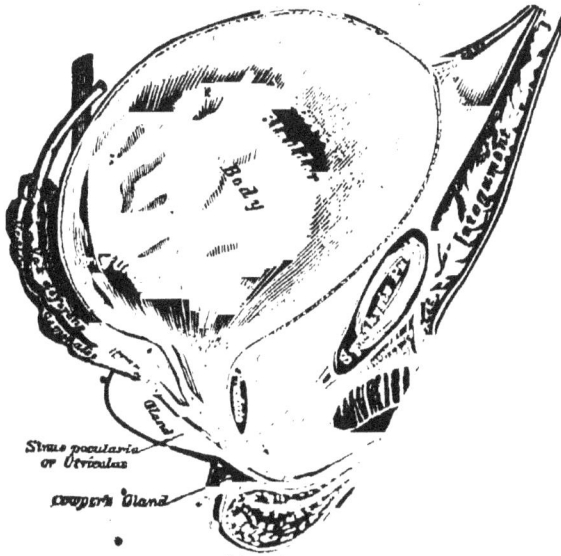

Fig. 28. Male Pelvic Organs.

Sinus pocularis
or Utriculus

Cowper's Gland

Body

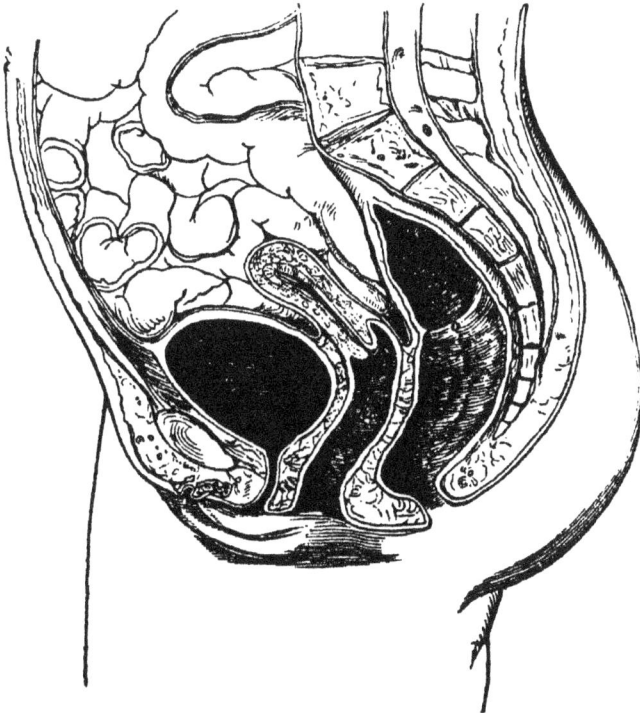

Fig. 29. Female Pelvic Organs.

PLATE XIV.

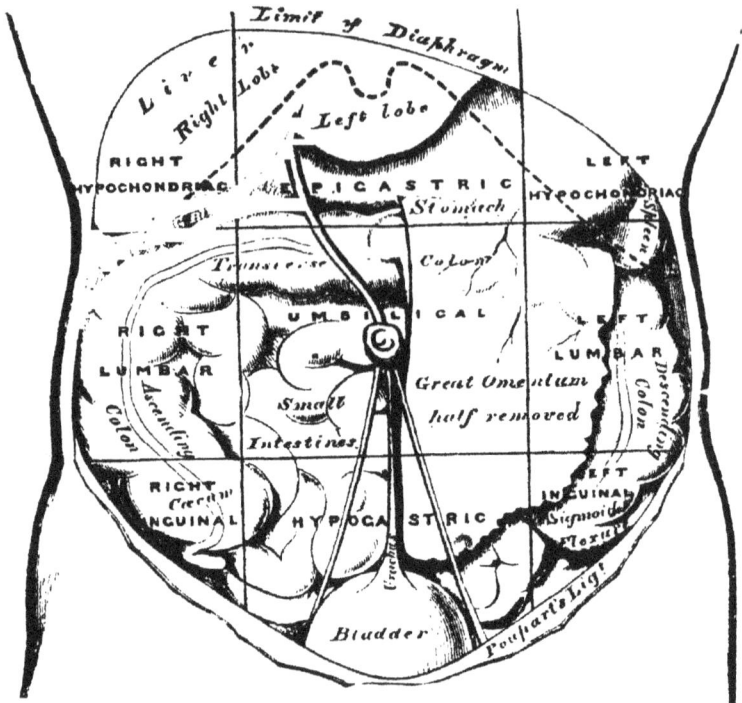

Fig. 30. Regions of the Abdomen.

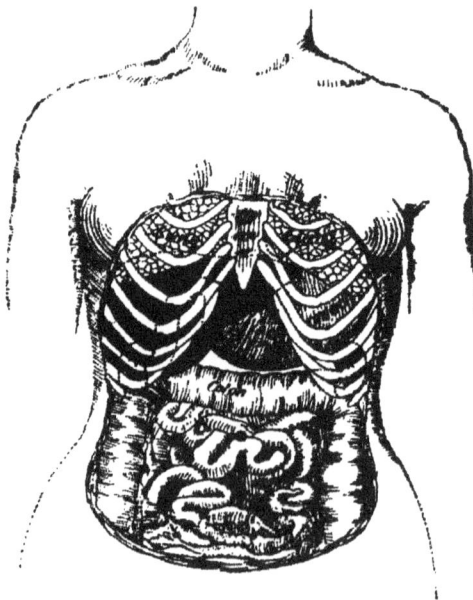

Fig. 31. The Viscera in Normal Position.

PLATE XV.

THE THERAPEUTIC APPLICATIONS OF MASSAGE.

As it is not the purpose of this work to enter into an exhaustive consideration of all the different applications of massage, we shall scarcely do more than mention briefly those maladies in which this therapeutic measure has been found most conspicuously useful. It is, in fact, hardly necessary to devote any very great amount of space to the general considerations which alone may be appropriately treated of under this head, since the concise *résumé* of the physiological effects of massage which has already been presented, will, for the intelligent practitioner, serve as the best possible index to its therapeutic applications; while for the masseur, the more specific directions given in connection with the individual measures of massage will be of greater practical use.

Disorders of Nutrition.— Ancient as well as modern 96 physicians have regarded massage as a measure by which the general nutritive processes of the body may be influenced in a most powerful degree. The value of massage as a therapeutic means arises from its remarkable influence upon the circulation (**42**), the direct and indirect stimulation of the nerves and nerve centers (**6, 10**), and its remarkable modifying influence upon assimilation, disassimilation, and all the processes of secretion and excretion.

Anæmia and chlorosis are more rapidly and permanently 97 cured by massage than by any form of medication which has been proposed. In connection with a properly regulated dietary and suitable hydropathic measures, massage must be considered as the treatment *par excellence* for these maladies.

98   The writer has seen excellent results in a number of cases of myxœdema in which massage was the leading therapeutic agent employed. If not capable of effecting a radical cure in this disease, it must at least be accredited with the power to prevent a further advance of the malady, and as a means of securing a very decided symptomatic improvement.

99   In cases of exhaustion from excessive mental, nervous, or muscular work, general massage secures the,most marked and satisfactory results, relieving the sense of fatigue in a most wonderful manner, and in cases of muscular exhaustion, restoring muscular power in a remarkably short space of time (31).

.00   Massage also exerts a decidedly quieting influence upon the nervous irritability and insomnia so commonly accompanying cerebral and nervous exhaustion (12).

.01   The restorative effects of general massage act with much efficiency as a means of retarding the encroachments of old age, as well as in relieving the infirmities incident to that period. It may be justly considered as a very excellent means of prevention against arterio-sclerosis, especially if employed in conjunction with suitable exercise.

.02   **Diathetic Disorders.**—While not a substitute for regimen in the treatment of those maladies having their foundation in a morbid diathesis, of which obesity, chronic rheumatism, and diabetes are the three leading types, massage is certainly a valuable adjunct in the management of this important class of disorders. It is of special value in the treatment of obesity, particularly at the beginning of a course, when the patient is too feeble muscularly to undertake the active exercises necessary to effect a change in his nutritive processes.

03   Massage is equally useful in cases of rheumatism in which exercise is impossible in consequence of pain, stiffness, or deformity, and also as a means of relieving pain occasioned by the first attempts at exercise.

.04   Of equal value is massage in the treatment of diabetes accompanied by great weakness or exhaustion, rendering the amount of exercise necessary for the burning up of the surplus sugar (**64**) impossible to the patient on account of the feeble condition of his nervo-muscular apparatus. Finkler reports a large number of cases of diabetes mellitus in which great improvement was secured by massage. Zimmer has shown that vigorous muscles, even when at rest, destroy more sugar than do feeble ones, a fact which is easily understood when we remember that the muscles are the furnace of the body, and are the chief seat of the vital combustion by which glycogen, or sugar, is consumed (**65, 66**). Large and vascular muscles will naturally consume more sugar than feeble and anæmic muscles, just as a large furnace with a good draft will consume more fuel than a small furnace with a poor draft. Under the influence of either massage or exercise, the blood is made to go through the muscles; while in a state of rest it goes round rather than through them. Bouchard also has shown that exercise of the muscles increases the consumption of sugar, and thus diminishes the amount of sugar found in the urine in cases of diabetes. I have often had opportunity to confirm this observation in my own experience in the treatment of this disease.

In the treatment of muscular rheumatism, massage not **105** only relieves the pain accompanying the disease, but also antagonizes the muscular atrophy which is one of its most constant results.

In the treatment of articular rheumatism, massage relieves **106** the pain through its derivative action, and also promotes the absorption of effused inflammatory products, and restores lost mobility. Other observers as well as the author have found massage useful in arthritis deformans, and it has given excellent results in the arthritic neuroses which are so often the result of acute or chronic inflammation and injuries to the joints.

The consecutive or secondary fatigue which is so apt to **107** occur in the employment of exercise in these maladies is more readily relieved by massage than by any other means (**31-37**).

108　**Disorders of the Circulatory System.**— Oertel has employed massage of the heart in cases of cardiac weakness with great success.

109　Massage and joint movements are of special advantage in cases of chronic diseases of the heart, by aiding the circulation and thus relieving the heart of a portion of its work, whereby it is afforded an opportunity to rally and its nutrition is improved (**42, 43**).

110　Centripetal friction of the extremities is the most powerful of all means of aiding the venous and lymphatic circulations in œdema and allied conditions (**54-58**).

111　When the heart and blood vessels are excessively active, as after violent exercise, the circulation may be quieted by centrifugal friction. This measure is useful in cases of insomnia from cerebral congestion, over-compensation through excessive development of the heart muscle as the result of valvular disease, or obstruction to the pulmonary circulation arising from disease of the lungs (**50, 51**).

112　In Raynaud's disease, or local asphyxia, massage affords a measure of treatment of great importance (**44**). There is, in fact, no single means which can be relied upon as of greater value than local massage systematically employed in the management of this very remarkable malady.

113　**Diseases of the Muscular System.**— Although disease of the muscles is usually accompanied by disorder of the controlling nerves, the application of massage directly to the muscles is of the highest value in the treatment of most cases of muscular paralysis and paresis.

114　In spasmodic diseases, such as chorea, most excellent results have been obtained through the improvement of the muscular tone resulting from suitable applications of massage (**29**), especially when combined with gymnastics.

115　In muscular atrophy, whether resulting from neuritis or from disease of the cord, massage of the muscles, especially friction and petrissage, is a measure of the highest value (**22-24**), affording, in fact, the best of all known means by which the nutrition of a muscle may be maintained while regeneration of the connecting nerve structures is taking place.

Even in fatty degeneration of the muscles, massage may **116** still prove of value. It is not to be expected, of course, that muscles which have undergone complete fatty change will be regenerated; but through the increased nutritive activity set up by judiciously administered massage, those muscular fibers remaining intact may be developed to such an unusual degree that they are able to perform in a very satisfactory manner the functions of the entire muscle or muscular group.

In pseudo-hypertrophy of the muscles, massage furnishes **117** the most satisfactory of all means of combating the morbid process which, left to itself, ultimately results in tissue degeneration and corresponding loss of function.

Diseases of the Nervous System.—There is cer- **118** tainly no class of disorders in which massage has won greater triumphs than in diseases of the nervous system, especially those which are purely functional in character. In the various forms of neurasthenia, massage has, in connection with a suitable regimen, often accomplished results little less than marvelous, as is illustrated not only by the cases published by S. Weir Mitchell, who first systematized the use of massage in this class of nervous disorders, but also by the experience of hundreds of other physicians who have witnessed the effects of massage upon an emaciated, neurotic invalid, when applied by a person thoroughly skilled in its employment.

Chorea, writer's cramp (**550-555**), blepharospasm, wry- **119** neck, and other maladies in which irregular muscular action, or spasm, is a leading symptom, are more amenable to this measure of treatment than to any other therapeutic means (**12-14**). Such other painful disorders as facial neuralgia, lumbago, sciatica, crural neuralgia (**339, 547-549**), and even migraine, also yield to general and local applications, and often in a most surprising manner (**12-16**).

The curative effect of massage in migraine is due to the **120** fact that it may be employed in such a way as to influence the sympathetic (**160**) as well as the central nervous system, since this disease has been clearly shown to be dependent upon a disordered state of the sympathetic, and probably in most cases to a disturbance of the abdominal sympathetic. In rare cases there are found in connection with the disease, and apparently sustaining a causative relation to it, points of induration or thickening in the trapezius and scaleni muscles. Massage locally applied is of special benefit in cases of this kind.

121   The various forms of headache are in a high degree amenable to treatment by general and local applications of massage, especially the different forms of headache from which neurasthenic and anæmic individuals so commonly suffer (**429-431, 155**).

122   Even in the treatment of neuritis, massage proves a serviceable measure, provided it is properly employed. It must, of course, be used derivatively in the first stage, and be wholly suspended in the second stage of the disease, while in the third stage, direct and vigorous applications are most effective.

123   Anæsthesias, hyperæsthesias (**153**), and the various forms of paræsthesia — numbness, tingling, crawling, burning, prickling, and other morbid sensations — when of functional origin, quickly yield to suitable applications of massage.

124   Even such structural maladies as locomotor ataxia, spinal sclerosis (**309, 341**), infantile paralysis, and progressive muscular atrophy, not infrequently make more improvement under massage than can be secured by any other means. The writer has seen, in cases of this sort, results which were truly surprising, and far beyond the most sanguine expectations.

125   **Disorders of the Digestive Organs.**— In the treatment of the various forms of indigestion, massage, general and local, is second in value only to diet and hydrotherapy. In certain classes of cases, indeed, massage can hardly be said to be second to the important therapeutic agents mentioned, especially in cases in which dilatation of the stomach, prolapse of the stomach or bowels, or other mechanical or static derange-

ments of the viscera are chiefly responsible for the symptoms present (**439-450**). We need not dwell further upon this point, however, as the application of massage in this class of disorders is considered at length elsewhere in this work (**389-424**).

Diseases of the Liver.—Although the liver is one of **126** the most important organs concerned in the digestive function, it performs so many and such varied functions that it is proper to consider it by itself. While organic diseases of the liver are only to a very slight degree benefited by massage, nearly all its functional disorders are capable of being very directly and beneficially influenced by appropriate applications of massage and joint movements. In acute inflammatory affections of the liver, massage and joint movements of the legs, carefully administered, are of great value as a means of relieving the general visceral congestion which results from hepatic inflammation, as well as the congestion of the liver itself.

In those conditions of the liver commonly termed torpidity, or sluggishness, massage of the liver itself is a measure of the greatest value. Vigorous percussion over the region of the liver, and kneading of those portions of the organ which are accessible to the hand of the masseur, are of very great value; but even greater value must be attached to general abdominal massage and chest massage combined with breathing movements, by which the stagnating circulation of the liver may be accelerated.

In cases of gallstones, massage has often proved a valuable measure, furnishing a means whereby the gall bladder may be made to discharge its contents into the intestinal canal. Manipulations of this sort must be employed with the greatest discretion, however, and should be trusted only to the hands of a trained masseur acting under intelligent medical direction.

Renal Disease.—Massage is undoubtedly of value in the **127** treatment of certain forms of renal disease, although in this class of cases it is necessary that it should be used with great care and discretion. This is especially true as regards acute inflammatory conditions of the kidneys, in which the throwing into the circulation of a great quantity of waste matters — leucomaines — by means of massage, might overtax the disabled kidneys.

Massage affords an excellent means of relieving the œdema sometimes present in renal disease, although, of course, it is not to be expected that a radical cure will be effected in all cases of this sort.

128   In displacement of the kidney (**447, 448**), massage locally and skillfully applied is of paramount importance, and in cases of renal insufficiency, massage may often be used with excellent results.

129   **Disorders of the Pelvic Organs.**— In diseases of the uterus and ovaries, massage often affords relief which cannot be obtained by any other means (**457-488**). While cures can seldom be expected in cases of chronic retro-displacement, displaced ovaries may often be restored to position by skillful manipulation; and even in cases in which the uterus and ovaries cannot be permanently replaced, so great improvement in the nutrition of the parts may be effected by massage as to relieve the patient from the distressing symptoms which had previously made life miserable.

130   Employed in connection with hydrotherapy, especially the sitz bath, the vaginal douche, and the moist abdominal girdle, with judicious applications of electricity and carefully graduated exercise, general and local massage may often be made to secure the most wonderful results. It is almost always necessary as a supplementary mode of treatment in cases in which an operation has been performed for shortening the round ligaments as a means of correcting retro-displacement. The neglect to employ massage and other curative means in these cases often results in failure to accomplish what might otherwise be effected in a most satisfactory manner, in the

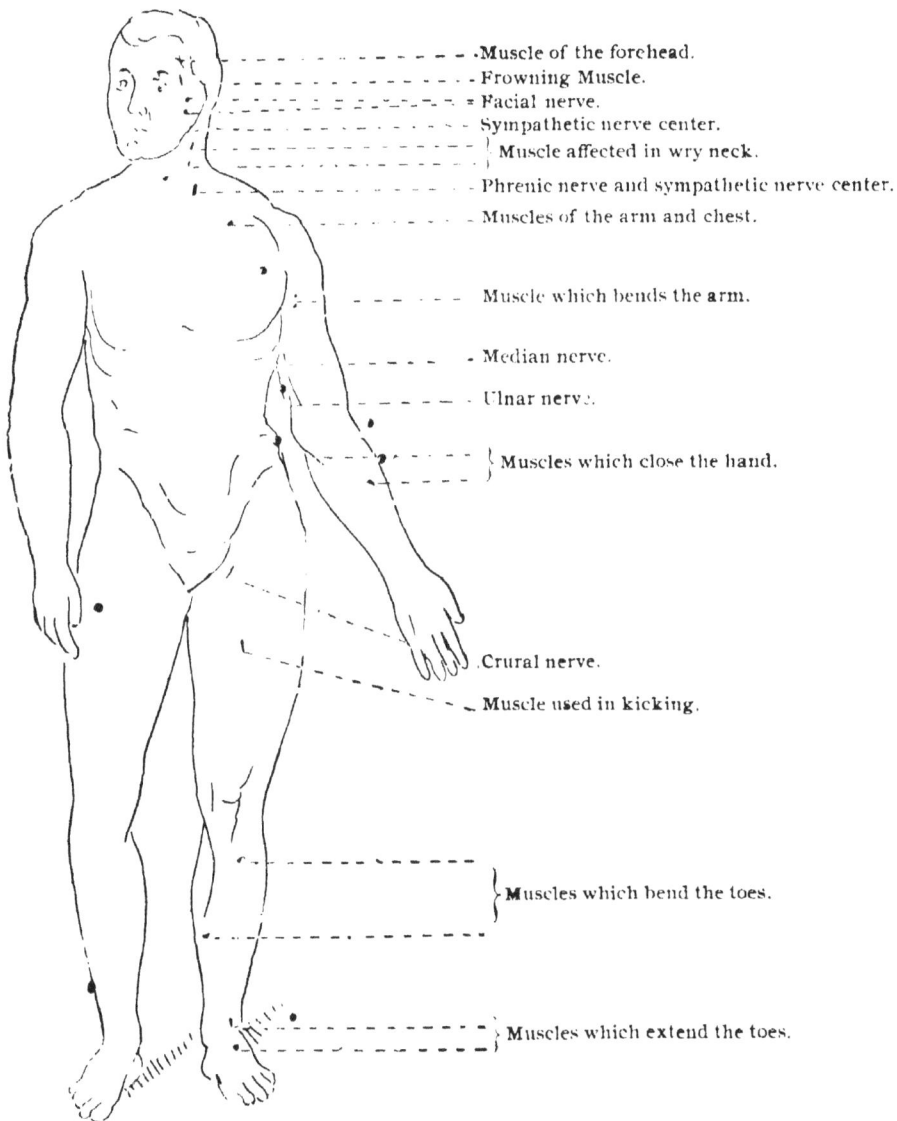

Muscle of the forehead.
Frowning Muscle.
Facial nerve.
Sympathetic nerve center.
Muscle affected in wry neck.
Phrenic nerve and sympathetic nerve center.
Muscles of the arm and chest.

Muscle which bends the arm.

Median nerve.

Ulnar nerve.

Muscles which close the hand.

Crural nerve.

Muscle used in kicking.

Muscles which bend the toes.

Muscles which extend the toes.

Fig. 32. Motor Points — Anterior View.

PLATE XVI.

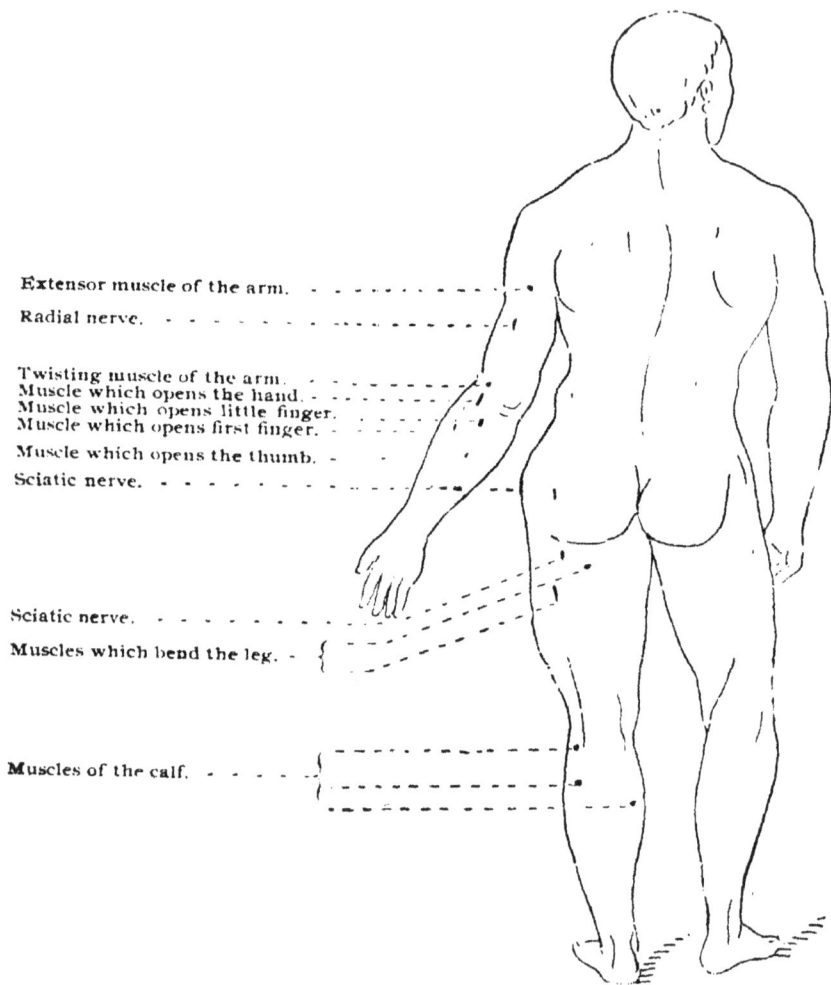

Extensor muscle of the arm.
Radial nerve.

Twisting muscle of the arm.
Muscle which opens the hand.
Muscle which opens little finger.
Muscle which opens first finger.
Muscle which opens the thumb.
Sciatic nerve.

Sciatic nerve.
Muscles which bend the leg.

Muscles of the calf.

Fig. 33.   Motor Points — Posterior View.

PLATE XVII.

reliet of this most obstinate, and with ordinary means incurable, class of maladies.

Amenorrhœa and dysmenorrhœa are often more effectively **131** treated by massage than by any other therapeutic means. Massage is useful not only in cases in which the menstrual pain is due to a morbid condition of the uterus, but also in ovarian dysmenorrhœa. In the latter class of cases, indeed, the writer has witnessed the most satisfactory and even remarkable results.

Subinvolution, and many other morbid conditions following **132** childbirth, are most efficiently treated by pelvic massage **(457-484).**

Among intelligent medical practitioners, massage of the **133** breast (**541-543**) has almost wholly replaced the old-fashioned breast pump, which has been responsible for so much mischief in cases requiring artificial emptying of the breast in nursing women.

Massage of the prostate (**485**) has afforded valuable results **134** in certain cases of recent enlargement of this organ as the effect of inflammatory action. In chronic enlargement from hypertrophy, however, very little result can be expected.

Spinal Curvatures.—In the treatment of spinal curva- **135** tures (**510-517**), massage is an extremely important adjunct to exercise and electrical applications, although it can hardly be said to be a substitute for either of these. By the combination of these three remedies, however, results which seem little less than marvelous may be obtained in suitable cases, but little can be expected when fatty degeneration of the muscles and structural changes of the vertebræ have taken place. In the last-named cases, mechanical support of some kind must be employed.

Pulmonary Disorders.— Massage is of value in va- **136** rious forms of pulmonary disease, especially in chronic pleurisy accompanied by serous exudate. Poliakow reports most excellent results in the treatment of cases of pleurisy with

4

exudation, absorption having taken place in eight to twenty days in each of the ten cases treated by this method.

137 In the application of massage to the thorax to promote absorption, the manipulations should be in the direction of the lymphatics, which run toward the axilla (**380-384**).

138 All of the different procedures of massage of the chest should be employed, but special attention should be given to friction and hacking movements.

139 Massage, in cases of this sort, is much to be preferred to blisters and other forms of counter-irritation, for the reason that the mild effects which it produces may be daily repeated, and it is accompanied by other results of even greater importance.

140 In emphysema, massage may be so employed as to relieve pulmonary congestion and aid expiration (**381**).

141 In phthisis the writer has seen excellent results from the use of massage, but it should be remembered that massage, as well as exercise, must be suspended during febrile conditions, as the heat-regulating functions of the body are seriously interfered with in phthisis as well as in acute febrile states. Massage, administered in such conditions, will increase the production of heat, and out of all proportion to the vigor of the treatment, just as so slight an amount of exercise as sitting up in bed will sometimes produce a relapse in cases of typhoid fever after convalescence is well established. The only form in which massage can be employed with advantage, or without risk of injury, is that of light friction. Both centripetal and centrifugal friction (**193, 194**) may be employed. As a rule, centrifugal friction should conclude the seance in all cases in which there is so slight an amount of temperature rise as one or two degrees Fahrenheit, and the patient should rest for at least two hours after the treatment. The best time of day for applying massage in cases of pulmonary disease, is soon after breakfast, or before the daily temperature rise begins. Massage of the chest is especially useful.

Sprains and Fractures (533-537).—The general **142** plan to be pursued in the employment of massage in the treatment of fractures is the following: When the fracture is reduced, place in an immobilizing apparatus. After three or four days, remove each day and apply massage to the whole limb, taking care to avoid displacement of the fragments. After the massage the splints or other immobilizing apparatus must be carefully replaced.

The massage of the portion of the limb adjacent to the fracture should at first be very gentle, consisting of centripetal friction and fulling movements, the pressure being gradually increased from day to day, deep massage being introduced not later than eight or ten days from the date of the fracture. Light percussion of various sorts may be applied to the whole limb. Deep massage may be applied to the uninjured portions of the limb from the start. The author has found it advantageous to use hot fomentations and alternate hot and cold compresses in connection with massage. At each treatment, the joints which are confined by the splints should be carefully flexed, so as to maintain perfect mobility.

The attention of the profession has been especially called to the value of massage in fractures by Schode, Mezger, Lucas-Championnière, and Berne.

Diseases of the Eye and Ear.— Muscular asthenopia, **143** glaucoma, corneal ulcer, corneal opacity, and various other affections of the eye, have been successfully treated by massage (**498-500**).

Certain forms of deafness, particularly deafness due to ca- **144** tarrhal disease of the Eustachian tubes, may be not only temporarily relieved but permanently benefited by massage of the ear, neck, and throat (**501-503, 432-438**).

Even acute and chronic nasal catarrh is improved under **145** careful applications of massage to the face (**489-497**) and neck.

THE PROCEDURES OF MASSAGE.

146   All the different useful procedures in massage may be classified under seven heads, as follows : —

    1. Touch.
    2. Stroking.
    3. Friction.
    4. Kneading.
    5. Vibration.
    6. Percussion.
    7. Joint Movements.

Under each of these heads we have several subdivisions, which must be separately considered.

TOUCH.

147   The touch of massage is not simply an ordinary touch or contact of the hand with the body, but is a skilled or professional touch.   It is a touch applied with intelligence, with control, with a purpose; and simple as it is, is capable of producing decided physiological effects.   This procedure has three different forms of application ; viz., *passive touch, pressure,* and *nerve compression.*

148   **1. Passive Touch** (Fig. 34).—This consists in lightly touching the part operated upon with one or more fingers, with the whole hand, or with both hands.

Physiological Effects.—The physiological effects of simple touch are :—

149   (1) Elevation of the temperature of a part by the communication of animal heat.

150   (2) A subtle influence upon the nervous system—the so-called hypnotic effect, not due to any occult force exerted or mysterious qualities possessed by the operator, but simply the reflex influence through the cutaneous nerves upon the centers of the brain and cord, of the gentle contact of a warm, soft hand with the skin.

(3) It is possible that certain electrical effects may result **151** from simple contact of the hand of the masseur with the body of the patient (**38**).

The effects of simple touch are quite remarkable. Some **152** persons seem to be especially sensitive to its effects, and feel, or imagine they feel, a peculiar influence emanating from the operator, to which the term "magnetism" has sometimes been applied. The hypnotic state is produced in some very susceptible individuals by simple passive touch. The peculiar influence attributed to the touch of certain persons is due, not to any occult power, but to subtle qualities of manner, a peculiar softness of the hand, or some other personal quality not easy to describe.

Therapeutic Applications.— Touch is often remark- **153** ably effective in relieving hyperæsthesias, especially in the region of the head and joints. Pain is lessened, and numbness, tingling, and other sensations are made to disappear. Sleeplessness may also be relieved, and nervous irritability quieted, by simple contact of the hand with the head.

In applications of touch for therapeutic purposes, it is important that the utmost quiet should be preserved. The patient should be required to shut his eyes, if the application is made for the relief of insomnia or general nervous irritability, and should not be allowed to speak, neither should he be spoken to. All noises and disturbing causes should be suppressed, as it is desirable that the patient's mind should become as quiet as possible, and that the sensorium should be protected from the disturbing influence of sensory impressions of every sort.

2. Pressure.— This consists in making light or heavy **154** pressure with the whole of one or both hands or with one or more fingers, upon the head, a joint, or some swollen or irritated part, or upon any portion of the body.

155   Physiological Effects and Therapeutic Applications.—The effect of pressure is to diminish swelling and congestion, and thus to relieve pain. Violent headache or pain in a joint may often be relieved in this way. A person suffering from severe toothache involuntarily makes firm pressure against the painful part. Pressure relieves pain, doubtless both by emptying the blood vessels and by benumbing the nerves.

156   3. Nerve Compression (Fig. 35).—In this procedure strong pressure is made upon a nerve trunk at some point in its course. The points usually selected for pressure are the so-called "motor points," which are located upon the surface where large nerve trunks are readily accessible, lying just beneath the skin. The accompanying cuts (Figs. 32 and 33) show at a glance the points at which the principal nerves may be most easily reached. The spinal nerves are compressed by placing one finger on each side of the spine and making firm pressure opposite the spaces between the vertebræ.

157   Physiological Effects.—The physiological effect of light pressure upon a nerve trunk is that of stimulation. The slight irritation produced by the pressure is transmitted to the nerve centers which give rise to the nerve operated upon, and thus both the nerve trunk and its centers may be, by repetition of the pressure, excited to almost any degree desired. A good illustration of the stimulating effect of pressure upon the nerve trunk is afforded by the coughing produced by light pressure upon the pneumogastric nerve in the neck, just above the sternum.

158   Firm, deep pressure, continued for some little time, produces numbness and may even paralyze the nerve trunk, thus giving rise to a sedative effect. An illustration of this is found in the well-known sensation resulting from a blow upon the ulnar nerve at the point where it comes near the surface, just behind the elbow. The numbness of the little finger and of the inner side of the fourth finger thus induced may last for some minutes, if the pressure or blow has been sufficiently severe.

Stimulation of the pneumogastric nerve is produced by **159** pressure at either side of the larynx just above the upper end of the sternum, the finger being carried backward and slightly below the level of its top, until resistance is felt by the compression of the tissues against the spine. This, however, is a measure which must be used with the greatest care. It should never be employed except under the advice of a physician. Sufficient pressure might easily be applied to produce grave symptoms in a sensitive patient (Fig. 35).

One of the most interesting and striking illustrations of the **160** sedative effects of nerve compression is to be found in the application of this measure to the abdominal sympathetic when in a hypersensitive or hyperæsthetic state. For this purpose the application should be made as follows : With the patient lying upon the back, the knees drawn up and the feet supported, the head — not the shoulders — resting upon a pillow, so as to relax the abdominal muscles, pressure is made at three points respectively, two inches on each side of the umbilicus, and two inches below this point. The tips of the fingers should be placed upon these points in succession, and pressed firmly and steadily toward the spinal column until resistance is felt. Sometimes the surface is so sensitive that the patient contracts his abdominal muscles so firmly that but slight impression can be made upon the tense abdominal wall. In such a case it is necessary to divert the patient's attention from his abdominal muscles. This can be done by making him breathe deeply and regularly. With each expiration, carry the fingers a little deeper into the tissues, until they are pressed against the anterior surface of the spine. The patient will experience some pain when the pressure falls, as it should, directly upon the lumbar ganglia (one on each side of the umbilicus) or the subumbilical ganglion or lumbo-aortic plexus, located two inches below the umbilicus (Fig. 76).

Without making hard pressure, the ganglia, when found, should be rubbed and pressed intermittently for half a minute, at intervals of two or three minutes. After a few applications the sensitiveness will be found to have disappeared either wholly or in part, unless the cause still continues active. Too great pressure must not be applied at first, as nausea, faintness, and even prolonged pain may thereby be produced.

161 **Therapeutic Application.**—Pressure is extremely useful in connection with joint massage, affording a means of emptying the veins and lymph spaces and vessels. It should be employed in connection with friction and kneading as a means of emptying the large veins and 'lymph vessels which are found in the region of the joints.

162 Nerve compression is either stimulating or sedative, according to the manner in which it is applied. By a repetition of stimulating applications to the nerve trunk, important alterative effects may be produced, rendering this mode very valuable in many cases of sciatica accompanied by structural changes in the nerve trunk, also in paralysis.

163 Nerve compression is one of the most valuable means of arousing the activity of the nerve centers, through the indirect stimulation induced by this procedure.

164 In the application of nerve compression in cases of paralysis, the pressure should be light and intermittent, repeated four or five times, the pressure lasting not more than two or three seconds, with an interval of five or six seconds.

165 For general stimulation of the spine, make firm pressure with the thumbs close to the spinous processes and opposite the spaces between the spines, or between the ribs near the spine.

166 In facial neuralgia, pressure may be made upon the seat of pain or at the nearest point at which the affected nerve is accessible from the surface.

167 Intercostal neuralgia is relieved by pressure applied to the intercostal space at the seat of pain, the pressure being directed toward the lower border of the uppermost rib.

168 In sciatica and crural neuralgia, pressure may be applied to the affected nerves (Fig. 25). In sciatica, pressure should be made at the points along the junction of the sacrum and

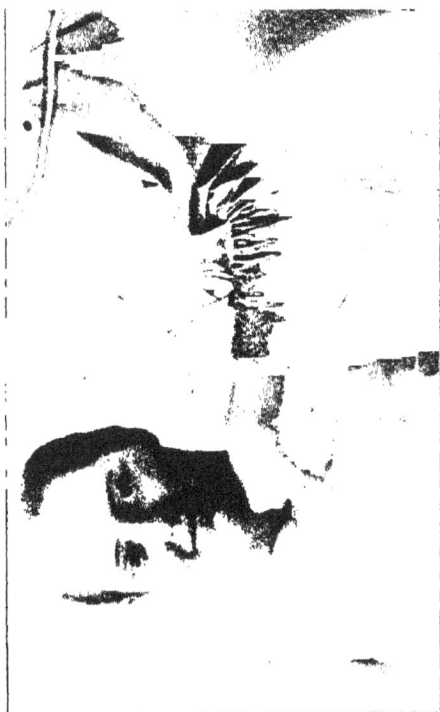

Fig. 35. Nerve Compression.

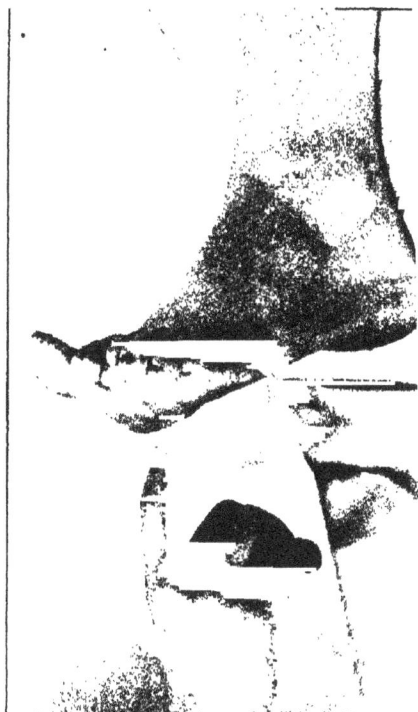

Fig. 34. Passive Touch.

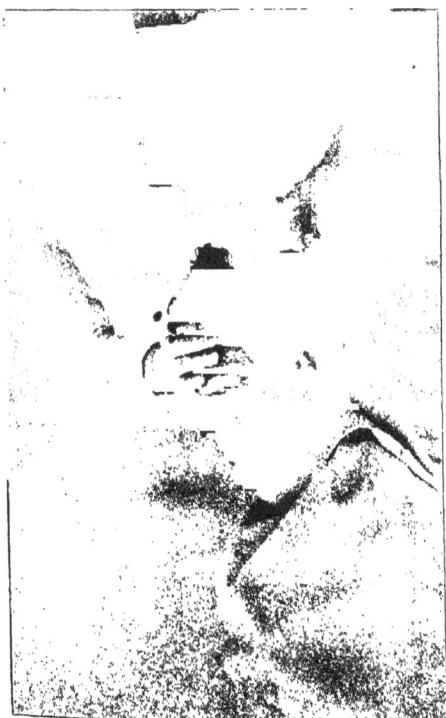

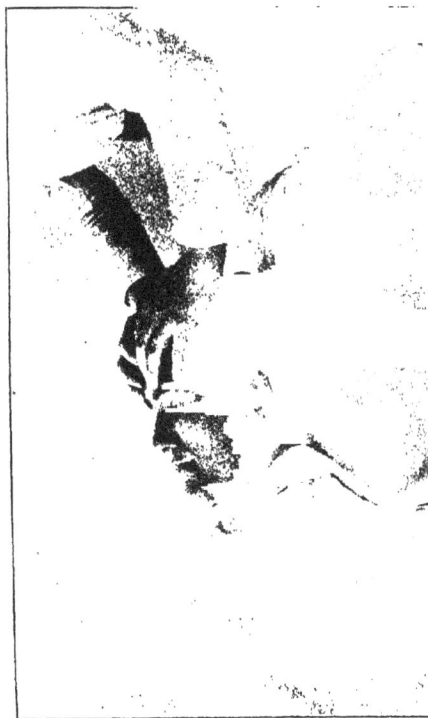

PLATE XVIII.—Touch.

ilium, as well as over the sciatic nerve in the hollow of the thigh. The pressure should be sufficient to cause some pain, and should be continued until the pain ceases or the nerve becomes numb.

Pressure is uniformly made, in nerve compression, upon the points at which nerve trunks are most easy of access. This procedure is one that needs to be employed with very great discretion.

STROKING.

This procedure (Fig. 36) is simply touch combined with **169** motion. The tips of two or three or of all the fingers, or the entire palmar surface of one or both hands, should be moved gently over the skin with light contact. In gentle stroking, not even the full weight of the hand is allowed to rest upon the surface, the contact being made as light as possible.

The direction of the strokes, or passes, in application to **170** different parts of the body, is as follows : —

Head, from before backward, starting at the center of the forehead, and from above downward, starting at the vertex.

Back, from above downward and from the median line outward.

Chest, from the sides toward the median line.

Abdomen, upper part, from the sides inward and upward ; middle part, toward the median line ; lower part, from below upward and inward.

Arms, from the shoulders toward the hands.

Legs, from the hips downward.

Feet, from the toes toward the heel.

The wrist must be flexible, and the movement even and slow, and perfectly uniform in relation to pressure and time.

Rate of Movement.— The number of passes per minute **171** will, of course, depend upon the extent of surface covered by each stroke, but the hand should not be allowed to move at a more rapid rate than one or two inches per second. The stroking may be repeated many times upon the same place — from two or three minutes to half an hour, or until the desired effect is produced.

172   Stroking is always done in one direction only, never to and fro.   As a rule, the direction of stroking should be that of the blood current in the arteries, outward or downward from the heart.   The direction, as a rule, is the opposite of that of friction.   When applied to hairy surfaces, the stroking should be in the way the hair lies, not against the hair, as in " rubbing a cat's back the wrong way."

173   There are several forms of stroking : —

    1. With the finger tips, *digital stroking.*
    2. With the palm of one or both hands, *palmar stroking.*
    3. With the knuckles, *knuckle stroking.*
    4. *Reflex stroking.*

174   **Digital Stroking** (Fig. 36).— The tip of one finger may be used, or the tips of all the fingers of one or both hands.   The fingers are held very slightly apart, a little curved, and in a flexible condition, so that all the fingers will fall lightly in contact with the surface.   Stroking with the finger tips is used chiefly for the forehead and spine.

175   **Palmar Stroking.**—In this procedure the whole or a part of the palm of one hand, or the palms of both hands, should be applied to the surface.   It is used for broad, fleshy parts, about the joints and for the soles of the feet.

176   **Knuckle Stroking.**— In this procedure the hand is closed, and the knuckles of the second joints of the fingers are applied to the surface. It is seldom used except in massage of the back.

177   **Reflex Stroking** (Fig. 37).— In this form of stroking, which, so far as the writer knows, has not been previously described, or systematically employed by others as a therapeutic measure, applications are made exclusively to those parts of the body which have been described by physiologists as areas which may be employed in developing the so-called cutaneous, or skin, reflexes.   Light stroking applied to these surfaces produces muscular contraction as the result of the formation of a reflex arc through the spinal cord.   These reflexes are

exceedingly well marked in those persons who are said to be
ticklish. The reflex is developed by gently stroking the sensitive part with the finger nail. The end of a lead pencil, a wooden toothpick, or the head of a pin may also be
employed.

Reflex Areas.—The principal areas which have been de- **178**
scribed as particularly susceptible in producing reflex influences, are the following : —

(1) The skin of the back between the scapulæ, or shoulder
blades ; (2) The sides of the chest between the fourth and
sixth ribs ; (3) The skin of the abdomen in the mammary
line ; (4) The surface at the upper and inner portion of the
thighs ; (5) The skin overlying the gluteal muscles ; (6) The
sole of the foot. The writer will venture to add to this list, as
the result of his observations, another reflex area ; namely,
(7) The skin of the axillary region, which in some persons is
exceedingly sensitive.

The various reflexes are named partly from their location **179**
and partly from the muscular effects produced reflexly by their
stimulation, as follows : —

Interscapular.

Epigastric (produces movement at the epigastrium).

Abdominal (causes contraction of the abdominal muscles
on one side).

Cremasteric (causes contraction of the cremasteric muscle in
males, and probably of the round ligament in females). The
writer has noticed that stimulation of the skin of the cremasteric area in girls and women causes a muscular contraction
just above Poupart's ligament and in the region of the inguinal
canal. This same reflex was observed in the case of a young
man whose development had assumed the feminine type in
consequence of arrest of development of the testicles.

Gluteal.

Plantar (causes contraction of the muscles of the thigh).

A seventh may be termed the *axillary.*

These reflexes affect not only the cutaneous nerves and **180**
muscles which are seen to act as a result of the local surface

stimulation, but necessarily also the nerve centers. The particular portions of the cord acted upon in connection with the several reflexes are as follows : —

Interscapular, sixth to eighth cervical and first dorsal segments.

Epigastric, fifth to seventh dorsal.

Abdominal, eighth to twelfth dorsal.

Cremasteric, first to third lumbar.

Gluteal, fourth and fifth lumbar.

Plantar, fifth and sixth sacral.

The *axillary* reflex, if admitted, is in relation to the second, third, and fourth dorsal, or that portion of the spinal cord lying between the areas excited by the interscapular and the cremasteric.

181   It is a curious fact that firm pressure upon the reflex areas does not develop the reflex, whereas very light stroking may produce so powerful a reflex that one or both limbs will be suddenly drawn up. The reflex is also excited by cold.

182   **Physiological Effects.**— Digital and palmar stroking, when properly applied, have a decided sedative effect ; but it is important that the application should be made in a proper manner,— with very light contact, and in the direction of the blood current in the arteries.

183   In friction, the purpose is to increase the circulation of the skin and excite activity, hence the movement is in the direction of the venous blood current. The purpose of stroking is the opposite ; namely, to diminish the blood supply. The race horse is always rubbed *down* after violent exercise. The athlete also has himself rubbed in the same manner, after a contest.

Stroking, even when very light, also produces a peculiar effect upon the cutaneous nerves, the action of which, when applied to certain regions at least, seems to be strongly sedative and remarkably quieting.

184   Knuckle stroking is stimulating. It might, perhaps, be more properly called friction than stroking, as it is applied with more pressure than ordinary stroking. The purpose, when applied to the back, is to excite the posterior branches of the spinal nerves, and thus stimulate the spinal centers.

Reflex stroking is certainly a most powerful means of stimu- **185** lating the centers of the cord. It must not be supposed that the muscular actions induced by reflex stroking are the sole effects produced. Very active reflex relations exist between the entire cutaneous surface and internal parts. The reflexes named are especially designated for the reason that the muscular effects produced are so apparent as to render them easy of observation and study. The same nerve centers which send branches to the muscles involved in these reflexes, also send branches to internal parts.

It must not be forgotten that the organic reflexes, those **186** concerned with the genito-urinary functions and those of defecation, as well as those of secretion and motion as concerned in digestion, have their seat in the spinal cord, so that the same stimulation which excites the gluteal and cremasteric reflexes must also excite, more or less, the nerve centers which control the digestive and the genito-urinary functions.

Therapeutic Applications.— Gentle stroking of the **187** forehead in many cases affords relief from sleeplessness. It is not an uncommon thing for a patient to fall asleep under what might be termed the hypnotic influence of gentle digital or palmar stroking of the head. Palmar stroking of the feet will in many cases produce the same effect, especially when employed in connection with stroking of the limbs.

Stroking may also be employed advantageously after other **188** procedures in massage, for the purpose of lessening an excessive degree of cutaneous congestion or stimulation which may have been produced. It is especially useful for this purpose when applied about a joint. It is also of value as a means for relieving hypersensitiveness, even when accompanied with inflammation. Certain forms of nervous headache may frequently be controlled in a most decided manner by gentle stroking of the head.

189 Neuralgic pains, likewise, are sometimes much alleviated by this means, as are numbness, formication, and a great variety of neurasthenic pains and paræsthesias. Stroking of the forehead produces in some persons a hypnotic effect which is more or less pronounced according to the temperament of the individual. This effect is rarely ever pronounced except in hysterical cases. It is due not to any magnetic or occult influence on the part of the manipulator, but simply to the reflex influence of the nerves involved, acting upon the volitionary centers.

190 *Reflex stroking* is applicable to a variety of conditions, especially the following : —

1. *Interscapular stroking*, used advantageously in spinal anæmia.

2. The *epigastric reflex*, excited advantageously in hypopepsia and motor insufficiency of the stomach.

3. *Abdominal reflex stroking*, especially useful for the relief of constipation and a relaxed condition of the abdominal muscles. It should always be used in connection with abdominal massage.

4. *Gluteal and cremasteric reflex stroking*, advantageously employed in cases of loss of tone in the rectum or the bladder, or in weakness of any of the genito-urinary functions.

5. *Plantar stroking*, usefully employed in cases of the last named sort, as well as in all others in which it is especially desired to improve the innervation of the muscles of the lower extremities.

FRICTION.

191 In this procedure the whole or a part of the hand is moved over the surface with a considerable degree of pressure, the amount varying in different parts — heavy over thick, fleshy masses, light over bony surfaces and thin tissues. The amount of pressure, however, should never be such that the hand will not readily slip over the surface, nor so great as to interfere with the movement of the blood in the arteries.

The principal effect of friction is upon the superficial veins, **192** the large venous trunks, and the lymph spaces and vessels. In the application of friction, the thumb only, or the whole or a greater part of the palmar surface of the hand, is brought in contact with the part operated upon.

Five different forms of friction may be described as follows : —

Centripetal friction (Fig. 38), in which the movement **193** is in the direction of the blood current in the veins, chiefly applicable to the extremities, the movement being from below upward, and from the hands and feet toward the body, the thumb or palmar surface of the hand being employed.

Centrifugal friction, in which the movement is opposite **194** to that of the blood current.

Circular friction (Fig. 39), applicable to the extremities. **195** The limb is grasped by both hands, which make an alternate wringing or twisting movement, beginning at the hand or foot and extending upward.

Spiral friction (Fig. 40), a sort of combination of the pre- **196** ceding, executed with one hand, which progresses from the lower, or distal, to the upper, or proximal, end of the part with a sort of spiral movement.

Rotary friction (Fig. 41), in which the hands are made to **197** move over a broad surface in an elliptical, circular, or semicircular direction ; especially applicable to such fleshy areas as the hip and that portion of the back lying above the spines of the scapulæ. In applying rotary friction, it is often necessary for one hand to support the tissues while the other hand is executing the movements.

Rate of Movement. — The rate of the movement will nec- **198** essarily vary according to the length of the stroke, and hence differs in different parts of the body. The rate may be varied from thirty to one hundred and eighty strokes per minute.

Direction of Movement. — The direction of the move- **199** ment in friction must necessarily vary more or less, according to the part operated upon. The general rule is to follow the large veins. Special care should be taken, in the treatment of the extremities, to follow the large venous trunks, making firm pressure directly over the large veins with the thumbs, passing from below upward.

200   In the treatment of the forearm, the masseur will give special attention to the *radial vein*, which runs along the outer and anterior portion of the forearm ; the anterior and posterior *ulnar*, which course along the anterior and posterior aspect of the inner border of the arm ; and the *median*, which lies along the middle of the anterior surface of the forearm (Figs. 23 and 24).

201   In the upper arm, special attention will be given to the *cephalic* along the outer side, and the *basilic* along the inner side, of the arm (Fig. 23).

202   In applying friction to the leg, the thumb should at first be passed with firm pressure over the *long saphenous*, the course of which is from the instep along the anterior and inner portion of the leg to the groin ; and the *short saphenous*, the course of which is from below the outer malleolus along the outer and posterior portion of the leg to the bend of the knee (Fig. 25).

203   Friction is applied to the following parts in the direction designated : —

Head, from before backward, and above downward.

Neck, downward.

Back, above shoulder blades, circular ; from shoulder blades to sacrum, down ; in the region of the loins, from the sides toward the spine.

Hips, circular.

Chest, from the sternum toward the axilla.

Abdomen, upper part, from above downward and outward ; lower part, from the median line downward and outward.

Arms and legs, from below upward.

204   *To promote absorption*, rub toward the heart (centripetal friction).

205   *For sedative and derivative effects* upon the viscera and nerve centers, rub downward (centrifugal friction).

206   Rubbing upward, or in the direction of the venous blood current, *increases the activity* of the circulation.

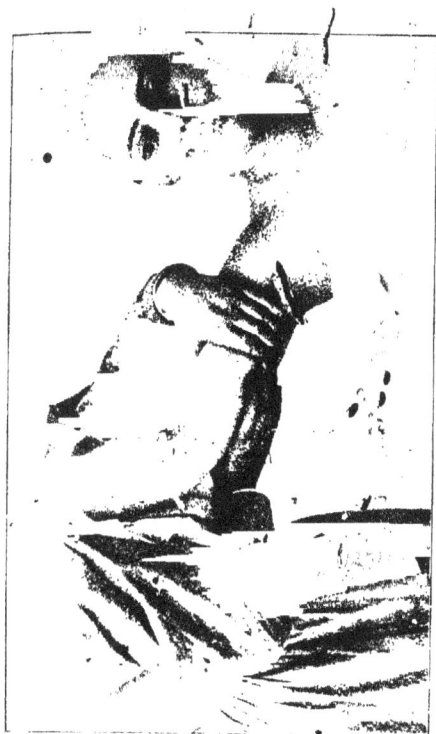

Fig. 39. Circular Friction.

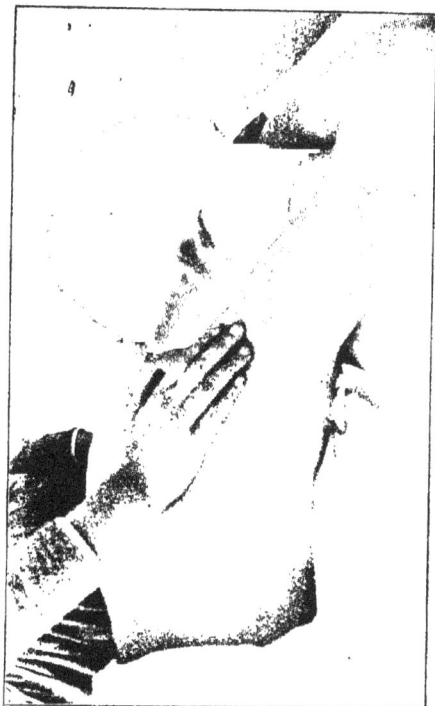

Fig. 41. Rotary Friction.

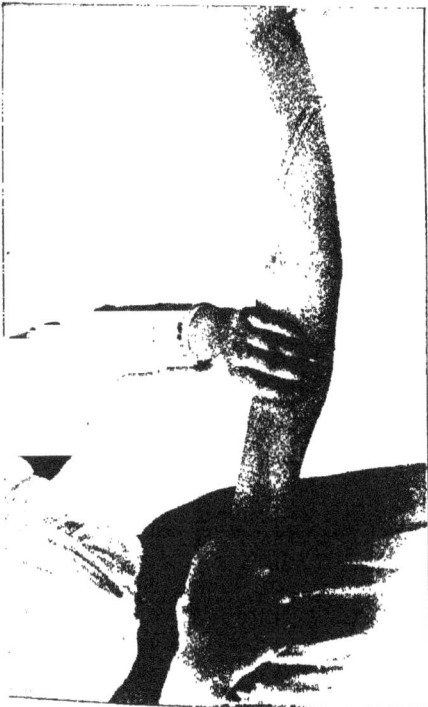

Fig. 38. Centripetal Friction.

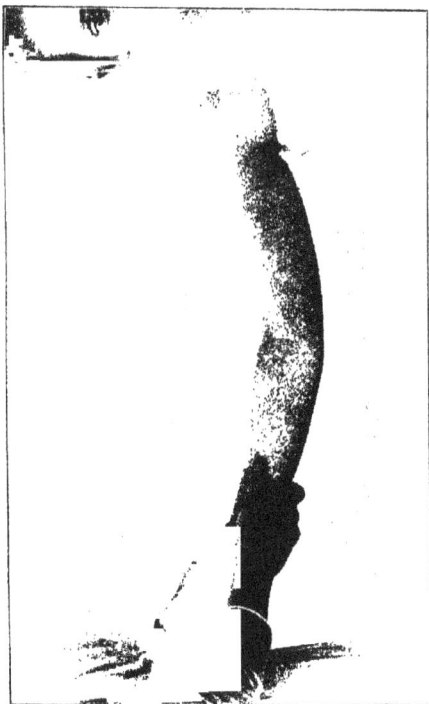

Fig. 40. Spiral Friction.

PLATE XIX.—Friction.

Rubbing downward *decreases vascular activity.* **207**

In the application of friction, pressure should always be **208**
uniform for the part operated upon, and should be carefully
graduated to meet each particular case.

As a rule, some lubricant should be used. Fine vaseline, **209**
cocoanut oil, cacao butter, and talcum powder are the best
lubricants.

Friction is applicable to all parts of the body, but is espe- **210**
cially useful to the limbs, head, and neck. It should always
be used at the beginning of the application of massage, if the
surface is cold.

In the application of friction to large parts, both hands **211**
should be used, either together or in alternation. In the
treatment of a part which is small, it may be steadied by one
hand while being treated by the other.

Mode of Applying Friction to Different Parts. 212
— A systematic order and method is essential in the application of friction to different parts of the body, which
may be described for the chief divisions of the body as
follows : —

The Hand.— The patient's extended hand being allowed to **213**
rest in one hand of the operator, with the dorsal surface up,
the masseur holding the fingers of his other hand firmly extended, applies the tips of his fingers to the patient's hand in
such a way that they will fall into the grooves between the adjacent fingers and metacarpal bones. The fingers are then
pushed along in these grooves from the roots of the nails to
the wrists. After repeating the movement several times on
the back of the hand, the patient's hand is turned so that the
palmar surface will be up, and the same movement repeated as
before, with the modification that the fingers are carried a little
farther up the wrist until the heel of the operator's hand rests
in the hollow of the patient's hand, when slight rotary movement and firm pressure should be made, for the purpose of
compressing firmly and emptying the numerous veins of the
fleshy portion of the palm.

The movements upon the back of the hand should be at the rate of sixty a minute; on the palmar surface a smaller number of movements will be executed per minute on account of the pause for three or four seconds in making rotary friction in the palm after each centripetal stroke.

214 *The Forearm.*— With the arm of the patient half flexed, the masseur, facing the patient and operating with both hands, should make strokes from wrist to elbow, first with one hand upon one side and then with the other hand upon the other side of the arm, in such a manner that each hand will include one half the circulation of the forearm, both thumbs resting upon the front of the arm. The operator may, if he prefers, stand with his back to the patient, making the strokes alternately with the two hands, as before.

215 The masseur should keep constantly in mind the fact that firm pressure is to be made only with the ascending friction stroke. The hand is allowed to glide lightly over the surface in the descending or stroking movement, as a soothing measure, and not for the purpose of applying friction.

216 In the treatment of very feeble persons the patient may be too much fatigued if the operator works with both hands at once, thus leaving him to support his own arm. In such case the patient's arm should be supported by the masseur, who will grasp the patient's right hand with his own right hand, or the left hand with his left, applying spiral friction (Fig. 40) with the other hand upon the front side of the arm, then changing hands to operate upon the back of the arm.

217 *The Arm.*— Work the arm in a manner similar to that described for the forearm.

218 *The Shoulder.*— In applying friction to the shoulder, the masseur faces the side of the patient, operating with the two hands in alternation, following the surface of the joint, and always taking care to work centripetally; that is, toward the heart or toward the center of the body, and taking pains to follow the irregularities of the surface. The under as well as the upper side of the shoulder should receive attention.

The Foot.—Begin as with the hand, by friction with the **219** ends of the fingers upon the dorsum of the foot, the operator standing in such a position as to face the sole of the foot. After finishing the dorsal surface, change the position so as to face the side of the foot, and make alternate transverse movements with the two hands on both sole and dorsum, working vigorously from toes to heel and instep. Lastly, extend the friction movements to the ankle, working with both hands, and following up the grooves on each side of the tendon Achilles.

The Leg.—With the leg half flexed upon the thigh, stand- **220** ing facing the patient, the masseur applies friction to the calf of the leg from ankle to knee, making eight or ten strokes, then turns his back to the patient, and operates upon the front of the leg by means of the thumbs working in alternation.

The Thigh.—Standing with his back to the patient, the mas- **221** seur grasps the leg in such a manner that the fingers fall behind and the thumbs in front, and makes very firm but rather slow strokes from knee to groin, not forgetting to give the knee due attention.

The Chest.—The patient's arms should be separated a little **222** from the sides, so as to straighten the outer portion of the pectoral muscles. The masseur, standing at one side, and facing the patient's feet, makes strokes from the insertion of the pectoral muscles at the humerus toward the median line, beginning at the upper border just below the clavicle. The two sides may be operated upon simultaneously, or in succession, both hands being employed upon one side, one hand following the other in the movements. In progressing downward, the movement should be reversed below the pectorals, and the hands should be carried as far around the sides as convenient, care being taken to work toward the axilla above, and to follow the direction of the ribs and cartilages, until the whole surface has been covered from the clavicle to the lower borders of the last ribs.

The Abdomen.—Facing the patient, the masseur first makes **223** long strokes from the upper to the lower portion of the abdomen, one hand following the other over the recti muscles, the two hands operating simultaneously over the lateral portions. After covering the whole surface six or eight times in this manner, strokes should be made more exactly in the direction of the veins, as follows : At the upper part of the abdomen, make strokes downward and outward, following the direction of the lower cartilages ; for the middle portion, make strokes from the median line outward, reaching around as far as possible ; for the lower portion, make the strokes downward and outward, in the direction of the hip joints.

224   *The Neck.*—Facing the patient, place the hands one on each side of the head in such a manner that the little finger will rest in the groove behind the lower jaw, the other fingers resting upon the mastoid processes, and the inner border of the heels of the hands touching. Move the hands downward, and at the same time rotate them inward, so as to bring as large a portion of the palmar surface as possible in contact with the neck. At the lower border of the neck, move the hands outward toward the shoulders. After a few strokes, carry the hands a little farther back around the neck, so that as they move downward, the thumbs will rest one on each side of the larynx, thus compressing all the veins of the neck, both the superficial and the jugular, which lie deep). Finish with a few strokes applied to the back of the neck, starting at the occiput, and carrying the strokes downward and outward to the point of the shoulder.

225   *The Face.*—Standing facing the patient, the operator places the palmar surface of his hands in contact, then applies them to the patient's face in such a manner that the little fingers touch the forehead at the median line. Separating the hands at the ulnar border, they are gradually spread out as in opening a book, until the little fingers rest upon the temples and the tips of the thumbs fall at the middle of the forehead.

Fixing the thumbs at this point, the outer borders of the hands are moved downward by lateral flexion at the wrist until the forefingers fall at a level with the eyes. The whole hand is then moved downward in such a way that the nose is grasped and compressed between the thumbs while the palms of the hands and the fingers cover the cheeks. The movement is continued downward, and finished by bringing the hands together below the chin. The object kept in view should be to bring as much of the hand as possible in contact with the face, and to touch every portion of its surface.

The Head.—With the patient sitting or half reclining, and **226** the masseur standing behind, the ends of the fingers and thumbs, with the fingers slightly flexed, are placed firmly in contact with the scalp, and a movement executed similar to that employed by a barber in shampooing. The mistake must not be made of applying the friction to the hair instead of the scalp. The movement begins at the vertex, gradually extending to the borders of the hairy scalp.

The Hip.—In friction of the hip a very considerable amount **227** of pressure is admissible, as the muscles and fleshy masses are very thick and firm. In applying friction to the hips, the masseur may face either the head or the feet of the patient.

1. Make rotary friction upon the two sides simultaneously or in succession. In very fleshy persons it will be found necessary to support the tissues with one hand while operating with the other, on account of the great mobility of the muscular mass and the roughness of the skin so frequently encountered in this region of the body.

2. Apply centripetal friction, working from the great trochanter toward the crest of the ilium, and along the crest of the ilium from behind forward.

The Back.—The patient lies upon his face, the masseur **228** facing his head.

1. A few light strokes are first applied from the occiput to the sacrum, along the center of the back, one hand following the other. The lateral surfaces are then covered by the two hands working simultaneously from above downward, and rotary friction is administered with greater pressure to the fleshy mass lying above the shoulder blade. The two sides may be treated simultaneously or in succession, one hand being

used to support the tissues.   The latter method is usually necessary in very fleshy persons.

2. From the shoulder blades to the hips, lateral strokes are made, the masseur standing with his left side to the patient, facing his feet, the hands being placed as far around the sides as convenient, and simultaneously drawn toward the spine, the movement ending with the hands in contact.   Great care should be taken to follow the ribs in the region of the thorax, which will give the movements a semicircular direction.

3. Separating the index and middle fingers of the right hand, place one on either side of the spinous processes, and making firm pressure, move the hand downward from the occiput to the sacrum.   The object should be to crowd the ends of the fingers as deeply into the tissues as possible on either side of the spinous processes, so as to influence the dorsi-spinal veins.   If necessary, the left hand may be used to increase the pressure.

4. Finish the back by a few light strokes from above downward, using both hands simultaneously, covering as much surface as possible with the fingers in contact with each other.

229   Physiological Effects.— The physiological effects of friction are somewhat complex.   They may be briefly stated as follows : —

1. Reflex effects upon the vasomotor centers, resulting in dilatation of the small vessels of the skin and increased activity of the peripheral circulation.

2. Mechanical aid to the movement of fluid in the veins and lymph spaces and channels.   The beneficial effects obtained are largely due to the existence of valves in the veins and lymph channels, by which the fluid displaced toward the heart is prevented from returning.

3. Friction, which, when applied in a skilled and proper manner, is capable of producing powerful derivative effects.

230   *Reflex or stimulating effects* may be increased by using no lubricant of any kind — in other words, making friction upon the dry skin.

Mechanical effects are increased, and the reflex or irritant **231** effects decreased, by lubrication of the skin.

The principal object in the application of friction is to **232** empty the veins and lymph spaces and channels, thus encouraging the circulation. By thus accelerating the flow of the blood and the lymph, vital exchanges are encouraged, and the tissues are freed from the waste matters which they contain. On the whole, friction is one of the most valuable of the various methods of procedure in massage.

All the functions of the skin are especially stimulated by **233** friction. Under the application of friction, a dry skin becomes moist and oily through the increased activity of the perspiratory and sebaceous glands. It is also a common observation that friction promotes the development of the hair upon the parts to which it is applied. Professor Winternitz and his students have shown that by the application of friction to the skin, the amount of moisture thrown off may be increased sixty per cent and the dissipation of heat more than ninety-five per cent. Under the influence of friction the temperature of the skin is raised to a very marked degree, both through the dilatation of the surface vessels, which brings more blood to the surface, and by increased production of heat. This is, of course, the cause of the increased heat dissipation under the influence of friction.

Therapeutic Applications.—Friction is usually em- **234** ployed therapeutically in conjunction with kneading and other movements, being used in alternation with other procedures.

The reflex or stimulant effect of friction is useful in all **235** cases in which the peripheral circulation is defective. Care must be taken in the employment of friction for stimulative effects, that the skin does not become abraded by too long manipulation without lubrication. From five to eight minutes is as long a time as it is safe to apply friction to the dry skin.

The mechanical effects of friction, by aiding the venous **236** and lymph circulations, are among the most valuable of all the results to be obtained by massage. It is by the acceleration of the circulation, by means of which a larger supply of white blood corpuscles is brought to the affected parts, thus encouraging phagocytosis (85), that friction is of great value in the treatment of inflammatory exudates, such as usually occur about joints. When used for this purpose, the friction should be applied in alternation to the affected part and to the tissues between it and the heart.

237   Friction is especially useful in general dropsy, and in all forms of local swelling, whether due to inflammation or to congestion resulting from a mechanical cause acting upon the circulation. Its efficiency in promoting absorption renders it of great value in sprains, chronic joint enlargements from various causes, sciatica, rheumatism, gout, and even in glandular enlargements. In the treatment of such affections, massage should first be applied to the diseased part and then friction, by the centripetal method, to the tissues between it and the heart.

238   The *derivative effects* of friction are of great value in the treatment of inflamed joints, painful sprains, pelvic pains, insomnia, and local congestion of various sorts." In cases of local inflammation the application should not be made directly to the affected or inflamed part, but between it and the heart. By this means the part may be drained of its surplus blood, and the inflammatory process thus be rendered less active or checked altogether. In the case of an inflamed joint or muscle, friction, by operating upon the superficial vessels, diverts the blood from the affected part, causing it to go round instead of through it.

239   Pelvic pain may often be alleviated by friction of the lower part of the back. Headache may be relieved by friction of the spine. Cerebral congestion, and the insomnia resulting from it, may often be relieved by centrifugal friction applied to the extremities. The rubbing should be in a direction away from the heart, thus impeding the flow of venous blood and so retaining a considerable amount of blood in the lower extremities, and thereby affording relief to the congested brain.

240   In *cerebral congestion* the rubbing should always be downward. In *anæmia* of the brain, rub upward.

Friction is of value in all conditions of the skin in which its **241** normal activities are impaired. "Hidebound" skins, and conditions in which the skin is dingy, tawny, jaundiced, cold, or otherwise inactive, are benefited by the application of massage.

KNEADING.

This is, perhaps, the most important of all the different **242** manipulations in massage, and of all the various procedures is that to which the term *massage* is most appropriately applied, since the meaning of the word is to knead, as a baker kneads dough. In all its varieties, this procedure consists essentially in the application to the tissues of alternate and intermittent compression, by grasping the tissues or by compressing them against underlying bony surfaces. Kneading differs essentially from friction in that the skin of the parts grasped or compressed is held in firm contact with the surface of the hand of the operator, the hand not being allowed to slip along the surface of the skin, as in friction.

The different forms of kneading may be divided into two **243** classes; viz.: (1) *Superficial* and (2) *Deep*. There is but one mode of applying superficial kneading, viz., pinching or fulling, but deep kneading may be applied in a variety of ways, the most important of which are *petrissage, rolling, wringing, chucking, palmar kneading, fist kneading*, and *digital kneading*.

1. Superficial Kneading, or Fulling (Fig. 42).— In **244** this procedure the skin is grasped between the thumb and the last two phalanges of the first finger, or in cases in which the skin is very thick, the terminal phalanges of the first and second fingers may be used in opposition to the thumb. The procedure is essentially a pinching movement which acts exclusively upon the skin and the loose cellular tissue underlying it. The skin is simultaneously compressed between the thumb and finger and lifted from the underlying bone or muscle, being released at the moment when the strain is the greatest, so as to secure the maximum effect in emptying and refilling the blood vessels and lymph spaces and channels.

The two hands are used in alternation, one hand picking up the tissue as the other drops it, and so following along over the surface in a systematic manner. The direction of the movement in relation to the veins is not important, as this form of manipulation is commonly used in alternation with centripetal or spiral friction movements.

245 **Physiological Effects and Therapeutic Applications.** — Superficial kneading stimulates powerfully all the functions of the skin, and hence is useful in all cases in which any of the functions of the skin are impaired. It is especially indicated in jaundice, and in cases in which the skin is dry or "hidebound."

246 **2. Deep Kneading.** — In deep kneading the object is to act upon the muscles. There is no procedure in massage which requires so much skill, discretion, and anatomical knowledge as deep kneading, since it is necessary to keep constantly in mind the quality of the tissues acted upon, the general condition of the patient, the form of the muscle or muscular group under treatment, and the outline of the individual bone underlying the parts undergoing treatment. The location of the large blood vessels and nerves must also be accurately known and kept in mind, as these structures may easily be injured by the application of too much force.

247 Comparatively little pressure should be used in kneading thin tissues; thick, firm tissues admit of much greater pressure. It is also important to remember that a tolerance of pressure is established by prolonged treatment; so that while very gentle pressure only should be applied at the beginning of treatment, the force may be gradually increased until almost the whole strength of the operator may be employed without injury to the patient.

248 *Petrissage* (Fig. 49). — By this term is designated that form of deep kneading in which the muscular structures are grasped by the hand very much as a baker grasps a mass of dough. The tissue is not grasped between the ends of the thumb and fingers, but the skilled masseur employs as large a portion as possible of the palmar surface of the hand, taking care to keep the fingers close together. The fingers should not be opposed by the end of the thumb but by the thenar eminence, or the fleshy portion of the thumb. By this means the force employed is spread out over a large surface, and so is transmitted to the deep tissues instead of being expended upon the skin, as would otherwise be the case.

Great care should be taken to prevent slipping of the skin **249** between the fingers. The movement of the tissues should be in the deeper parts, but so great pressure should not be applied as to prevent the deeper parts from gliding easily over the still deeper-lying structures or bones.

In petrissage the parts should not only be squeezed or com- **250** pressed in the hand, but should be lifted from the bone or underlying tissues, rolled and stretched, always in an upward direction in operating upon the limbs, or *from* the point of insertion. Each time a muscle is grasped, it should be at the same time dragged outward from the median line, by which means it will be lifted from the bone, and the underlying tissues will be stretched. The grasp should be released when the strain is at its maximum, so as to encourage to the highest degree the flow of fluids toward the parts operated upon.

The movements of petrissage should not be executed too **251** rapidly ; the rate of movement should be about thirty to ninety per minute. Movements are naturally more rapid in the treatment of small parts, such as the fingers, hand, and forearm, than of such large parts as the thigh.

After the area under treatment has been gone over until **252** each part has been grasped, squeezed, rolled, and stretched four to six times, three or four strokes of centripetal friction should be applied, then the petrissage repeated, so alternating three or four times ; then proceed to another part.

The greatest care should be taken to individualize muscles **253** or groups of muscles, so far as possible. This is important, since the blood and lymph circulation of large muscles or muscular groups is to a considerable degree independent, indicating the necessity for separate treatment.

254   Either one or both hands may be used in petrissage; generally the two hands are used in alternation, one hand following the other, or working upon the opposite side.

255   *Rolling* (Fig. 43).— In this procedure the tissues are compressed against the deep-lying structures, and rolled by a to-and-fro movement. In rolling, the fingers are extended and held close together. Rolling may be applied with either one or both hands. One alone is used, being, if necessary, reinforced by pressure with the other hand, in the treatment of broad, fleshy surfaces. In the treatment of the limbs, both hands should be used.

256   If the patient is lying upon the back, the arm will be extended upward, the masseur grasping the arm between the two hands pressed against the sides. The movements should begin at the shoulders, the hands of the operator being slowly carried toward the hand of the patient, and moved in alternation in such a manner as to roll the tissues upon the bone. The pressure should be of sufficient firmness to prevent the hand from slipping upon the skin.

257   In rolling of the leg, the limb should be placed in a half-flexed position, the movements being applied first to the thigh and then to the leg in the manner described for the arm.

258   **Rate of Movement.**— The movement should be executed rapidly — at the rate of two hundred to four hundred per minute. The movement should proceed from above downward, and should alternate with centripetal friction movements; that is, after the whole limb has been rolled from axilla to wrist, or from groin to ankle, three or four centripetal friction strokes should be executed from the lower end of the limb upward.

259   The degree of pressure used should be considerable — in fleshy persons it may be as much as the masseur can apply by lateral pressure of the hands with the arms extended.

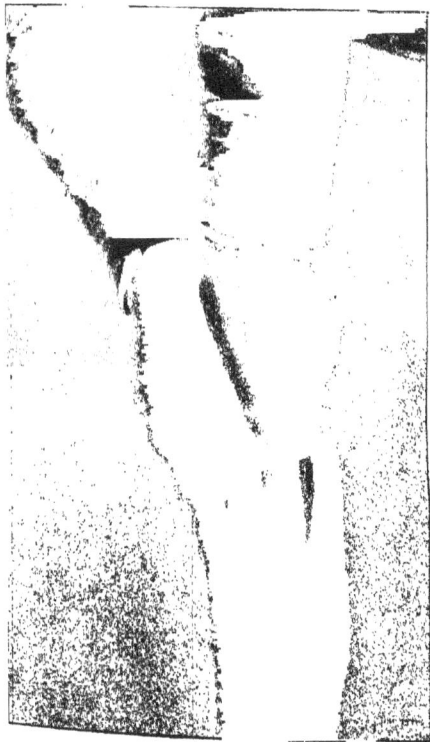

Fig. 46. Kneading Fingers.

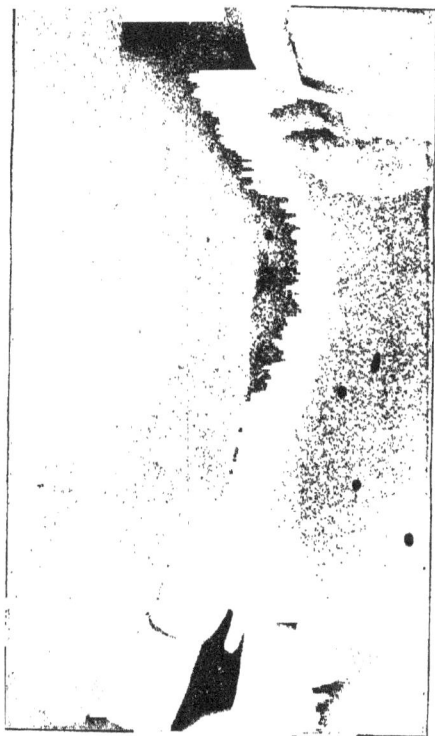

Fig. 47. Kneading Hand.

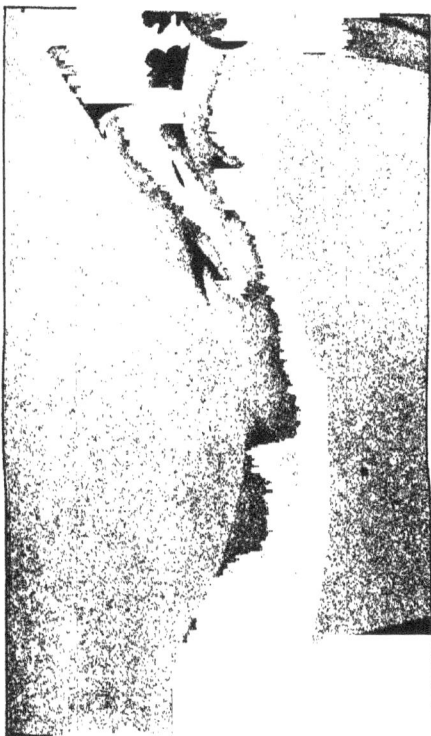

Fig. 48. Kneading Forearm.

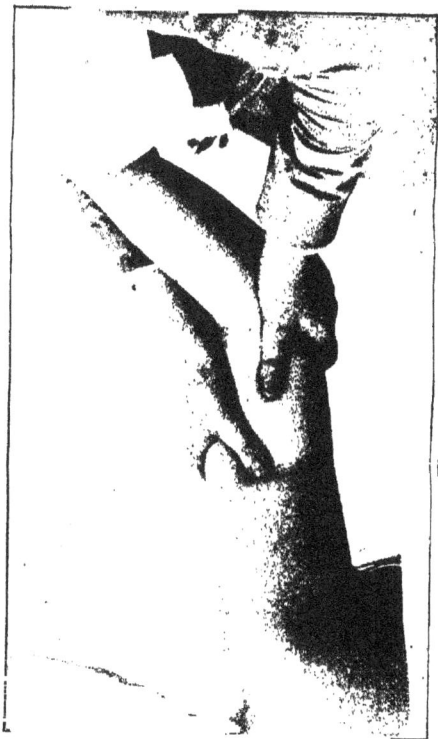

Fig. 49. Kneading Arm.

Rolling is especially useful in masseing the upper portion **260** of the back, the hips, arms, and legs.

Wringing (Fig. 44).—This procedure is executed by grasp- **261** ing the limb with the two hands placed on opposite sides and close together.

Wringing or twisting movements are executed by the hands **262** either simultaneously in the same direction or in alternation. If alternate movements are executed, the hands must be separated a little. Sufficient pressure is employed to prevent the hands from slipping over the surface, as in circular friction.

The movement begins at the shoulder or groin and pro- **263** gresses downward to the wrist or ankle, or it may be made to extend only from one joint to another. This is a very vigorous form of massage, but is obviously applicable only to the arms and legs, and will seldom be called into use.

The movements must not be too rapid; the rate should **264** not exceed thirty per minute.

Chucking (Fig. 45).—In this procedure the limb is sup- **265** ported by one hand while the other firmly grasps the fleshy portion and drags it first upward and then downward in the direction of the long axis of the limb. These movements are executed two to six times, the hands traveling along the surface until the whole limb is operated upon. This application is especially useful in overcoming muscular rigidity and in stretching contracted muscles. It acts powerfully upon both blood vessels and nerves. When employed for the scalp, either one or both hands may be used.

Palmar Kneading (Fig. 53).—This movement is executed **266** either with the heel of the hand or the whole palmar surface, as may be required. When much force is to be employed, the heel of the hand only is used. When a large mass is to be masséed, as in mass-kneading of the abdomen, the whole palm may be employed. It is chiefly used in kneading the back, chest, and abdomen.

Fist Kneading (Fig. 78).—This procedure is used only **267** in kneading the abdomen. It consists in compression of the deep tissues by the knuckles of the closed fist. Pressure is made along the course of the colon, beginning in the right groin. The advantage in fist kneading is that the greatest degree of force can be employed, and pressure may thus be communicated to the deepest parts.

268   *Digital Kneading* (Figs. 51, 54).— In digital kneading, the ends of the fingers or thumbs alone are employed, the tissues being rubbed and pressed against the underlying bony surfaces; it is used also for operating upon the contents of the colon in abdominal massage. The tip of the thumb or of one finger may be employed alone, or the ends of all the fingers may be used together, the fingers being held close together and extended. Digital massage is chiefly used in masseing the joints, the spine, the head and face, and the abdomen.

269   **Physiological Effects.**— The physiological effect of kneading is to stimulate all the vital activities of the part operated upon. The nerves, blood vessels, glands, also the cell exchanges and other tissue processes are stimulated. By the alternate compression and relaxation, blood and lymph vessels are emptied, and fresh blood drawn into the parts, thus effecting a sort of suction or pumping process by which the old blood and poison-laden tissue juices are forced onward, and a new supply of pure and well-oxygenated blood drawn in. Dilatation and quickened activity of the blood vessels are also induced by reflex nervous action. It is the most effective of all means for producing alterative effects and general vital renovation. Under the influence of massage, the parts operated upon become reddened through the increased blood supply, and acquire a higher temperature, both from the introduction of an increased supply of blood and from a stimulation of the heat-making process in the muscles.

270   Kneading acts more powerfully than any other procedure in massage, in stimulating heat production.

271   **Therapeutic Applications.**— Under the influence of deep kneading, weak muscles increase in size and firmness, demonstrating the value of the method in paralysis and paresis,

and in all cases of tissue weakness and relaxation. By its use, also, enlarged, stiffened, and painful joints return to a normal condition, and inflammatory exudates are broken down and absorbed.

There is no remedy more valuable in the treatment of mus- **272** cular and joint rheumatism, sciatica, various forms of neuralgia, general defective development, neurasthenia, writer's cramp, convulsive tic, locomotor ataxia, various forms of chronic spinal disease, and in the opening up of closed lymph and blood channels. It is also of great value in the treatment of fractures and sprains. Superficial kneading is especially indicated in dropsy, œdema, jaundice, and all other forms of disease in which the skin is inactive, or in which the functions of the skin are defective.

Mode of Applying Kneading to Different Parts. 273 — Begin either with the hands or the feet. If with the hands, proceed as follows : —

The Hand.— The manipulator grasps between his thumb **274** and finger the terminal phalanx of a finger at the root of the nail. Intermittent compression is then applied, while the thumb and forefinger of the manipulator creep along up the finger to its junction with the hand. A sort of pushing and twisting movement is executed at the same time, and attention is given to the sides of the finger, as well as to the palmar and dorsal surfaces. The thumb and each of the fingers may thus be treated in succession, or both hands may be employed at the same time (Fig. 46).

After finishing the fingers, the manipulator places the **275** patient's hand in one of his own, with the dorsum up, and with the tips of the fingers of his other hand, works thoroughly between the bones of the patient's hand from the fingers to the wrist ; then, turning the palm of the hand upward, he grasps each side of the palm, and compresses, twists, and rolls the hand in such a way as to draw the tissues away from the median line, to move all the bones, and put a gentle strain upon every muscle and ligament.

276   In masseing the wrist, it is seized between the thumb and finger of each hand, the thumbs and fingers following all the irregularities of the carpal bones and the lower extremities of the bones of the forearm, the hand in the meantime being slightly moved in various directions to facilitate the process.

277   *The Forearm.*— In kneading the forearm (Fig. 48), both hands are used, one grasping the inner, the other the outer, side of the arm, the fingers and thumb of each hand operating together in such a way as to secure thorough squeezing and manipulation of all the soft parts.   The two thumbs should follow the median line of the anterior surface of the forearm.   The movement is gradually extended from the wrist to the elbow with a rolling, spiral movement, concluding with special attention to the supinator group at the outer part of the arm just below the elbow.

278   *The Arm.*— In masseing the arm (Fig. 49), one hand grasps the extensor group of the back of the arm, while the other manipulates the flexors of the anterior region.   In masseing these fleshy parts, it must be borne in mind that the chief purpose of the manipulation is to empty the parts of their blood, and to quicken the circulatory processes by which blood and lymph are conveyed through them.   This process may be assisted by grasping the muscles of the anterior and posterior portions of the arm in such a way as to drag the tissues away from the large blood vessels which pass through the arm just beneath the inner border of the biceps muscle (Fig. 16).

279   *The Shoulder.*— The deltoid is masséed by seizing it just below the point of the shoulder, the two thumbs grasping the central portion while the fingers work the edges of the muscles. The movement is carried up over the point of the shoulder, and then repeated.

280   Attention should also be given to the supraspinatus and infraspinatus muscles, and also to the teres muscles, which help to form the posterior boundary of the axilla.   The supraspinatus and infraspinatus muscles must be masséed by the ball of the thumb or the ends of the fingers ; the teres muscles,

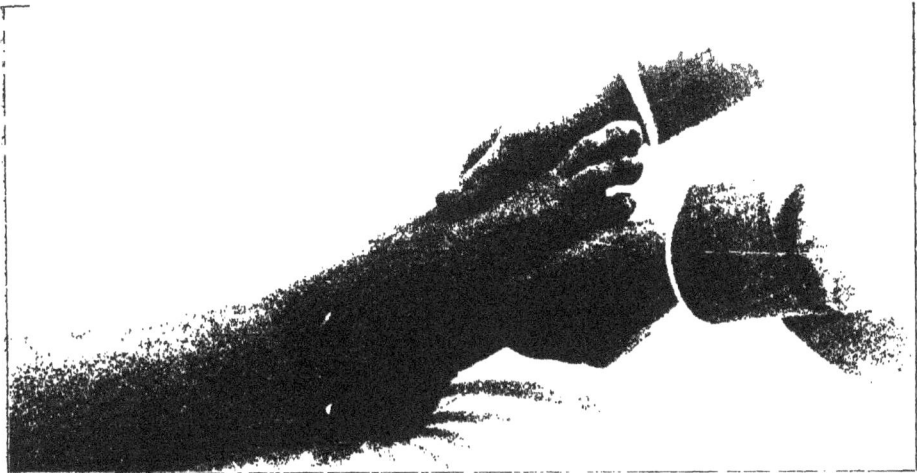
Fig. 50. Kneading Foot.

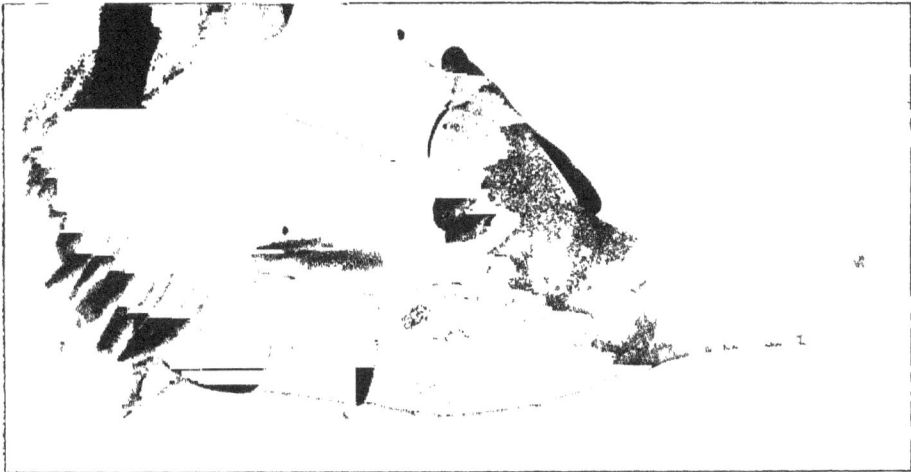
Fig. 51. Kneading Ankle.

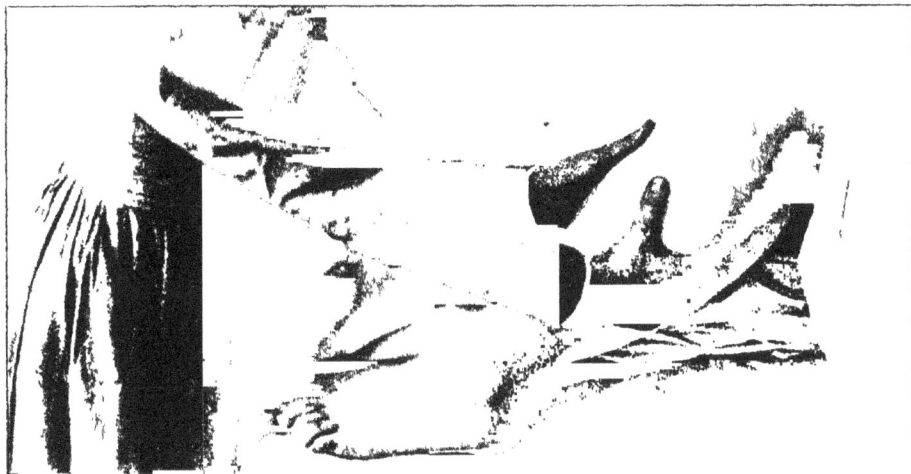

by grasping between the thumb and fingers the soft tissues beneath the arm which form the posterior boundary of the axilla, or armpit. It is important that these muscles should not be neglected, as they act an essential part in holding the shoulders back, and are generally weak through neglect to bring them into active use by the maintaining of a proper poise in sitting and standing.

The Foot.—The feet are manipulated (Figs. 50, 51) in essen- **281** tially the same manner as the hands. The dorsum of the foot and the ankle are masséed with the ends of the fingers ; the tissues of the sole are stretched in the same way as those of the hand. The foot should be rolled by compression of the sides between the two hands in such a manner as to act upon the ligaments and excite activity of the circulation in the deep structures. These manipulations are especially important in cases of flatfoot, or cases in which the instep is low, indicating a tendency to the development of flatfoot.

The foot is finished by grasping the heel in the palm of the **282** hand, rolling and compressing it, and working about it with the ends of the fingers and thumbs.

The Leg.— The leg is manipulated (Fig. 52) in essentially **283** the same manner as the arm, one hand seizing the fleshy mass of the inner and posterior region, the other the outer and an- terior, working from the ankle up to the knee. The thumbs should be well worked between the different muscular groups, special attention being given to the peronei muscles at the upper and outer part of the leg, by pressing the tips of the thumbs down between this group and the tibialis anticus. The tibialis anticus lies in such close relation to the tibia that it is not easy to grasp it between the thumb and fingers, and thus lift it from the bone. A similar effect may be obtained, however, by rolling the muscular masses which lie upon the anterior and outer side of the tibia away from the crest of the bone by pres- sure with the thumbs.

The Thigh.— Grasp the quadriceps with one hand, and with **284** the other grasp the adductor muscles which lie along the inner

6

side of the thigh, working the two groups simultaneously, but with alternate movements of the hands.

Changing hands, grasping the quadriceps with one, and the biceps, or outer hamstring muscles, with the other, a similar manipulation is carried along the outer side of the leg from the knee to the hip.

Then, grasping the whole limb between the two hands, the thumbs running along the anterior surface, while the fingers are applied to the posterior region, the whole mass of tissue of the posterior region may be manipulated with the fingers. Care should be taken to drag and stretch the muscles away from the large blood vessels which pass down along the inner border of the quadriceps.

285   In manipulating the thigh, unless the patient is very feeble, a considerable amount of force may be employed, as the skin is thick and the mass of tissue great.

286   *The Back* (Fig. 53).— The patient should lie upon the face, with the hands crossed under the forehead.. This position secures good separation of the scapulæ without rendering the rhomboid muscles too tense to prevent manipulation of the large masses of muscular tissue beneath.

287   Starting from the base of the skull, work downward, stretching the tissues by pressure of the thumb upon either side of the spinal column, employing the fingers at the same time as much as possible upon the more superficial tissues lying at a distance from the spine. These movements should be made in alternation, not together, since when made together there is danger of excessive stretching of the skin over the line of spinous processes.

288   In persons with thick, rigid tissues, manipulation of the back may be performed by the flat surface of the hand pressed firmly upon the tissues, the pressure being increased, if necessary, by reinforcement with the other hand.

289   After manipulating the large muscular masses of the back from the base of the skull to the sacrum in the manner directed, make deep pressure alongside of the spinous processes

with the ends of the fingers, thus crowding the large muscular masses away, and bringing pressure to bear upon the dorsispinal veins and upon the ligamentous structures which bind the vertebræ together. Work down first one side of the spine, then the other.

290 Another manipulation (Fig. 54), which is very effective and should not be forgotten, is a form of digital kneading which consists in placing the ends of the fingers on each side of the spine in such a manner that the fingers are parallel with the spinal column, and then making short but steady and uniform movements to and fro in the direction of the spine, working from above, downward.

291 Still another valuable form of kneading is executed as follows: Place the two hands, one upon each side of the spine, at the lower part of the back, and work the fingers in such a manner as to make the finger tips creep up the spine in a hitching fashion, dragging the heels of the hands after them. Return by an opposite movement, the heels of the hands leading.

292 Similar movements may also be executed from the spine outward, following the direction of the ribs. In these movements, the thumbs, the fingers, or the heel of the hand may be the fixed point.

293 Another form of digital kneading is administered thus: Facing the side of the patient, place the thumbs upon the spine, the fingers reaching over upon the opposite side, the wrists slightly raised. First make firm pressure with the ends of the fingers, then drag the tissues toward the median line. Apply this movement from the occiput to the sacrum and back upon one side, and then treat the opposite side in the same manner.

294 An effective manipulation of the extensor muscles of the back consists in working the heels of the hands from the sacrum to the base of the skull, then working down, applying the knuckles of the closed hand with a vibratory movement.

295 Avoid too much pressure over the spinous processes, as it will be likely to injure the skin and produce unpleasant abrasions. It should be remembered that the skin of the back is much less sensitive than that of other portions of the body, so that injury may easily be done without eliciting complaint on the part of the patient.

296   *The Chest.*—The tissues of the chest are extremely sensitive, hence care must be taken to avoid bruising them. This region is masséed by rolling movements effected by the flat of the hand pressed firmly upon the tissues, by intermittent compression, and by ordinary deep kneading with the thumb and fingers, executed with care to avoid pinching. Much less force should be used upon the chest and abdomen than in masseing the back. The tissues may be gently dragged away from the median line by the hands placed one on either side, the traction being from the origin toward the insertion of the pectoral muscles.

297   Many neurasthenic patients present tender points between the ribs, especially in the axillary line and near the sternum, and also, in some instances, in the region of the heart. Care must be taken to avoid painful pressure upon these points.

The Abdomen.—Kneading of the abdomen involves so many special procedures that a particular description will not be given under this head, the subject being more fully dealt with farther on. The same remark applies to kneading of the head, face, neck, and several other special regions.

VIBRATION.

298   This procedure consists of fine vibratory, or shaking, movements communicated to the body through the hand of the masseur. One or both hands may be placed against the surface, or may grasp some part of the patient, as the hand, the foot, or the head. Sometimes one hand and sometimes both hands are employed. Vibratory movements may be communicated to the body in a variety of ways. The following are those which may be most conveniently and efficiently employed : —

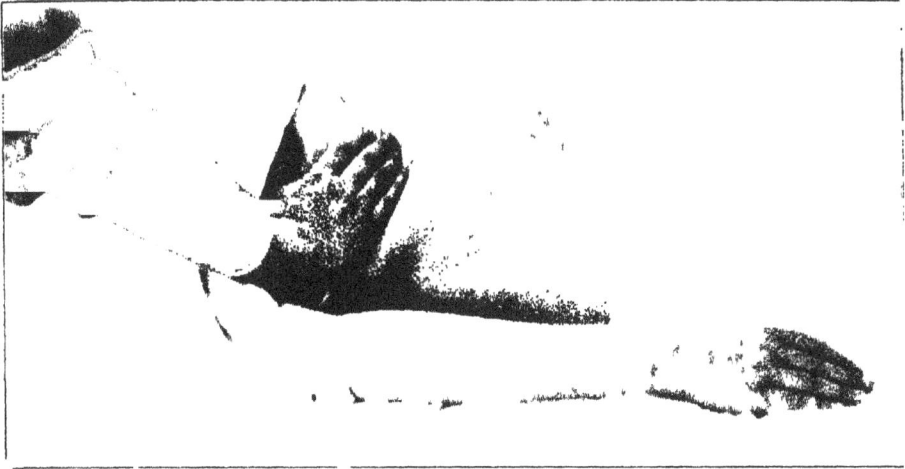

Fig 55   Deep Vibration

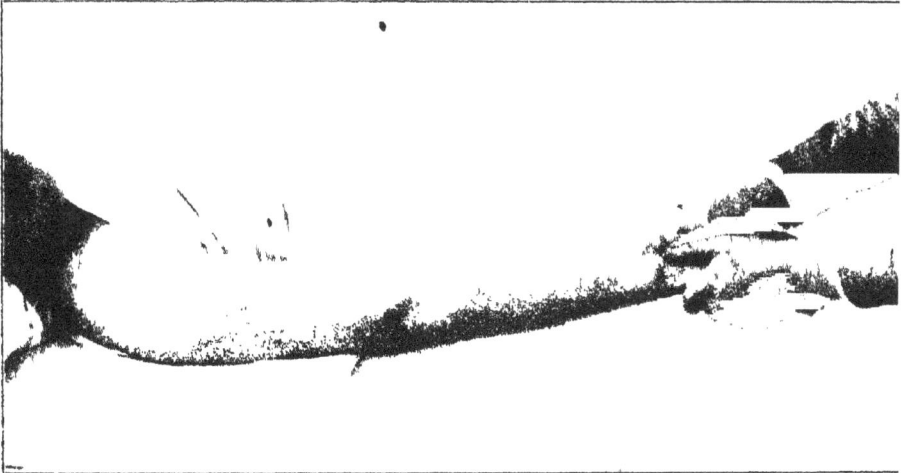

Fig 56   Shaking.

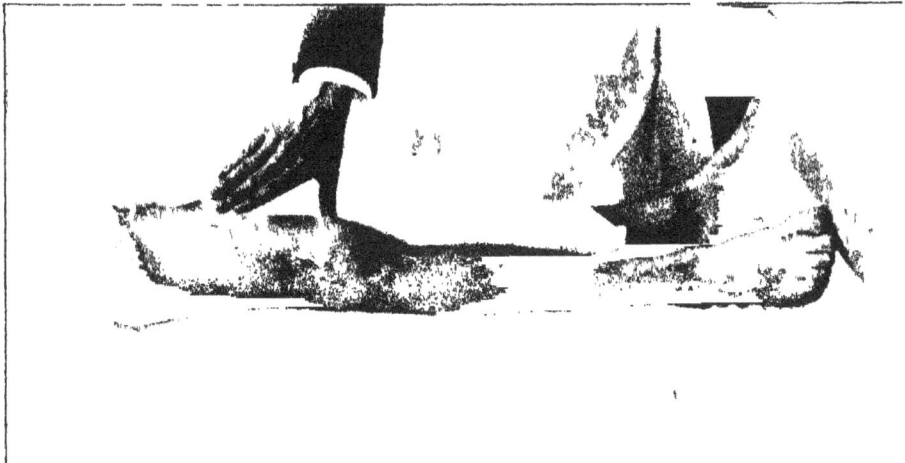

Lateral Vibration.—The palmar surface of the hand being **299** held upon the skin with sufficient firmness to prevent slipping, the hand is moved laterally to and fro. The movements should be as rapid as possible—at the rate of at least six to ten per second. It is used chiefly in applications to the head, the joints, and the abdomen. The finger tips alone are used for the head and joints, the palm of the hand in abdominal and pelvic massage.

Knuckle Vibration.—The knuckles of the closed hand are **300** placed in contact with the skin, and moved slowly over the surface, a vigorous vibratory movement being executed at the same time.

Superficial Vibration.—One or both palms being placed **301** upon the surface, they are made to move slowly over the area to be operated upon, a fine trembling movement being executed at the same time. Much practice is required to enable the masseur to execute this movement with sufficient vigor to produce an effect.

Deep Vibration (Fig. 55).—The palm of the hand or the **302** closed fist being placed firmly upon the surface of the part to be acted upon, the arm is held straight, and a fine jarring or trembling movement communicated to it by an action of the flexor and extensor muscles of the upper part of the arm. This movement is difficult to produce, requiring long practice on the part of the operator, and is extremely fatiguing; but it is one of the most valuable of all the vibratory movements, as by means of it motion can be communicated to the most deeply seated parts.

Shaking (Fig. 56).—The part to be operated upon is grasped **303** firmly by both hands and shaken with a rapid vibratory movement. This movement is especially applicable to the extremities and the head.

Digital Vibration (Fig. 57).—The end of the thumb or **304** of one or more fingers being placed upon the part to be operated upon, the arm of the operator is thrown into violent vibrations, which are communicated through the thumb or fingers to the patient.

305   **Physiological Effects.**—The special effect of vibration is that of stimulation. When applied with sufficient vigor, it is one of the most stimulating of all the procedures of massage. Deep vibration may be made to act forcibly upon the most deeply situated organs. The effect of rapid vibration is somewhat similar to that of electricity; it is capable of causing muscular contraction, even producing tetanus when applied with sufficient vigor. Very rapid vibration produces a pleasurable, tingling sensation in the parts acted upon, akin to that produced by electricity, but more agreeable, which affords sufficient evidence of the effect of this procedure upon nerve structures. Under the influence of vibratory movements, the activity of the circulation increases, the blood vessels dilate, the temperature of the part rises, and a pleasurable glow and sensation of well-being pervades the part.

306   Profound effects may be produced by the application of vibration to nerve trunks and nerve centers, as has been shown by Mortimer Granville, Charcot, and others.

307   The most pronounced effects of vibration can be obtained only by the aid of proper mechanical appliances, several of which the writer has had in use for a number of years. (Figs. 115–119).

308   **Therapeutic Applications.**— Vibration is useful in cases in which stimulation is required, and is only contra-indicated in cases in which there is marked hyperæsthesia, acute inflammation, febrile action, morbid growths, or some active morbid process, such as suppuration. It is valuable in most forms of paresis and paralysis. As an application to nerve trunks, it is also valuable in neuralgia and neurasthenia and in most functional nerve disorders accompanied by diminished activity.

309   Applied to the spinal column, it is of special value in sclerosis and other degenerative affections of the spinal cord, as has been well shown by Charcot. The violent trembling

of patients suffering from spinal sclerosis is often greatly relieved. Vibration of the extremities is one of the most excellent means of relieving coldness arising from spasm of the small vessels due to vasomotor disturbances, numbness, tingling, and various other morbid sensations.

PERCUSSION.

This procedure consists of blows administered in various **310** ways and with varying degrees of force. The two hands are used in alternation. The movement is always from the wrist joint, which gives to the blow the quality of elasticity. The inexperienced operator holds the wrist rigid, and pummels the patient much as a pugilist would do, thus producing disagreeable and painful effects. A dexterous and experienced operator maintains a flexibility of the wrist which adds greatly to the good effects of the treatment.

A stiff blow bruises the surface tissues without producing **311** any beneficial effect upon the deeper structures, the force of the blow being expended upon the surface. An elastic blow, executed in the manner described, penetrates deeply without injuring the superficial structures. A skilled masseur gives springy blows, the movement being almost wholly from the wrist. As a rule, the hand should strike the body transversely with relation to the muscles.

The effect of percussion is increased by placing the muscles **312** upon the stretch. This is accomplished upon the back by having the patient bend forward in a standing or sitting position, and for the abdominal muscles by having the patient raise the head without assistance while lying on the back.

The following are the principal modes of applying percussion, or *clapotement*, as this procedure is termed by the French : —

Tapping (Fig. 58). — This is a form of beating in which **313** the tips of the fingers alone are employed. Either one or all of the fingers of one or both hands may be employed. It is chiefly used for the head and the chest.

314   *Spatting* (Fig. 59).—This consists of percussion with the palmar surface of the extended fingers held rigid. This is the form in which percussion is most frequently employed. It is applicable to most parts of the body. It should be used before the application of other procedures when the surface is cold, or when the patient complains of chilly sensations. It is much used in connection with hydropathic applications as a means of promoting reaction.

315   *Clapping* (Fig. 60).—In this procedure, the whole hand is employed, the palmar surface being so shaped as to entrap the air as it comes in contact with the skin, producing a sort of explosive effect and a loud sound. It is used on fleshy parts when strong surface stimulation is desired.

316   *Hacking* (Fig. 61).—In this procedure the ulnar, or little-finger, border of the hand alone comes in contact with the skin. The fingers are held slightly apart, but loosely, so that they are made to come successively in contact by the force of the blow, thus giving a peculiar vibratory effect. This form of percussion is exceedingly useful. It is chiefly employed in applications to the chest, spine, and head. It may also be employed upon any other part of the body.

317   *Beating* (Fig. 62).—In this procedure the body is struck by the palmar surface of the half-closed fist, the dorsal surface of the terminal phalanges of the fingers and the heel of the hand alone coming in contact with the body. This mode of percussion is chiefly useful for applications to the lower part of the back and the fleshy portion of the thighs. It is a powerful means of stimulating the genito-urinary system. When applied to the sacrum, the patient stands upon the feet, bending slightly forward. Muscle beaters may be very efficiently used for beating (Fig. 136).

318   **Reflex Percussion.**—By this term is meant percussion movements to the so-called reflex areas, which have been fully described under the head of "Stroking." The well-known "knee-jerk" is an illustration of the effect of even so gentle a percussion as a slight tap with the finger tip in provoking

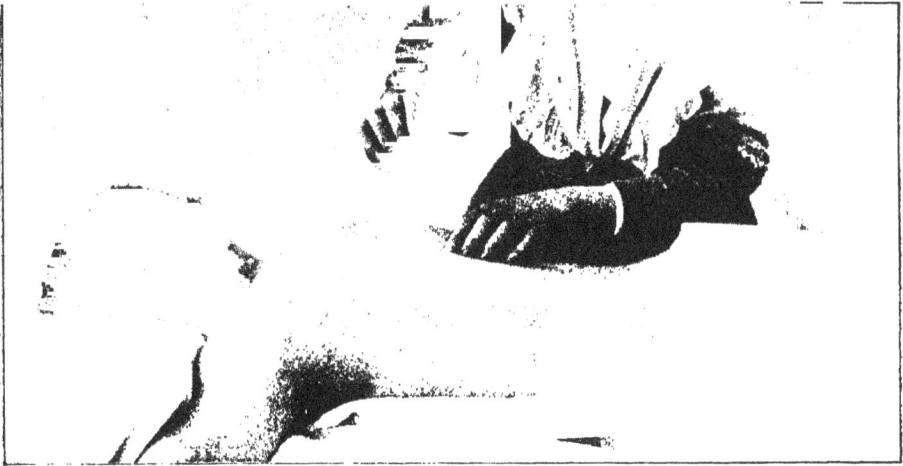

Fig. 58. Tapping

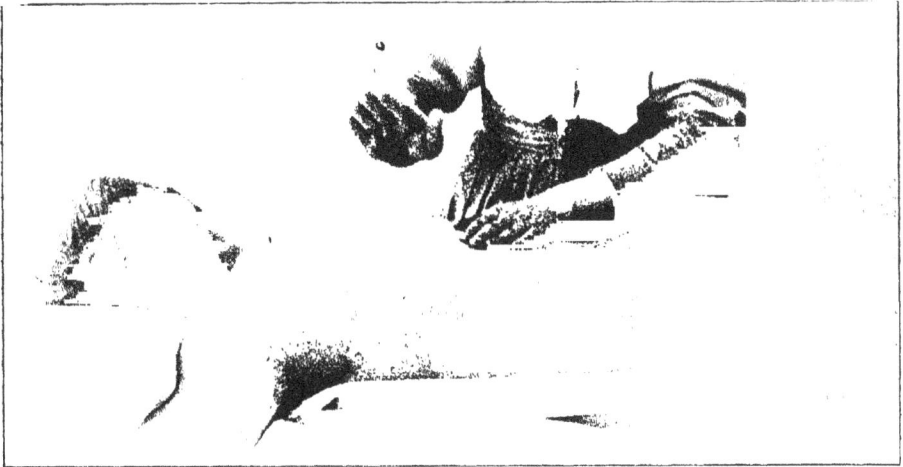

Fig. 59. Spatting.

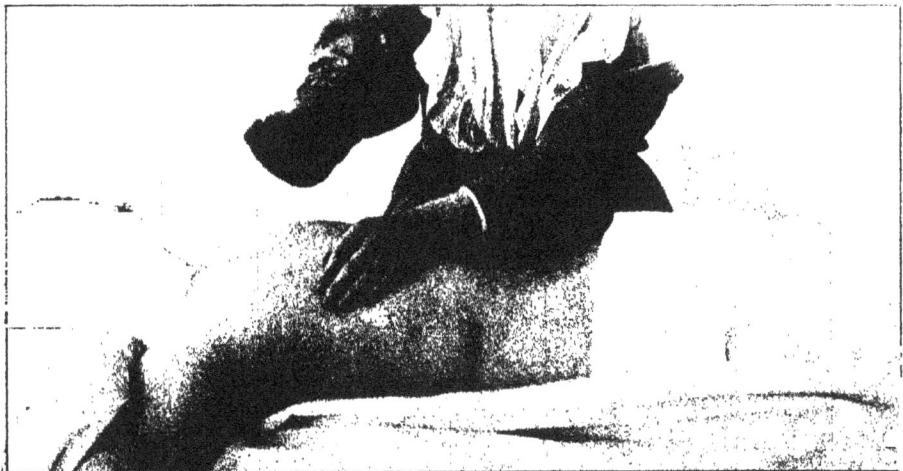

Fig. 60. Clapping.

reflex action, which, of course, involves the stimulation of one or more nerve centers and nerve trunks, as well as of the acting muscle or muscles. Percussion of any part of the body doubtless gives rise to reflex activities of varying degree, but the most pronounced effects necessarily follow the application of this procedure to those surfaces which are in most direct relation to definite centers in the spinal cord.

The principal reflex areas which may be named, and the proper mode of stimulation, are as follows: —

Interscapular Area.—The application is best made with the **319** patient sitting with the arms folded in front, and bending slightly forward. The masseur, standing behind, applies percussion — hacking and spatting—to the space between the scapulæ, or shoulder blades. The interscapular reflex has relation to the sixth, seventh, and eighth cervical, and first dorsal, segments of the spinal cord.

Epigastric Area.—The patient lying upon the back, tap- **320** ping, hacking, spatting, or beating movements are applied to the sides of the chest between the fourth and sixth ribs. This area is in relation to the fifth, sixth, and seventh dorsal segments.

Abdominal Area.—With the patient lying upon the back, **321** tapping, hacking, spatting, or clapping movements are applied to the sides of the abdomen in the mammary line. This application stimulates the eighth, ninth, tenth, eleventh, and twelfth dorsal segments.

Cremasteric Area.—Hacking and percussion of the inner **322** portion of the upper half of the thigh stimulates the first, second, and third lumbar segments.

Gluteal Area.— With the patient lying upon the face, hack- **323** ing, spatting, clapping, or beating movements are applied to the fleshy portions of the hips, thereby stimulating the fourth and fifth lumbar centers.

Plantar Area.—Spatting and hacking movements applied **324** to the sole of the foot stimulate the five sacral segments of the cord.

325   **Tendon Reflexes.**— Percussion of the tendon of a muscle, and sometimes percussion of the muscle itself, gives rise to
muscular contraction. This is best illustrated in the knee in
what is called the "knee-jerk," or "patellar reflex." With
one limb crossed over the other, a light tap upon the tendon
just below the patella gives rise in most persons to contraction
of the quadriceps extensor, as evidenced by a movement of the
foot. To be effective, it is necessary that the blow should be
applied when the tendon of the muscle is tense.

The principal points at which tendon percussion may be
advantageously employed, and the nerve centers which are
stimulated at the several points na.ned, are as follows : —

326   *Back of the Neck.*— With the patient sitting with the head
flexed forward as far as possible, apply hacking movements
from the *vertebra prominens* to the *occiput*, striking the muscles
transversely. This application stimulates the first, second,
third, and fourth cervical segments.

327   *Wrist Tendons.*— Grasping the patient's hand with the
palmar surface up, and extending it as far as possible, so as to
render tense the tendons at the wrist, make light tapping or
hacking movements across the front of the wrist. In many
cases a decided muscular contraction may be noticed after each
blow. Percussion at this point stimulates the fourth, fifth,
sixth, seventh, and eighth cervical segments of the cord.

328   *The "Knee-jerk"* (Fig. 63).— The patient sits with one leg
crossed over the other, so as to render tense the tendon of the extensor muscles of the thigh. Tapping the part of the tendon just
below the patella with the tip of the middle finger, or applying
a transverse blow with the edge of the hand, will usually give
rise to strong contraction of the quadriceps and thrusting of
the toe forward. In some persons this reflex may be developed
with the patient lying with the limbs extended, by placing one
finger just above the patella and crowding it down as far as
possible, then striking the finger with the middle finger of the
other hand. This reflex involves all five of the lumbar segments of the cord.

The Ankle Reflex.— With the patient lying upon his face, **329**
the limbs extended, grasp the foot with one hand and forcibly
flex it upon the leg so as to render the tendon Achilles as tense
as possible. Tapping or hacking movements applied to the
stretched tendon will often give rise to contraction of the muscles of the calf and extension of the foot. This application
stimulates the first, second, and third sacral segments.

The tendon reflexes are all rendered more active by divert- **330**
ing the patient's attention. This may best be accomplished by
causing him to contract forcibly a muscular group in some other
part of the body than that which it is desired to operate upon.
For example, in testing the ankle and knee reflexes, the patient
may be caused to close his hands as firmly as possible; when
operating upon the wrist or the back of the neck, the patient
may be made to forcibly flex or extend his foot.

Percussion is sometimes applied by means of rubber balls **331**
attached to reed or whalebone rods, or by elastic rubber tubes
attached to a handle,— the so-called "muscle beater" of
Klemm. These instruments are worthy of mention, as they
afford a means by which the patient can apply percussion
to himself (Fig. 138).

Point Percussion.— Percussion applied at the motor points **332**
is sometimes a most effective means of producing muscular contraction, as at these points the motor nerves may be directly
stimulated by the mechanical force applied. Tapping and
hacking are the most efficient means of applying point percussion. Usually the best effect will be obtained by placing
one finger upon the motor point, pressing firmly upon the
nerve, and then tapping the finger with the fingers of the
other hand.

Physiological Effects.— Percussion is a powerful ex- **333**
citant, acting not only upon the skin, but upon the tissues
beneath. A short, light application produces spasm of the
superficial vessels, which may be easily demonstrated by tapping a point upon the back of the hand with the finger for
a few seconds, and noting the decided pallor which results.

Strong percussion, or a prolonged application of light blows, gives rise to dilatation of the surface vessels, as evidenced by marked redness of the skin. Strong percussion may even produce paralysis of the blood vessels.

334   Reflex percussion is certainly a most powerful means of stimulating those nerve centers which may be brought under the influence of this special mode of application, which include, to a greater or less extent, all the segments of the cord. The lumbar and sacral portions of the cord especially may be acted upon in a powerful manner by this procedure. The therapeutic value of this special form of percussion will be recognized at once when it is remembered that the important functions of the bladder, rectum, and sexual organs are largely controlled by centers located in the lower portion of the cord.

335   The direct application of percussion to the spine is one of the most powerful means of stimulating the vasomotor centers and the nutritive functions of the viscera which are controlled by the splanchnics. The cervical splanchnics which emanate from that portion of the spine included between the first cervical and the fourth dorsal segments, control the circulation of the heart, stomach, and lungs; the second group of splanchnics, leaving the cord between the second dorsal and the second lumbar, controls the great vascular area of the intestines; while the third set of splanchnics, leaving the cord at the second and third sacral segments, controls the circulation and, through it, the nutrition and, to a large extent, the functions of the genital organs.

336   It is thus apparent that vigorous vibratory movements communicated to the spine, especially by means of hacking and beating, which act most effectively upon deep-seated structures, may be the means of powerfully influencing the functions of all the viscera of the trunk, as well as the genital organs, though the latter are partly internal and partly external.

337   Point percussion produces powerful motor effects, inducing vigorous contraction of the muscles to which the nerve operated upon is distributed. The results produced by point

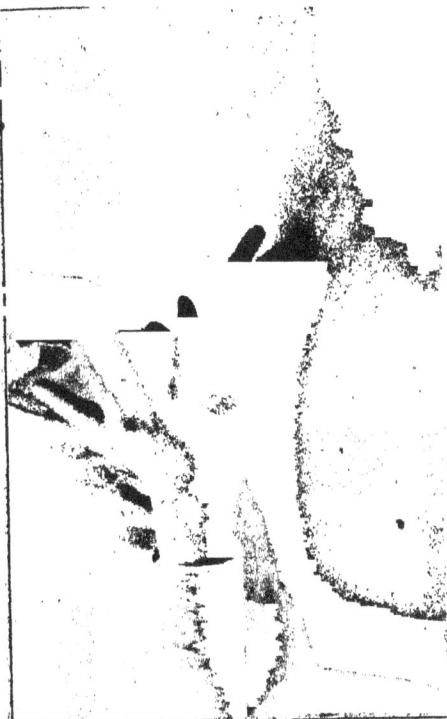
Fig. 61. Hacking.

Fig. 62. Beating.

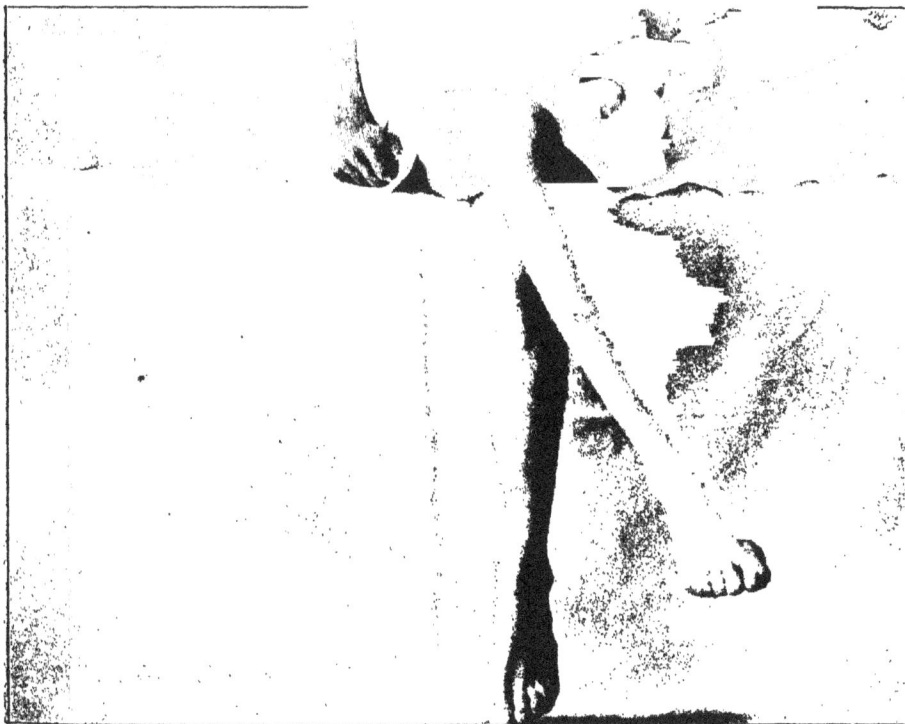

percussion are often more marked than those obtained from faradization, especially in cases in which the excitability of the muscle is modified by disease.

Therapeutic Applications. — Percussion, especially **338** spatting and clapping, is much used in connection with hydrotherapy as a means of promoting reaction after cold applications to the surface. This procedure is useful in all cases in which stimulation of the skin is desirable, either for derivative effects or for direct influence upon the skin. It is consequently useful in all cases of functional inactivity of the skin, as in jaundice.

In chronic sciatica, lumbago, and coldness of the extremities, **339** percussion has a decidedly favorable influence, as also in passive congestion of the liver and spleen, in which cases it is employed over the region of these organs. In constipation, it may be applied over the abdomen as a means of stimulating general peristaltic activity, and over the sacrum to stimulate activity of the lower bowel.

Beating the sacrum is valuable in atony of the bladder and **340** in impotence or sterility from loss of sexual vigor. The ancient Romans practiced whipping of the buttocks for relief of impotence in man and sterility in women. Vigorous spanking has sometimes been employed by libertines for the same purpose; and the writer has met one or two cases in which whipping had given rise to involuntary action of the genital organs in a boy, and one or two cases in men in which the same effect was produced by percussion of the lower portion of the back and upper thighs, thus clearly demonstrating the powerful influence of this procedure upon the centers of the cord.

Hacking of the spine is especially useful in sclerosis; and **341** hacking of the chest, in unresolved pneumonia, adhesions from chronic pleurisy, and in promoting absorption in cases of serous effusion into the pleural cavity.

JOINT MOVEMENTS.

342 The principal movements included under this head are : —
Flexion, extension, abduction, adduction, pronation, supination, circumduction, stretching.

Certain principles which apply to all the different forms of joint movements must first be considered before describing particularly the individual movements. The most important of these are the following : —

343 1. Joint movements may be either *passive* or *resistive*. In *passive* movements there is simple motion of the joint, effected wholly by the manipulator, and without any effort on the part of the patient. In passive movements, the effect is chiefly confined to the joint, involving its articular surfaces, the ligamentous bands by which the joint is supported, and the blood and lymph vessels connected with it. In *resistive* movements, not only the joint but the muscles acted upon, are involved, since both the patient and the masseur take part in the movement, the patient resisting the movements which the masseur endeavors to execute, or *vice versa.*

344 2. The *extent* of the *movement* in passive motion of the joint should be sufficient to produce a distinct feeling of resistance, the degree of which will indicate the extent to which the ligamentous structures of the joint are acted upon.

345 3. The *degree* of *resistance* employed in resistive movements should always be carefully regulated to the condition of the patient's tissues. Too great resistance is likely to leave the muscles sore, requiring several days' rest from treatment, and perhaps discouraging the patient. Slight soreness, however, may be expected at the beginning of treatment. This is due simply to the congestion of the muscle resulting from the afflux of blood, and will be followed by improved nutrition which will terminate in an increase of strength.

4. In *resistive* movements, resistance on the part of the **346** masseur should carefully follow the movements of the patient in flexion and extension. The ability to do this well can only be acquired by careful practice.

5. In case of great feebleness of the muscles, the move- **347** ments must sometimes be *assistive* rather than resistive, until the patient acquires ability to lift the limb, which may some-times be found lacking at the beginning of treatment, or until the connection between the will and the muscles, which has been at first interrupted, shall be restored. Sometimes the pa-tient fails to contract a muscle through lack of confidence. Assistive movements made in such a manner as to give the patient the impression that the movement is effected through his own volition, will overcome this obstacle with surprising readiness.

Every experienced gymnast is acquainted with the fact that when a muscle is once contracted to the extent of its capacity, much greater force is required to overcome the con-traction than the same muscle would have been capable of ex-erting in contracting against resistance. This fact may be utilized in the treatment of patients whose muscles are ex-tremely feeble, the resistance being made by causing the patient to first flex the limb or extend it, as the case may be, and endeavor to hold it in position while the manipulator applies force to change its position.

6. In *resistive* movements either the patient or the masseur **348** may initiate the movement. Usually the patient initiates the movement, and the operator, the instant the movement starts, begins to offer resistance, first very slight, but gradually increasing to the limit of the patient's strength, then diminish-ing, so as to allow the completion of the movement on the part of the patient; that is, the complete extension or flexion, ab-duction or adduction, supination or pronation, of the limb, as the case may be. If the muscle is very feeble, the patient

should completely extend, flex, abduct, adduct, supinate, or pronate the limb, before the resistance is begun, the masseur then making the attempt to execute the opposite movement, while the patient endeavors to retain the limb in the position in which it has been placed.

349   7. Patients often need to be taught how to execute a movement, especially those whose muscles have been long at rest. Sometimes the patient fails to move a limb as requested, because he contracts both the extensors and the flexors equally at the same time, producing a trembling oscillation between flexion and extension instead of a definite movement. This obstacle must be met by careful training, in which assistive movements may be at first required.

350   8. When it is desired to limit the motion to a single joint, the portion of the limb on the proximal side of the joint—that is, the side next the body—should be steadied so as to prevent motion of the next joint above, while the distal part of the limb is grasped and made to execute the movements required.

351   9. As a general rule in *resistive* movements, the *fingers pull* to resist flexion while the *heel* of the *hand pushes* to resist extension. The same principle applies to abduction, adduction, and other movements.

352   **Physiological Effects.**—The venous and lymph channels, especially the latter, are larger in the vicinity of the joints than in other parts of the limbs, a fact which is doubtless attributable to the great amount of absorption required to keep the articulating surfaces in perfect working order. This fact attaches very great importance to manipulations involving the joint or its immediate vicinity. On account of it, joint movements and manipulation of the joints are capable of producing very powerful derivative effects upon neighboring and more distal parts. Through the direct influence of movements and massage upon a joint, its nutrition may be modified to a very marked degree, as the result of the hyperæmia induced and the increased circulation of fluids in the blood and lymph channels. The influence of movements upon a joint is well illustrated in

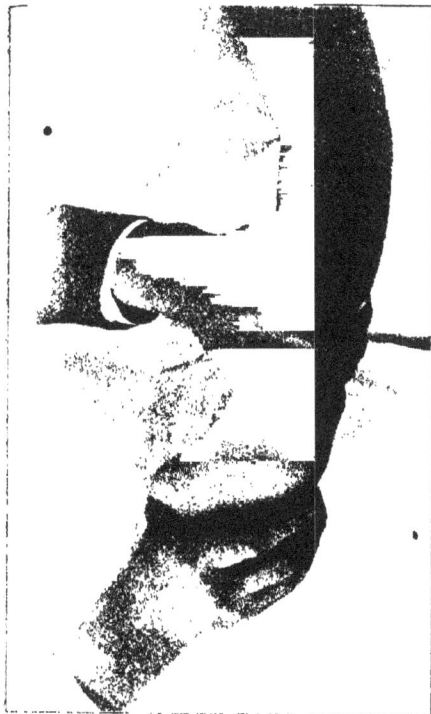

Fig. 65. Passive Flexion and Resistive Extension of Wrist.

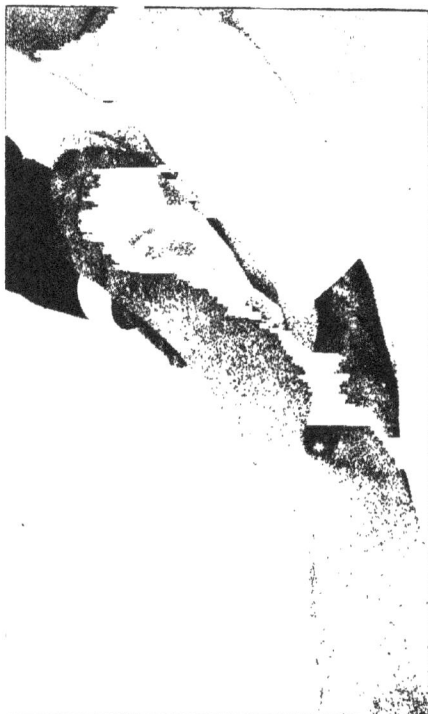

Fig. 67. Passive Supination and Resistive Pronation of Hand.

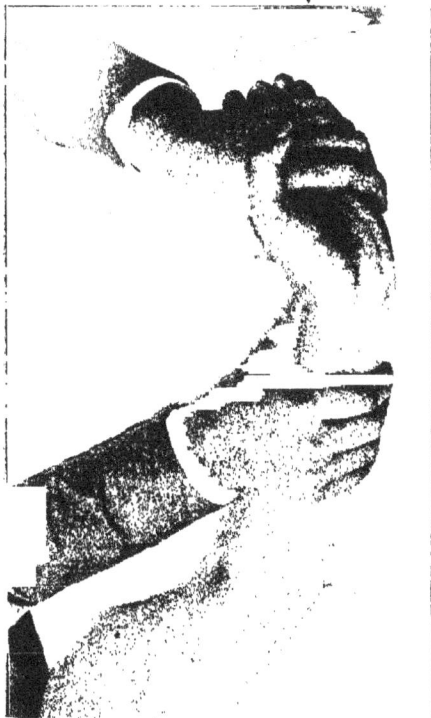

Fig. 64. Passive Extension and Resistive Flexion of Wrist.

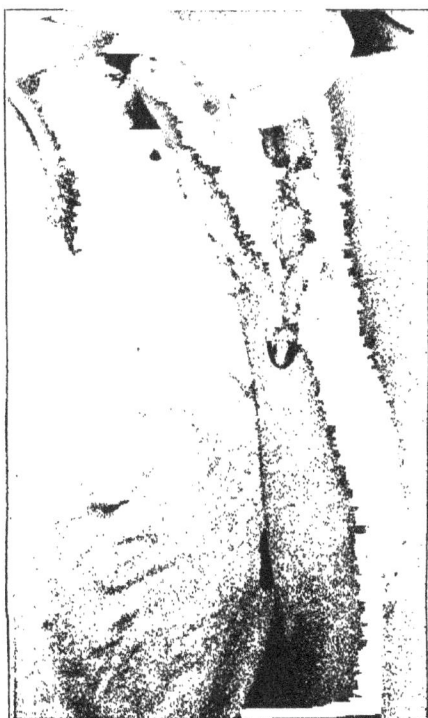

Fig. 66. Passive Pronation and Resistive Supination of Hand.

PLATE XXVII.— Joint Movements.

the large finger joints of artisans, especially those who use the hands in heavy lifting.

Therapeutic Applications.—Joint movements are of **353** special value in the various forms of chronic joint disease in which movement is lessened, as in the stiffening which arises from rheumatism, rheumatic gout, chronic synovitis, and the treatment of fractures and sprains by complete immobilization. Joint movements, cautiously employed, may also be of use in the derivative treatment of an acute inflammatory process in a neighboring and more distal joint. It should be remarked that great care is necessary in treatment by the application of joint movements in neuroses of the joint, such as are frequently left after attacks of inflammation arising from injury or otherwise. Even the gentlest manipulations are sometimes very badly borne in these cases. Often derivative friction practiced upon the joint above and the neighboring soft tissues will alone be tolerated by these cases until after a very considerable degree of improvement in the nutrition of the parts and a lessening of the patient's general nervous irritability have been secured. It is sometimes necessary to postpone joint movements several weeks, and perhaps for two or three months. It is hence highly important that cases of this sort should be recognized at the outset, as otherwise the patient is likely to be made worse and, becoming discouraged by the treatment, give it up. Hydrotherapy and electricity are almost indispensable in the early stages of the treatment in these cases.

Flexion, Extension, Abduction, Adduction, Supination, Pro- **354** *nation, and Circumduction.*—Practically the same principles govern the application of these several different movements. The chief points to be considered, in addition to those already presented, relate to the special mode of executing the different motions for different parts, which may be briefly described as follows:—

Flexion and Extension of the Wrist (Fig. 64).—With the **355** forearm halfway between supination and pronation, take the

7

patient's hand as in shaking hands, right to right or left to left. The other hand should seize the forearm just above the wrist. In this position, *passive* movements of both *flexion* and *extension* may be executed. The same position is also used for *resistive* flexion.

356   For *resistive extension*, the patient's forearm should be pronated and the hand of the patient grasped by the masseur with his opposite hand ; that is, left to right and right to left. The other hand should steady the arm, by grasping it just above the wrist (Fig. 65).

357   *Pronation and Supination of the Hand.*— For passive pronation and resistive supination (Fig. 66), the masseur grasps the wrist of the patient with his opposite hand (right to left or left to right), in such a manner that the back of the wrist and the lower ends of the bones of the forearm fall into the hollow of his hand, the thick portion of the thumb resting just behind the lower end of the radius so as to control it. The other hand is placed beneath the elbow to support the patient's arm, care being taken not to hold the bones of the forearm so tightly as to prevent their free movement.

358   For *passive supination* and *resistive pronation* of the hand (Fig. 67), the masseur grasps the patient's right hand with his own right, supporting the arm with his left. With the patient's arm in pronation, the hand of the masseur should grasp the forearm in such a way that the palm of his hand will rest upon the front of the wrist, the fleshy portion of the thumb falling upon the front side of the lower end of the radius.

359   *Flexion and Extension of the Forearm* (Fig. 68).— The masseur grasps the wrist of the patient with his corresponding hand, and with his other hand seizes the arm just above the elbow and steadies it.

360   The same grasp serves for either *passive* or *resistive flexion* or *extension*, and may be employed for *passive pronation* and *supination*, *abduction* and *adduction*, and *rotation* of the *humerus*. All of these movements, with the exception of resistive flexion and extension, may be accomplished in making the wrist describe a circle.

Circumduction of the Arm.— The masseur stands behind **361** the patient, fixes the shoulder with his opposite hand, and with the other seizes the arm just below the elbow, and causes the lower end of the humerus to describe as great a circle as possible without too great resistance. The peculiar formation of the shoulder joint gives the greatest resistance at the upper part of the circle.

This same grasp is a suitable one for *resisting* the action of **362** the muscles which pull the arm forward and those which draw it backward.

Circumduction may also be performed by standing in **363** front of the patient and seizing the wrist with the corresponding hand, and the elbow with the other hand (the patient sitting).

Backward movements of the arm may be resisted by taking **364** the hand of the patient with the corresponding hand, and with the other hand grasping the arm above and behind the elbow.

The *deltoid* may be resisted by placing one hand upon the **365** shoulder and the other upon the outside of the arm near the elbow. It is most convenient for the masseur to stand behind the patient.

Movements of the Ankle (Fig. 69).— The masseur should **366** sit facing the patient, who sits with leg extended. Seize the foot with the corresponding hand at the junction of the toes with the body of the foot, the thumb falling upon the sole of the foot ; with the other hand grasp the leg above the ankle. This grasp is convenient for *passive* and *active flexion* and *extension*, and also *circumduction*. The pressure should be applied against the distal ends of the metacarpal bones, rather than upon the toes.

Movements of the Knee Joint (Fig. 70).— These movements **367** are usually combined with movements of the hip joint, as follows : The heel of the patient is grasped by the corresponding hand of the masseur, while the other grasps the calf of the leg. In *passive* movements the limb is simply pushed up, and allowed to return to extension by its own weight.

368   For *passive circumduction*, the assisting hand is placed upon the top of the knee instead of the calf, the knee being made to describe as large a circle as possible with moderate resistance.

369   In *resistive flexion* and *extension* of the *leg*, the leg and foot are grasped as in movements of the ankle. Considerable force must be used by the masseur in resisting extension, which may be done either when resting upon the knee placed upon the edge of the couch, throwing the body forward, or by standing with the back to the patient and clasping the hands across the sole of the foot beneath the instep.

370   *Abduction and Adduction of the Thighs* (Fig. 71).—The patient lies with the knees half flexed by drawing up the heels. *Abduction* is resisted by placing the hands against the outer side of the knees; *adduction*, by placing them against the inner surface.

371   *Resistive Flexion of the Thigh.*—The patient draws up the leg while the masseur makes resistance by placing the hand upon the anterior surface of the thigh, near the knee.

372   **Joint Stretching.**—This is a powerful means of stimulating the nutrition of a joint. Enlargement of the joint has long been noticed to be a consequence of "cracking" the fingers. Joint stretching is much practiced by the Turks in connection with the shampooing of the Turkish bath. Stretching may be applied as follows : —

373   *The Arm and Shoulder Joints.*—The patient lying upon the back, the head and shoulders slightly elevated and the arms extended upward, the masseur stands behind and seizes the hands of the patient in such a manner that the palmar surfaces of the hands are in contact, the thumb of the masseur passing between the thumb and the first finger of the patient, while his fingers pass around the fleshy portion of the thumb and the back of the hand of the patient. The grasp might be described by saying that the patient and masseur each grasps the other's thumbs with the corresponding hand. A series of vigorous elastic pulls are made, avoiding sudden

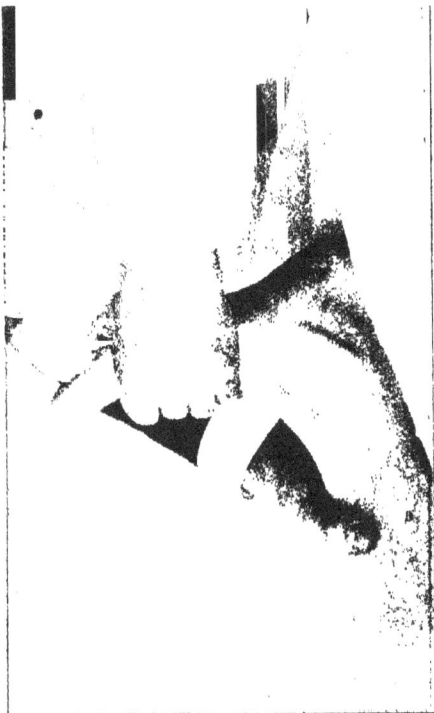

Fig. 69. Passive Flexion of Ankle.

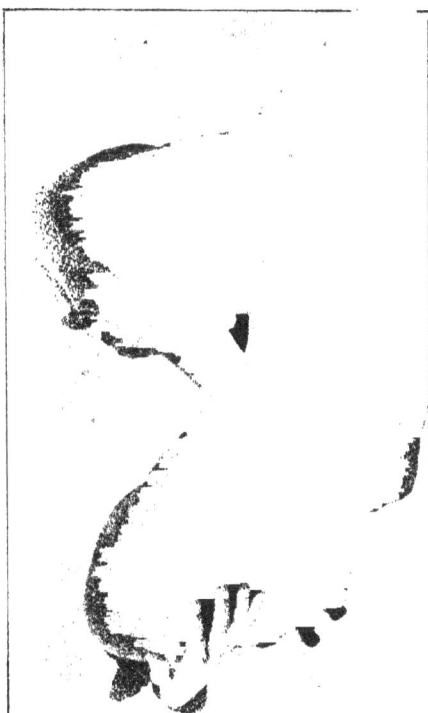

Fig. 71. Resistive Abduction of Thighs.

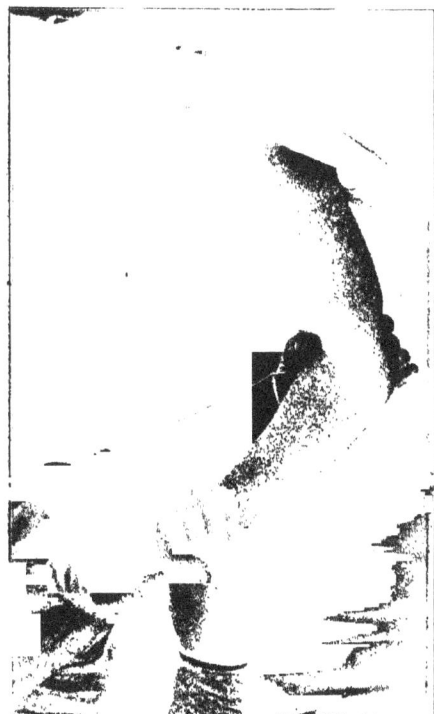

Fig. 68. Passive Flexion and Resistive Extension of Forearm.

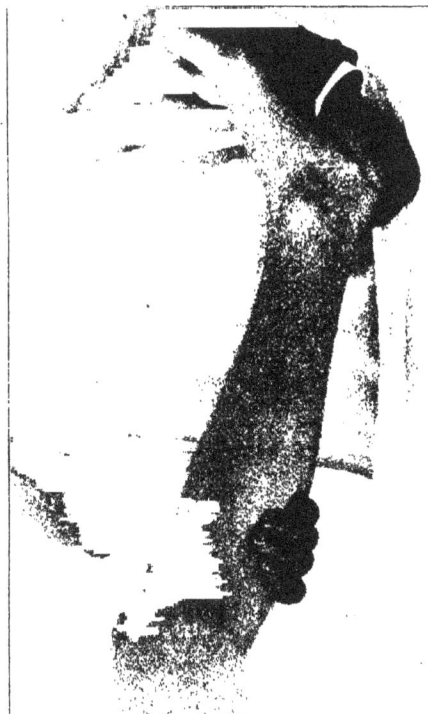

Fig. 70. Movements of Knee and Hip Joint.

PLATE XXVIII. — Joint Movements.

twitches. The application of the force applied should be gradual, the withdrawal sudden.

This movement not only acts upon the joints of the shoulders and arms by stretching them, but may be a powerful means of expanding the chest by making the patient inspire while the masseur stands in a chair behind him and resists the downward pull of his arms. As before stated, the pull should not be continuous, but should be intermittent, each strain lasting three to five seconds, the patient being allowed to take a breath during each interval.

The arm and shoulder joints may also be stretched as fol- **374** lows: The patient lying with the arm extended at the side, the masseur, facing the same side, grasps the patient's hand with his opposite hand, placing the other hand against the chest close to the axilla, and pulls with force graduated to the strength of the patient.

Stretching of the joints of the legs may be applied by seiz- **375** ing the foot and pulling in the line of the body. The toe joints are stretched by pulling each toe separately.

The Finger Joints. — Flexion, extension, and stretching **376** movements should be applied to the finger joints especially in the treatment of cases in which these joints are stiffened by disease or by improperly treated fractures of the wrist or forearm, and in writer's cramp.

MASSAGE OF SPECIAL REGIONS.

In the foregoing pages has been given a careful description of the various procedures employed in massage. I will now proceed to give more specific directions for the general and local application of massage in which the various manipulations are combined.

377   General Massage.— The order of application to different parts of the body in the administration of general massage should be as follows : —

(1) Arms ; (2) Chest ; (3) Legs ; (4) Abdomen ; (5) Hips ; (6) Back ; (7) Head.

In the application of the different procedures named below, it should be understood in general that the parts are to be gone over with each manipulation from four to eight times. For specific directions respecting the application of each of the various procedures, the reader is referred to previous pages, except in the case of such movements as are especially adapted to particular regions, directions for which will be given as may be required to make their application plain.

378   Massage of the Arm.— The several procedures are applied in the following order : —

1. Friction — light centripetal **(193, 199-201, 213-217)**.
2. Fulling **(244)**.
3. Friction — spiral and centripetal **(196)**.
4. Petrissage, or muscle kneading **(248-254)**.
5. Rolling **(255-260)**.
6. Friction — centripetal.
7. Wringing **(261-264)**.
8. Friction — centripetal.

9. Percussion — hacking (**316**), spatting (**314**), beating (**317**).

10. Joint movements (**343-348**) — flexion, extension, rotation, stretching, etc. (**355-365, 372-376**).

11. Vibration — shaking (**303**).

12. Stroking (**175, 169-172**).

In masseing the arm, centripetal friction and fulling are **379** first applied to the whole arm, beginning with the hand, as preliminary treatment. Friction and deep kneading are then alternately applied in sections, first to the hand, then the forearm, then the upper arm. Procedures 5, 6, 7, 8, 9, 11, and 12 are applied to the entire arm; joint movements (10) are applied in succession to the fingers, wrist, elbow, and shoulder; rolling, wringing, and stroking, from above downward; friction, from below upward; percussion, both from above downward and below upward. Shaking, or vibration, may be applied simultaneously with stretching.

Massage of the Chest.— Order of movements : — **380**

1. Friction — centripetal (very light) (**203, 222**).

2. Fulling (carefully) (**244**).

3. Friction.

4. Palmar kneading (**266**).

5. Percussion — tapping (**313**), hacking (**316**), spatting (**314**), beating (**317**), clapping (for very fleshy persons only) (**315**).

6. Assistive and resistive respiratory movements (**381-384**).

To *assist expiration*, compress the sides of the chest dur- **381** ing expiration, or raise the arms outward and upward with inspiration.

To *resist inspiration*, place one hand upon the abdomen, **382** causing the patient to lift it upward by the inspiratory movement, making at the same time a degree of pressure adapted to the patient's condition; or a shot-bag may be used instead of the hand (Fig. 72).

383   To *resist expiration*, have the patient breathe through a small tube (Fig. 72) or through a small opening in the lips.

384   In massage of the chest, great care should be observed that the patient breathes properly. The patient should be taught the proper mode of chest and waist expansion in breathing (Fig. 73). Few women know how to expand the lower part of the chest. Patients should be made to inspire through the nose, and to take deep and slow respirations.

385   **Massage of the Leg.**— The order of movements is essentially the same as for the arm, as follows : —

1. Friction — centripetal (**193, 202**).
2. Fulling (**244**).
3. Friction — spiral (**196**), circular (**195**), centripetal (**219-221**).
4. Petrissage, or muscle kneading (**248-254**).
5. Rolling (**255-260**).
6. Friction—centripetal.
7. Wringing (**261-264**).
8. Friction.
9. Percussion — hacking (**316**), spatting (**314**), beating (**317**), clapping (**315**).
10. Joint movements (**343-348**) — flexion, extension, abduction, adduction, circumduction, stretching (**366-372**).
11. Shaking (**303**).
12. Stroking (**175, 169-172**).

386   Movements 1 and 2 are preparatory ; 3 and 4 are applied successively to the feet, lower leg, and thigh ; 5, 6, 7, and 8 are applied in succession to the leg and thigh in connection with 3 and 4 ; 10 is applied successively to the toes, ankle, knee, and thigh ; 9, 11, and 12 are applied to the whole leg.

387   The principles laid down in relation to massage of the arm apply equally to the leg.

388   The muscular structures of the thigh are so massive in adults, and especially in very fleshy persons, that they cannot be so conveniently grasped as in the arm and lower leg, hence it is impossible to so perfectly individualize muscles and

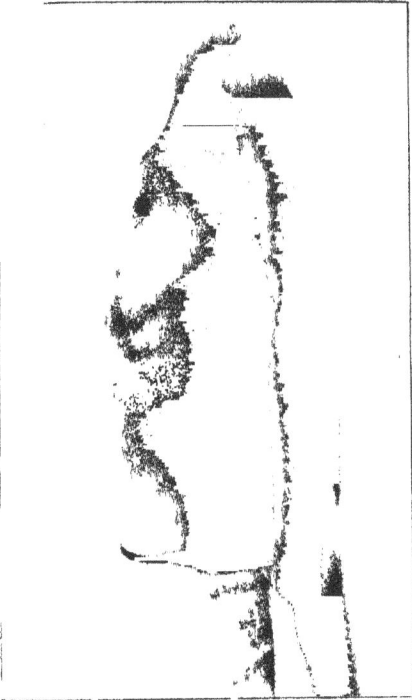

Fig 73. Full Breathing (Preliminary to Abdominal Massage)

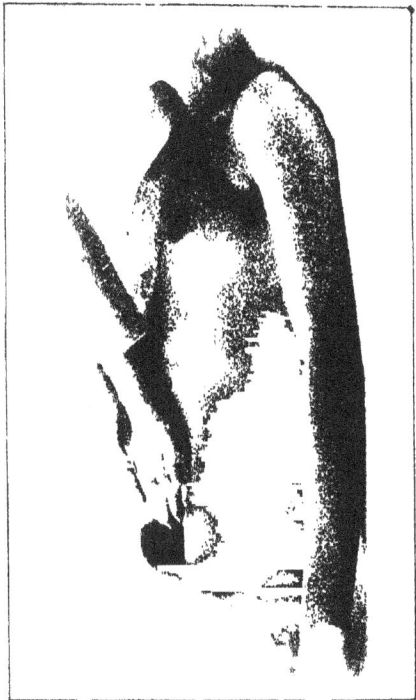

Fig 75. Lifting Viscera

Fig 72. Resistive Expiration and Inspiration (Using the Author's Expiration Tube).

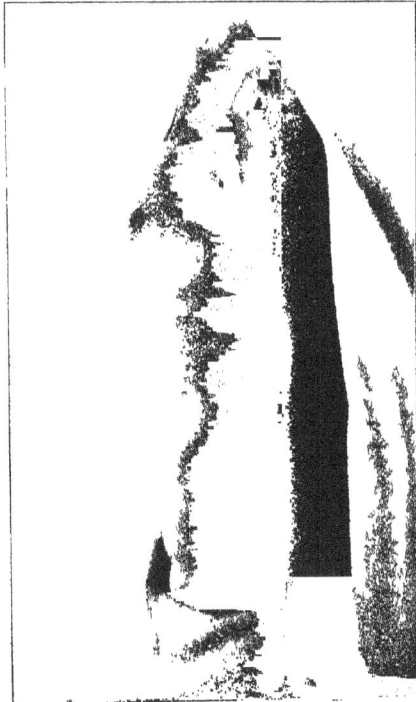

Fig. 74. Inspiratory Lifting of Abdominal Contents.

PLATE XXIX. — Abdominal Massage.

muscular groups in the manipulation. Rolling movements must, to a considerable extent, be substituted for petrissage. Special pains must be taken, however, to follow the general contour of the bones, so as to lift and stretch every muscle, working especially over the course of the great vessels which lie along the inner border of the extensors, and taking care to pull and stretch the muscular masses away from them on each side.

Massage of the Abdomen.— Order of movements :— **389**

1. Preliminary movements — deep breathing (**441, 461**); inspiratory lifting (**444, 445**); lifting the abdominal contents (**442**).

2. Reflex stroking (**395**).

3. Nerve compression (**160, 396, 397**).

4. Vibration — deep vibration, lateral shaking, circular shaking (**398-400**).

5. Percussion — tapping (**313**), spatting (**314**), hacking (**316**), beating (**317**), clapping (**315**).

6. Deep kneading — digital kneading of the colon (**404, 405**); kneading of the colon with the fist (**406-408**); kneading of the colon with the fingers and heel of the hand (**412-414**) ; kneading of the colon with the thumbs (**409, 410**).

7. Mass kneading of the abdominal contents (**411**).

8. Rolling (**415**).

9. Fulling (carefully) (**420**).

10. Petrissage, or muscle kneading (**421, 422**).

11. Stroking (**175, 170**).

12. Percussion of lumbar spine and sacrum (**315-317**).

13. Hips-raising and knees-separating exercises (**481, 482**).

The twelfth step may be omitted when massage of the abdomen is employed in connection with general massage, as it is included in massage of the back (**426**), and also the knees-separating exercise (13), which is included in joint move-ments of the legs (**385** (10), **366-371**).

The following rules should be carefully observed in abdomi- **390** nal massage : —

1. General abdominal massage should not be administered until two hours after eating.

2. The bladder should always be emptied just before abdominal massage.

3. In obstinate cases of fæcal accumulation, a coloclyster (large enema taken in right Sims's, or knee-chest, position) of warm water should be administered, the water being allowed to pass off before treatment.

4. The patient should be taught to relax the abdominal muscles, and to breathe deeply and regularly during treatment.

5. If the abdomen is very sensitive, apply a hot fomentation before giving the massage.

6. If the skin perspires very freely, render it firm and smooth by sponging with cold water.

7. Very "ticklish" patients require careful education by avoidance at first of superficial movements.

8. Pain and coldness of the extremities, or depression, after abdominal massage, is due either to bungling or violent treatment, or to extreme hyperæsthesia of the abdominal sympathetic. In such cases, employ fomentations and the moist abdominal bandage in connection with massage.

9. It is important in all manipulations of the abdomen to exercise great care not to excite pain. All movements should be executed in such a manner as to avoid sudden thrusts, thereby causing the patient pain or other disagreeable sensations, as such disturbances create rigidity of the abdominal muscles, thus seriously interfering with the effects of the manipulations.

10. In applying massage to the abdomen, the operator should stand over the patient, so as to aid his hands, as far as possible, by the weight of his body, taking care, of course, to graduate the pressure to the requirements of each individual case.

11. All deep-kneading movements in massage of the abdomen should be slower than for other parts of the body, to allow time for movement of the fæcal mass.

Therapeutic Applications. — Abdominal massage is **391** so important a therapeutic procedure, and is so much employed as a special measure of treatment, that the subject is worthy of further consideration and a more particular description of the several procedures enumerated, and of the conditions in which each is useful. Abdominal massage is useful for the following purposes : —

1. To relieve chronic constipation.

2. To aid stomach, intestinal, and liver digestion.

3. To promote the absorption of fluids and elimination by the kidneys in ascites and in cases of deficient renal action.

4. For the removal of abnormal deposits of fat.

5. To develop weak or relaxed muscles.

6. For the replacement of displaced viscera in enteroptosis. The stomach, general intestinal mass, colon, one or both kidneys, spleen, and liver when prolapsed may usually be replaced by proper manipulations.

7. Abdominal massage is a necessary accessory in the treatment of many forms of pelvic disease. Indeed, in most of these cases the primary seat of the disorder is the abdomen rather than the pelvis.

The most common and important use of abdominal massage **392** is as a means of relieving chronic intestinal inactivity. The general causes of constipation, as regards conditions of the bowels which may be relieved by massage, are the following:—

1. Relaxed abdominal muscles, resulting in prolapse of the bowels and other viscera, and consequent stasis of the intestinal contents, with resulting dilatation of the colon. The dilatation may exist either in the cæcum or the sigmoid flexure, or the entire colon may be affected. In consequence of delay to evacuate the bowels, the fæcal contents often form hard masses, as the result of the excessive absorption of fluid due to their prolonged sojourn in the colon.

2. Deficient production of bile, due to an inactive state of the liver, either as a result of inactivity in the portal circulation, or that condition of the liver termed by the French "hepa-

tism," in which there is some local functional derangement. This condition, commonly spoken of in this country as "torpidity" or "biliousness," is one in which the liver fails to perform its work effectively in destroying ptomaines which are received in the food or are formed in the alimentary canal, or to convert into less toxic forms the leucomaines, or tissue poisons, normally developed in the system and prepared by the liver for elimination by the kidneys. This condition is commonly present in rheumatism, gout, and the various conditions included under the term "uric acid diathesis."

3. Deficient activity in the nerve elements supplying the intestines and controlling the reflexes by which peristalsis is maintained, the contents of the bowels moved along the intestine, and the normal diurnal rhythm maintained whereby the residuum reaching the lower part of the colon is regularly discharged from the body.

393   The immediate indications in relation to the removal of these causes, so far as massage is effective to accomplish it, may be enumerated as follows : —

1. Increase of glandular activity by an increase of the activity of the blood current in the portal vein, and stimulation of the abdominal sympathetic ganglia, the splanchnics, and Meissner's and Auerbach's plexuses, the nerve mechanisms which control the motor, vascular, and secretory functions of the intestines.

2. Increase of peristaltic activity through a stimulation of the nervous reflexes by which this activity is maintained, and by an increased outflow of bile from the liver, the natural laxative by which rhythmical peristaltic activity is promoted.

3. Relief of passive congestion of the portal system and of the viscera under the influence of this branch of the circulatory system, especially the liver, spleen, stomach, and intestines, thus aiding the return of these structures to a normal state and a consequent restoration of their functions.

4. Mechanical dislodgment of the contents of the colon.

5. Development of the abdominal muscles, thereby increasing intra-abdominal tension, which favors expulsion of the intestinal contents.

6. Replacement of displaced viscera.

Not infrequently — in the majority of cases, in fact — all of these indications are found coincidently present.

The procedures offered by massage by which these indications are best met, are the following : —

1. *To stimulate the nervous reflexes, and hence the peristaltic,* **394** *glandular, and vascular activities, under control of the abdominal sympathetic.*

This may be accomplished by employing the following **395** measures : —

(1) *Reflex Stroking.*— With the ends of the fingers, make very light strokes in a circular or semicircular direction about the umbilicus. Begin very close to that point, gradually extending outward, then return and repeat. Also make vertical strokes along the sides in the mammary line, and parallel with the rectus muscle. Strokes may also be made over the fourth, fifth, and sixth ribs at the sides of the chest. In sensitive persons, one-sided contraction of the abdominal muscles or a twitching at the epigastrium will be noticed as the result of the so-called abdominal and epigastric reflexes. This procedure is strongly exciting ; some patients are not able to endure it. The profound reflex effect produced in patients who are very sensitive, or " ticklish," is evidence of the strong influence of this procedure upon reflex nervous activity.

(2) *Nerve Compression* (Figs. 35, 76).— The stomach and **396** the intestines are directly controlled by the *solar plexus* and the *lumbar ganglia* of the sympathetic. The solar plexus is at the epigastrium, just below the lower end of the sternum. The chief lumbar ganglia are situated on each side of the umbilicus, about two inches from it. Pressure upon these ganglia has a marked stimulating effect, because they send out energetic nerve impulses into the parts which they supply, which include not only the stomach and the intestines but all the abdominal viscera.

It should be remembered that these nerve masses lie beneath the abdominal contents, resting upon the bodies of the vertebræ. It is hence necessary to make a considerable degree of pressure in order to reach them. The tips of the fingers, being placed upon the points indicated, should be carried directly back toward the spinal column, the patient in the meantime being directed to take first a full breath and then to exhale as completely as possible. This diverts the mind of the patient from the procedure which is being executed, and also diminishes the abdominal tension, thus making it less difficult to bring pressure to bear upon the posterior wall of the abdominal cavity.

With patients who are extremely fleshy, and in cases in which the abdomen is greatly distended with gas, this procedure can be executed only in a very imperfect manner.

397   The position of the patient is a matter of great importance. The shoulders should be slightly raised and the knees well drawn up, the legs being supported, so that the anterior abdominal wall shall be relaxed as much as possible. The patient's hands should be by his side, and all the muscles of the body in a state of rest. Only gentle pressure should be employed, and the application should be continued only two or three seconds at each point. In many cases it will be found that extreme sensitiveness exists at the points indicated, which is evidence of an excited or hyperæsthetic state of the abdominal sympathetic. Continuous gentle pressure may be beneficial, even in these cases, however, acting as in other cases of abnormal nerve sensibility, as chronic sciatica, by setting up a series of vital activities which result in the restoration of the nerve to its normal condition.

398   (3) *Vibration.* — (*a*) Strong vibration applied to the abdominal contents has been shown to be one of the most powerful means of stimulating the nervous reflexes, circulation, glandular activity, and peristalsis, which can be employed for this part of the body. Either one or both hands may be used. The flat palm of the hand is applied to the surface, with the arm extended, and fine vibratory movements are executed in such a manner as to throw the whole abdominal contents into vibration. The same movement, which consists of a sort of trembling, as elsewhere described, may be beneficially applied to the liver (Fig. 55).

(*b*) A more vigorous shaking movement is communicated **399** to the abdominal contents by making intermittent pressure either with one hand, or with one hand reinforced by the other, or by both hands- in alternation, the movements being made with sufficient rapidity to produce a decided motion of the abdominal contents. The effect of this procedure is very marked in cases in which the abdominal walls are considerably relaxed.

(*c*) A third method of applying shaking is by placing the **400** palm of the hand upon the abdomen, the arm slightly flexed, then making a rapid rotary movement without allowing the hand to slide upon the surface. The direction of the movements is alternated, half a dozen in one direction and then an equal number in the opposite direction.

(4) *Percussion.*—This is unquestionably the most powerful **401** of all the stimulating means which can be applied to the viscera through the abdominal wall. All the different modes of percussion, viz., tapping, spatting, clapping, hacking, and beating, may be usefully employed. The mode of executing these movements has been elsewhere indicated.

2. *To produce mechanical effects by means of which stasis* **402** *of the intestinal contents may be overcome and accumulated fæcal matter dislodged at the same time that the circulatory and glandular activities are stimulated.*

For this purpose deep kneading is especially to be recom- **403** mended. This may be accomplished by a number of different procedures :—

(1) *Digital Kneading* (Fig. 77).—Standing face to the **404** patient's feet, and with the fingers very slightly flexed, place the finger tips, the hand being reinforced by the other hand placed above it, upon the abdomen, low down upon the right side. Crowd the finger ends backward, pressing with as much

force as possible without giving the patient much inconvenience, against the cæcum. Carry the hand upward in the direction of the ascending colon as far as permitted by the ribs. Repeat the movement four or five times. Execute similar movements on the left side, beginning above instead of below, pressing the fingers upon the abdominal wall at a point close under the ribs on the left side. Carry the hand downward, turning toward the median line at the conclusion of the movement, so as to follow as closely as possible the course of the sigmoid flexure of the colon.

405   In cases in which it is believed that a considerable amount of fæcal matter exists in the colon, the procedure should be somewhat different. It should begin with the left instead of the right side, and instead of placing the hand at the start close under the ribs, it should be pressed down at a point two or three inches above the point at which the movement terminates. After two or three movements starting at this point, the hands should be carried a little farther upward, the strokes repeated as before, and the hand carried at each stroke down to the lowermost point which can be reached.

After doing the left side in this manner, execute the same movements upon the right side, beginning at a point just below the ribs instead of at the lower end of the cæcum, and gradually increasing the length of the stroke from below upward until the lower end of the cæcum is reached. The above movements may be advantageously repeated with the patient lying in the right or left Sims position, the left side for the ascending colon, and the right side for the descending colon.

406   (2) *Kneading with the Closed Fist* (Fig. 78).— With the closed fists used in alternation, work along the whole course of the colon, beginning at the lower end of the cæcum, directing the movements upward to the lower border of the ribs on the right side, following the oblique border of the ribs to a point midway between the umbilicus and the sternum, at which the median line is crossed ; then down on the opposite side, end-

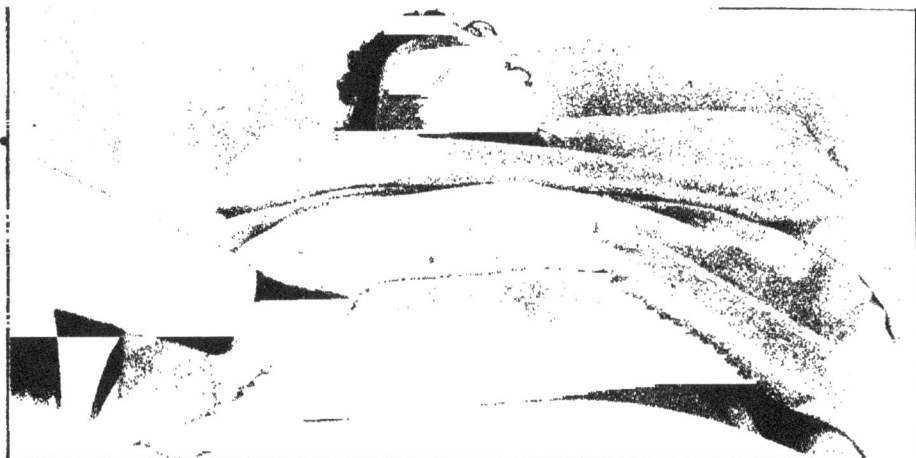
Fig. 76. Compression of Lumbar Ganglia of the Sympathetic.

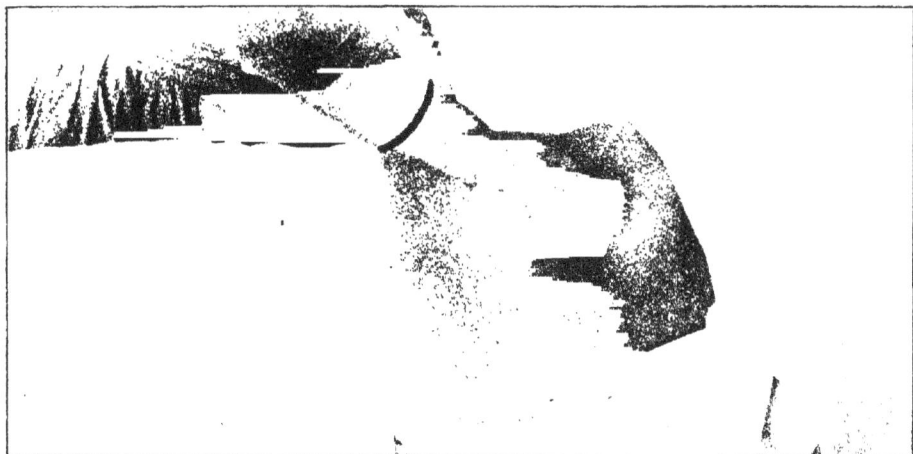
Fig. 77. Digital Kneading of Colon.

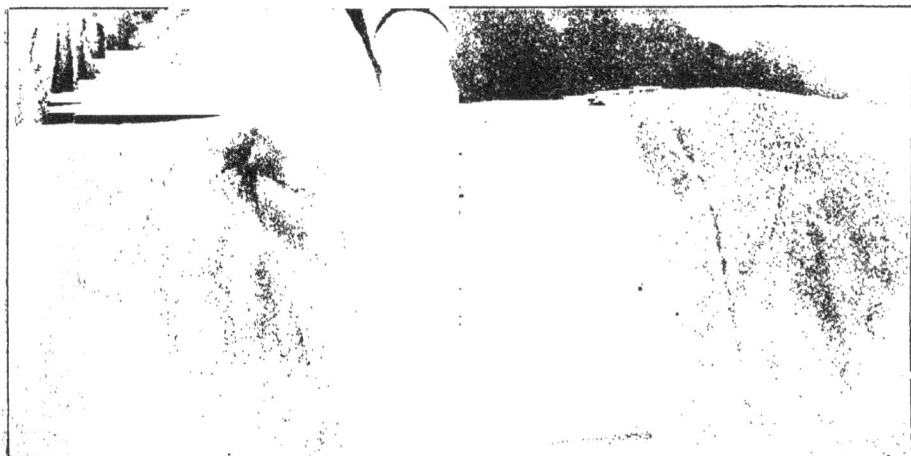
Fig. 78. Fist Kneading of Colon.

ing at a point close to the pubic bone, and just to the left of the median line.

It should be remembered that the colon lies much deeper at the sigmoid flexure than at any other portion of its course, so that in order to reach the lower part of the colon it is necessary to press the hand in as deep as possible without giving the patient too much inconvenience. The movements must be directed with great care and deliberation.

The *rate of movement* should not be more than thirty per **407** minute, or two seconds for each hand. Care should be taken not to release the pressure upon the bowels with one hand until the other hand has been placed in position just in advance and close to it. Care must also be taken to follow the curves of the colon.

In the directions given above, the colon is supposed to be **408** in normal position. This is by no means always the case, however. In the majority of women who have worn the ordinary dress, and in nearly all elderly women, the colon will be found more or less prolapsed. The prolapse usually involves chiefly the central portion of the colon, as this portion is more easily displaced than the points of junction of the ascending and descending colon with the transverse portion. The case shown in Fig. 95, a photograph of which was sent to the writer by Professor Meinert, of Dresden, Germany, will give a good idea of the unnatural conditions often found in these cases. Many cases equally bad have been encountered by the writer. A fairly correct idea of the location of the colon may be obtained by noticing the contour of the abdomen when the patient is placed in a sitting or standing position. The colon may be considered as lying along the line of greatest prominence. This may be observed with the patient standing or sitting, and marked with a soft sketching pencil or a bit of cotton moistened with tincture of iodine.

(3) *Kneading with the Thumbs* (Fig. 79).— With the fin- **409** gers behind and the thumbs in front, grasp the loin on each

8

side between the thumb and the fingers. The right hand should thus grasp the lower end of the cæcum, while the left hand grasps the upper part of the descending colon just beneath the ribs. Movements are then executed in an upward direction with the right hand, and a downward direction with the left hand, the operator facing the patient's feet.

410   In thin persons the ascending and the descending colon can be more efficiently manipulated in this way than in almost any other, as at least some portion of the intestine may by this procedure be actually seized between the fingers and the thumb, and the contents forced along. When the colon is loaded with fæcal matter, thumb 'kneading, as well as fist and palmar kneading, should begin near the ribs on the right side, and as low down as possible on the left side, working gradually downward and upward respectively, in such a manner as to clear the way.

411   (4) *Mass Kneading* (Fig. 80).—Still another procedure which is of value in abdominal massage, is what may be termed "mass kneading," in which the operator .endeavors to seize the abdominal contents with both hands, manipulating them precisely as a baker does a mass of dough, the fingers of one hand being used in opposition to the heel of the other hand, and the abdominal contents kneaded and manipulated between the two hands. In this procedure the heel of one hand of the manipulator operates upon the side of the patient nearest him, while the fingers of the other hand operate upon the tissues of the opposite side. Mass kneading is only applicable to cases in which the abdominal walls are considerably relaxed.

412   (5) *Palmar Kneading.*—Two movements, both of great value, may be executed with the heel of the hand, as follows:—

413   (*a*) Describe a circle about the umbilicus, the hands being used in alternation, the heel of one hand moving up on the right side, and the other moving down on the left side, the stroke on the left side being made to slightly overlap that of the right side. This acts especially upon the small intestines.

(*b*) Starting at the lower end of the ascending colon, work **414** the whole colon with the heel of the hand, carefully following its direction from the cæcum to the sigmoid flexure, one hand assisting the other by supporting the tissues to prevent over-stretching the skin. Or, knead the ascending colon with the heel of the hand, the transverse colon with the ulnar side of the hand, and the descending colon with the tips of the fingers. This method obviates the necessity of changing the position of the body during manipulation.

(6) *Rolling.* — When the abdominal walls are considerably **415** relaxed, they may be gathered between the hands placed parallel with the body, one on each side, and thus compressed, rolled, and shaken, together with the intestinal contents. Care must be taken to include the abdominal contents — not simply the skin and subcutaneous tissue or a mass of subcutaneous fat. The patient's position must be such as to secure very thorough relaxation of the abdominal muscles in order to make this procedure effective.

(7) *Massage of the Gall Bladder.* — The movement of the **416** bile from the liver toward the intestine may be assisted, and the liver be gently manipulated, by applying pressure with the left hand as follows : The operator, standing by the left side of the patient, places the left hand at the lowermost border of the ribs of the right side; a stroking movement is then executed along the lower border of the ribs of the right side in the direction of the epigastrium, the fingers being crowded up under the ribs as high as possible or until the lower border of the liver is felt. In this way it is possible to reach the gall bladder, and to facilitate the discharge of its contents into the intestine. The bile being a natural laxative, this is one of the most effective means of stimulating peristaltic activity.

Care should be taken to place the patient in such a posi- **417** tion as to completely relax the abdominal muscles, and he must be made to take long, deep inspirations during the procedure, so as to prevent, so far as possible, spasm of the abdominal muscles.

418   3. *To Strengthen the Abdominal Muscles.*

Massage alone is not sufficient as a means of developing the abdominal muscles, as is the case with all muscular structures. They must be brought into voluntary action by proper gymnastics, for which the Swedish gymnastics and the manual Swedish movements, or medical gymnastics, afford the most effective means. The application of electricity, particularly of the sinusoidal current, is the most efficient of all modes of passive exercise. This current, used with slow alternations, brings the muscles of the abdomen into vigorous contraction without producing pain or other sensation than that of motion. Much, however, can be accomplished by massage. The following procedures are the most effective : —

419   (1) *Kneading.*— As with other muscular structures, kneading is the most effective of the procedures afforded by massage, for stimulating development of the abdominal muscles. Both superficial kneading, or fulling (**244**), and deep kneading, or petrissage (**248-254**), may be employed.

420   (*a*) Apply fulling movements to the whole abdominal surface, working up and down in the direction of the recti muscles, and in circles about the umbilicus.

421   (*b*) In deep kneading, or petrissage, of the abdominal muscles, care should be taken, as in other regions, to include the individual muscles or groups of muscles in the grasp of the hand, as far as possible. The *recti* and the *external oblique* are the only muscles readily accessible to the hand. The outline of these muscles may be easily discerned by causing the patient to raise the head by forcible effort, and without the assistance of the arms. Forcible contraction of the recti muscles causes the external oblique to bulge at the sides, showing the outline of both sets of muscles. When the abdominal muscles are thoroughly relaxed by proper position, and in cases in which they are especially in need of this form of treatment, the recti muscles can be quite easily grasped and manipulated individually. The external oblique is less easily managed, but by a

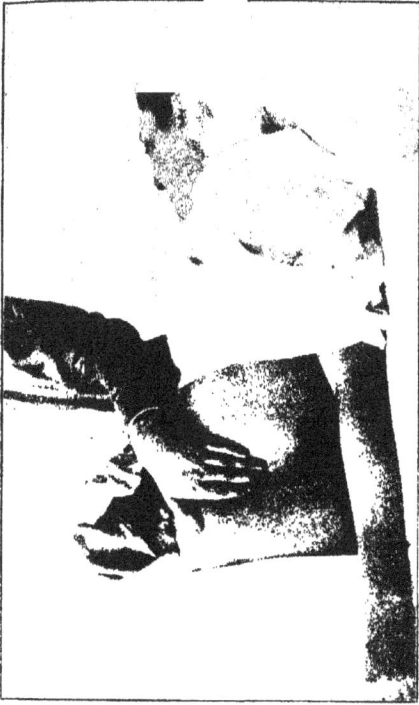

Fig. 80. Mass Kneading.

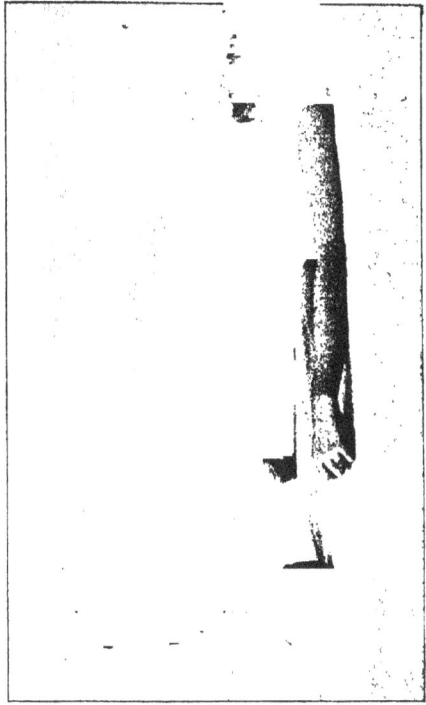

Fig. 82. Raising Hips.

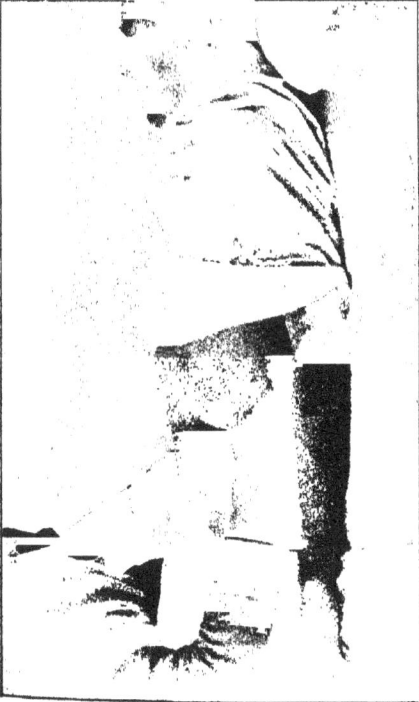

Fig. 79. Thumb Kneading of Colon.

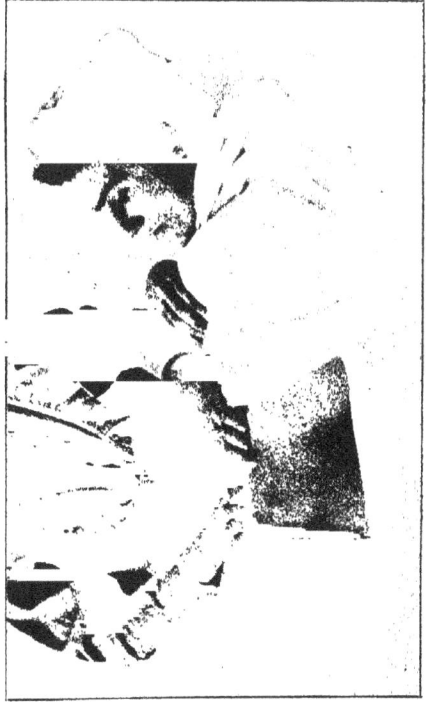

Fig. 81. Kneading of Abdominal Muscles.

PLATE XXXI.— Abdominal Massage.

painstaking effort the whole muscle can be subjected to a thorough manipulation.

A very effective mode of massing the recti muscles is to **422** cause the patient to raise the head (Fig. 81) ; then, with both hands placed upon the abdomen in such a manner that the thumbs rest upon the recti, the operator facing the patient, the muscles are rapidly manipulated by the thumbs, working from below upward.

In some patients these manipulations are apt to produce **423** excoriations of the skin in consequence of its thinness. This is especially the case when the skin becomes moist by perspiration. To obviate this difficulty, the surface should be well lubricated with cacao butter or talcum powder.

Replacement of the Abdominal Viscera.—This is neces- **424** sary in many cases of abdominal massage, as a preliminary procedure. It is especially required in women, since in the majority of invalid women some of the viscera are almost certain to be found displaced. The stomach is displaced from two to five inches below its normal position in nineteen out of twenty of all adult civilized women who have worn the conventional dress. A movable, or floating, right kidney is to be found in at least twenty-five per cent of women who are likely to require abdominal massage. The liver is also not infrequently found displaced. The methods employed in replacing the various viscera are given elsewhere (**439-450**).

Massage of the Hips.— With the patient lying upon **425** the back, the manipulations are applied to the fleshy portions of the hips, or the buttocks, the several procedures being administered in the following order : —

1. Light centripetal friction (**193**).
2. Fulling (**244**).
3. Circular friction (**195, 203**).
4. Petrissage (**248**).
5. Palmar kneading (**266**).
6. Centripetal friction.

7. Nerve compression along the sacro-iliac synchondrosis (junction of sacrum with iliac bones) and over the sciatic nerve (Fig. 35).

8. Percussion — hacking (**316**), spatting (**314**), beating (**317**), clapping (**315**).

9. Stroking (**175**).

426   **Massage of the Back.**— The patient lies upon the face, the forehead resting upon the crossed hands, the elbows well raised from the sides so as to spread the scapulæ and uncover as much of the back as possible : —

1. Centripetal friction (**193**).

2. Fulling of the neck, shoulders, sides, and loins (**244**).

3. Friction — circular (**195**), centripetal (**193**).

4. Deep kneading — palmar kneading, or rolling, above the scapulæ (Fig. 53); digital kneading, following the ribs (**292**); palm kneading up and down the spine (**288, 291, 294**) ; digital kneading of the spine (Fig. 54) (**287, 289, 290, 293**).

5. Nerve compression (**156**); spine stretching (**427**).

6. Percussion of spine and sacrum — tapping, hacking, slapping, beating, clapping (**313-317**).

7. Friction (alternating with kneading, as above) (**228**).

8. Stroking (**175, 170**).

427   *Spine stretching* may be applied in one of the following ways : —

1. Suspension by the head or the head and shoulders. By means of an improved form of apparatus which the writer has had constructed, and has used for several years, the tension upon the head and shoulders may be separately determined and proportioned with accuracy.

2. The patient lying upon his face, hips and chest supported by pillows, his head is strongly flexed by the masseur over the end of the couch.

3. The patient sitting with legs extended horizontally, leans forward while the attendant flexes his head strongly forward.

428   Massage of the back is a very agreeable procedure for most patients. The skin of the back is but little sensitive, and will bear the employment of considerable force. Percussion of the spine is one of the most powerful means of affecting the deep-lying nerve centers, and affects not only the spinal centers but, reflexly, the sympathetic centers also, and through the splanchnics, influences the circulation in the stomach and intestines. Pain in the spine is most often due to hyperæsthesia of the abdominal sympathetic, but is often due to anæmia which may be present, or the result of spasm of the vasomotor centers, having its origin in sympathetic irritation. The pain usually disappears under treatment when the force employed is graduated with sufficient care. Fomentations applied daily and the moist, or so-called, heating, compress worn at night are necessary adjuncts to massage in cases in which there is much tenderness of the sympathetic. Pain in the sacral region may be due to rectal, ovarian, or bladder disease. Pain in the lumbar region is usually due to hyperæsthesia of the abdominal sympathetic. Pain in the dorsal region originates in irritation of the solar plexus.

Massage of the Head.— Massage of the head and neck **429** is not usually included in general massage, but may often be advantageously added to the general manipulations as a means of quieting any slight excitement which may have been produced, and leaving the patient in a restful state. Head massage is especially valuable for the relief of headache, neurasthenic pains, baldness, the dullness and other uncomfortable sensations resulting from loss of sleep, cerebral anæmia, neuralgia, and migraine.

The procedures which I have found most useful are the **430** following, usually employed in the order given : —

1. Digital kneading, from forehead to occiput (Fig. 83) (**268**).

2. Hacking (**316**), from before backward.

3. Chucking (Fig. 45), one hand placed upon the forehead or the side of the head, the other opposite.

4. Tapping (**313**).

5. Hacking.

6. Head rolling, flexion, and twisting, both active and passive, repeated four to eight times.

7. Stroking from vertex to base of skull, down back of neck, and along the submaxillary groove.

8. Vibration — shaking (**303**).

9. Pressure.

10. Hypnotic stroking (**189**).

431 In cases of great immobility. of the scalp (a "hidebound" condition), when necessary, a better hold of the scalp may be obtained by grasping the hair between the fingers close to the roots. Care should be taken, however, not to give so great latitude to the movements as to produce unpleasant sensations from pulling the hair.

432 **Neck Massage.**—The purpose of neck massage is to withdraw blood from the brain. The circulation in the brain is so directly affected by the breathing movements that it is especially important that respiration should receive attention. The patient should sit with the head well raised, the arms extended downward as far as possible, so as to expose the neck to the fullest extent, and should be made to execute deep breathing movements for a few times before the manipulations are begun, so as to insure full respiration, and to distract his attention from the manipulations. The strokes should be made at the same time with inspiration, and with both hands simultaneously, except in cases in which the throat is so sensitive that irritation of the larynx and coughing result from compression of the larynx between the fingers or thumbs of the two hands, when the strokes should be made in alternation.

433 *Höffinger's Method.*— Massage of the neck may be applied in several ways. The following is known as Höffinger's method (Fig. 84): The patient sits upon a high seat, the operator standing behind. The hands are brought in contact with the neck in such a way that the little fingers fall into the groove beneath the jaw. The hands are then made to move downward, the arms rotating inward at the same time, the ends of the fingers pressing upon the jugular veins. After a few

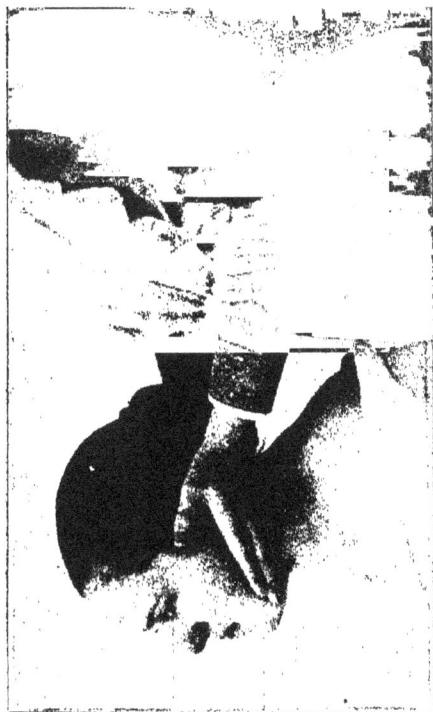

Fig. 84. Neck Massage (Hoffinger's Method).

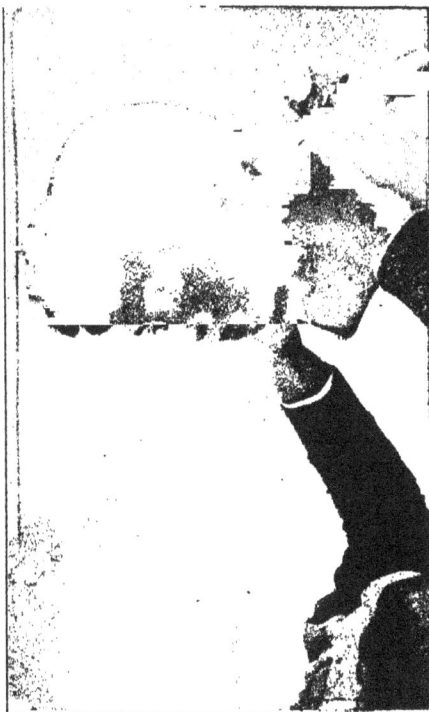

Fig. 86. Neck Massage (in Children).

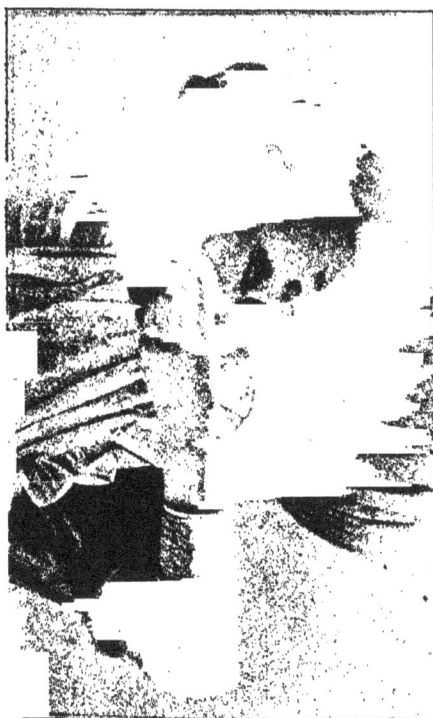

Fig. 83. Digital Kneading of Head.

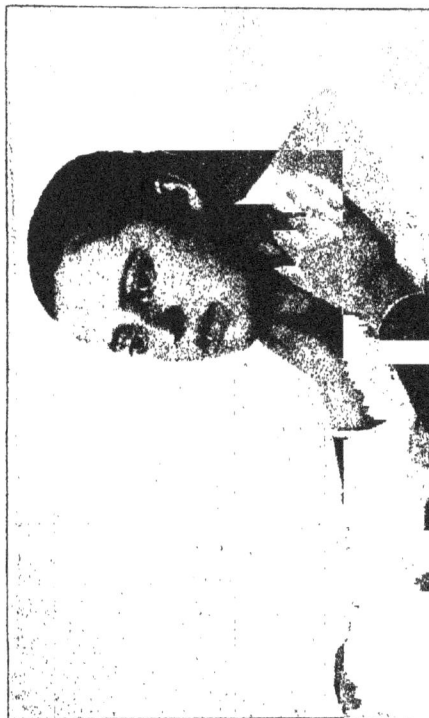

Fig. 85. Neck Massage (Gerster's Method).

PLATE XXXII. — Massage of Head and Neck.

strokes over the anterior portion of the neck, similar strokes are made with the thumbs over the back part of the neck. The deep breathing should be continued during the manipulation.

Höffinger employs only manipulations of the anterior por- **434** tion and sides of the neck. Experience has led me to employ also manipulation of the back part of the neck, extending from the occiput down on either side of the ligamentum nuchæ to the vertebra prominens. This manipulation powerfully influences the cervical sympathetic, and is of very great value in cases of occipital headache and the " neckache " so common with neurasthenics.

Gerster's Method. — Massage of the neck may also be **435** applied from the front — Gerster's method (Fig. 85). With the fingers extended and held close together, the palm upward, the little fingers are applied to the neck just below the ears. The hands are then moved downward and rotated inward, so that the tips of the thumbs fall on each side of the larynx. Friction is thus applied in such a manner that the fingers compress and empty the external veins, while the thumbs press upon the internal jugular veins.

In the case of children or persons with very small necks, **436** the thumb may manipulate the front part of the neck while the fingers are applied to the back of it (Fig. 86).

Author's Method. — I employ hacking and fulling, as well as **437** friction, and direct my manipulators to apply the following procedures in the order given :—

1. Gentle fulling of the skin of the neck (**244**).

2. Friction of the anterior portion of the neck (**433** or **435**).

3. Friction of the back of the neck (**434**).

4. Percussion — gentle tapping (**313**) and hacking (**316**) of the back of the neck from occiput to vertebra prominens.

5. Stroking from the forehead backward and down the back of the neck, and from the vertex downward and over the anterior portion of the neck.

438 Neck massage is an extremely useful procedure for the relief of insomnia and cerebral congestion, and is often effective in cases of migraine and other forms of headache. Some cases have been reported in which non-cystic enlargement of the thyroid gland has been improved by neck massage.

439 **Replacement of the Abdominal Viscera.**— Glenard, of France, first called attention to the great mischief arising from the condition which he terms *enteroptosis*, or prolapse of the viscera of the abdomen. A careful study of the subject for the last ten years has convinced the writer that displacements of the stomach, colon, kidneys, spleen, and liver are responsible for a much greater number of symptoms than is generally supposed, and is the real cause of suffering in a large proportion of cases, especially in women, which have been treated with little or no benefit for supposed disorders of the pelvis. The accompanying cuts (Figs. [1] to [11]) illustrate a few of the many cases of visceral prolapse which have come under the writer's observation within the last ten years. Fig. [1] represents a case in which the right kidney had become so diseased in consequence of its prolapsed condition that its removal by a surgical operation was necessary. In operating for its removal, it was found to contain a calculus weighing more than four ounces. This was a case in which massage would have been unavailing; but it would have been a measure of great value, had it been employed a few years earlier.

Figs. 87 to 95 illustrate the causes of visceral prolapse, and will suggest the means necessary to aid recovery in these cases, and the advantages which may be derived from massage. Gastric neurasthenia certainly owes many of its distressing symptoms to disturbance of the abdominal sympathetic resulting from displacements of the sort referred to. I have found the following the most effective means of replacing the abdominal contents, as a whole, and restoring the viscera to their normal position : —

[1] Visceral Displacement from Incorrect Standing and Corset Wearing.

[2] Displaced Viscera.

[3] Results of Corset Constriction (Woman of 30).

[4] Displacement of Spleen and Other Viscera from Corset Wearing.

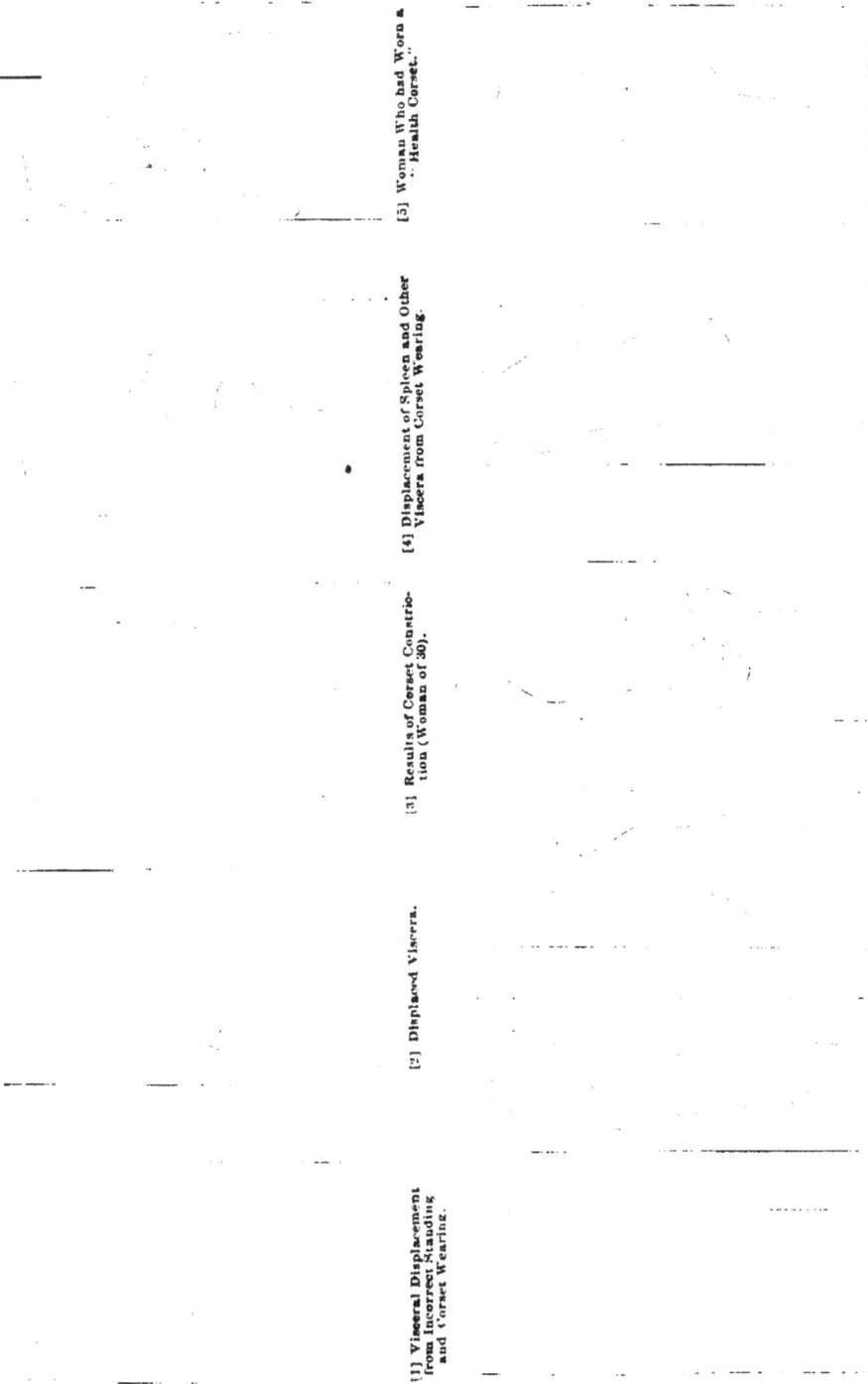

[5] Woman Who had Worn a "Health Corset."

[6] Bad Standing Corrected (Man).

[7] Bad Standing Corrected (Woman).

[8] Standing on One Foot Corrected.

[9] Results of Corset Constriction in a Young Woman of 30.

[10] Displacement of Spleen and Other Viscera from Corset Wearing.

[11] Woman Who had Worn a "Health Corset."

PLATE XXXIII.—Visceral Displacement.

Fig. 93. Young Woman of 22, with Weak Waist.

Fig. 94. Same Young Woman after a Year of Training.

Fig. 92. Same Young Woman a Year Later, Reformed.

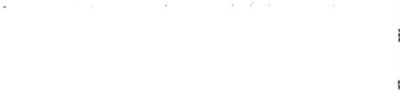

Fig. 91. Effect of Heavy Skirts and Bad Position in a Woman of 24.

Fig. 88. A Woman of Fashion.

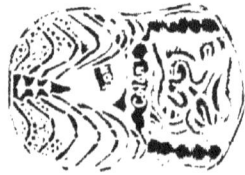

Fig. 90. Corset-deformed Figure, Internal View.

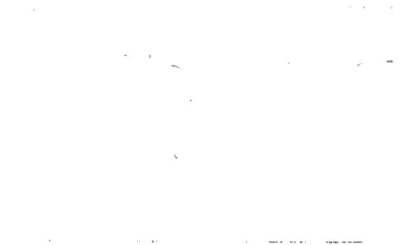

Fig. 87. Venus de Milo.

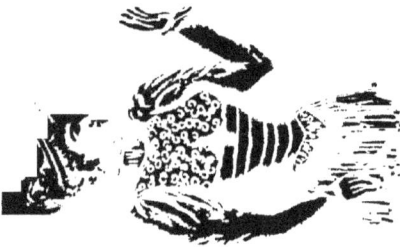

Fig. 89. Internal View of a Healthy Figure.

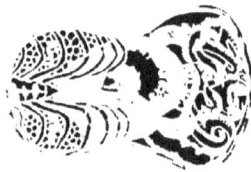

PLATE XXXIV.—Causes of Visceral Displacement.

The patient lies upon the couch with the head, not the **440** shoulders, elevated, and with the knees well drawn up so that the abdominal wall shall be as thoroughly relaxed as possible.

First of all, the patient is made to take several deep breaths, **441** care being taken to see that the abdomen is expanded well with each inspiration (Fig. 73). In women the reverse is likely to be the case.

The next proceeding is to lift the entire intestinal mass as **442** follows (Fig. 75): The masseur stands with his right side to the patient, facing the patient's feet, and places his hands one in either groin, the hands resting upon their ulnar borders (little fingers), and having the direction of Poupart's ligament. The hands are made to move slowly upward, the ulnar borders being at the same time crowded as deep as may be into the pelvis so as to grasp as much as possible of the abdominal contents, which are then drawn forcibly upward.

Shaking and rolling movements are valuable as a pre- **443** liminary measure, or used in alternation with the lifting movements, as a means of loosening up, so to speak, the abdominal contents, to prepare them for gliding easily into their normal positions. The lifting movements should be executed in alternation with rolling or shaking movements, from three to six times.

Inspiratory Lifting (Fig. 74).— I was led to adopt this **444** means of lifting the abdominal contents by a series of studies for the purpose of noting the influence of respiration upon intra-pelvic pressures. I observed that the ascent and descent of the uterus in respiration may be greatly increased by modifying the inspiratory and expiratory movements. For example, by directing the patient to take a deep breath and then asking her to force the breath downward, it was noticed that the pelvic contents were forced downward to a notable extent; while by causing the patient to completely empty the lungs, and then, with the glottis closed, to make a forcible inspiratory effort, the pelvic and abdominal contents were made to ascend in a very remarkable manner. In one instance it was noted that the uterus, which lay quite low in the pelvis, was drawn up more than an inch with each respiratory effort.

445 Inspiratory lifting is administered thus: The patient lying upon the back, with the hands at the side, so as to relax the abdominal muscles as much as possible, she is directed to take first a full breath, breathing as deeply as possible, then to completely empty the lungs. Then, instead of drawing in the breath as usual, the glottis is closed, and a strong inspiratory effort is made without the admission of air. By this method the whole inspiratory force is used in lifting the abdominal contents. In this movement the patient should be made to expand the chest, both the upper and the lower parts, as much as possible, as it is desired to suppress the action of the diaphragm so far as can be done voluntarily, while bringing into most active play those muscles of inspiration which act upon the ribs. This not only produces a powerful upward draft upon the abdominal contents, but at the same time enlarges the waist, and makes room for the viscera, so that their ascent is facilitated.

At the same time that the patient executes inspiratory lifting (**444, 445**), the abdominal contents should be lifted from below with the hands, as directed above. The patient should not be allowed to refrain from breathing more than ten or fifteen seconds. During this time, however, from three to five vigorous inspiratory liftings may be made. Then the patient may be allowed to take a few ordinary respirations, and finally a deep inspiration, followed by a complete expiration and a renewal of the inspiratory lifting. Repeat with the patient in the knee-chest position. This procedure is of special value in connection with pelvic massage.

446 **Replacement of the Stomach** (Fig. 96).— To accomplish this, lifting of the abdominal contents (**442**) is first executed ; then the operator, standing upon the right side of the patient and facing the side, places his right hand upon the left side of the abdomen in such a way that its ulnar border is in contact with the skin and lies in a transverse direction. With the fingers slightly flexed, the hand is first pressed backward, then carried upward and toward the median line in such a way that the tips of the fingers will sweep along the inferior borders of the false ribs, the movement ending at the epigastrium. The hand should be held at this point while the patient is asked to execute a deep breath ; the procedure is then repeated.

Replacement of the Right Kidney (Fig. 97).— Dis- **447** placement of the kidney is always associated with displacement of the stomach and bowels, hence lifting movements (**442**) and movements for the replacement of the stomach (**446**) should be employed in connection with those for the replacement of the kidneys.

To replace the kidney, after making movements to replace **448** the stomach and bowels, the operator proceeds as follows: Standing upon the right side of the patient, the fingers of the left hand are placed behind, while those of the right are placed' upon the abdomen; and by movements of the two hands the location of the kidneys is determined. While gently pressing the kidney upward, the patient is asked to take repeated deep breaths. With each exhalation, an effort is made to press the kidney up under the ribs of the right side by gentle pressure. As it moves upward and approaches its position, the right hand is shut, and the closed fist is made to follow the kidney and hold it in position while the patient makes a number of deep respirations.

Replacement of the Left Kidney and Spleen.— **449** The method employed is precisely the same as that for the replacement of the right kidney, except that the operator stands upon the patient's left side, and places the fingers of the right hand behind, manipulating the displaced organs with the left hand.

In all cases of enteroptosis, a proper abdominal bandage **450** must be applied after replacement of the prolapsed viscera, and means must be employed for strengthening the abdominal muscles,— gymnastics, massage, and proper applications of electricity, especially the sinusoidal current.

451   Massage of the Stomach (Fig. 96).—This is one of the most important applications of massage. Its objects are : —

1. To aid digestion by stimulating motor activity.

2. To aid digestion by increasing glandular activity.

3. To empty the stomach mechanically.

4. To restore the prolapsed stomach to its normal position.

452   The most important procedures to be employed are : —

1. Abdominal massage (**389**).

2. Standing upon the right side, and with the back to the patient, place the right hand upon the left side of the abdomen opposite the umbilicus ; with the fingers extended and close together, press the ulnar border of the hand backward, at the same time carrying it upward with a vibratory movement. Following along under the ribs of the left side, continue the movement upward to the epigastrium. At this point, before releasing the tissues, place the tips of the fingers of the left hand so as to support the tissues at the point to which they have been lifted by the movement of the right hand, making firm pressure ; then withdraw the right hand and repeat the movement. Continue for three or four minutes. If it is desired to empty the stomach, carry the strokes across the epigastrium and along under the lower border of the ribs of the right side.

3. When the object is to aid digestion, combine with these movements deep breathing movements (**441**) and inspiratory compression, obtained by having the patient take a deep breath and hold it for a few seconds while strongly contracting the abdominal muscles.

4. In cases of extreme prolapse of the stomach, in which patients suffer from flow of bile into the stomach, replace the abdominal viscera with the patient in the knee-chest position, standing with the back to the patient's head, grasping the abdomen near the pubic bone, and lifting toward the chest.

Firm compression of the stomach is an efficient means of suppressing vomiting and hiccough.

453   Massage of the Liver (Fig. 98).—This procedure is of great value in chronic cases of catarrhal jaundice, gallstones, and in numerous cases of so-called torpid liver, and is, in fact, valuable in all cases in which massage is indicated as a means of securing general improvement in nutrition, as in chlorosis, anæmia, emaciation, and impaired digestion. Increased activity of the liver aids digestion, and promotes especially the fat-making processes and blood formation. Massage of the liver is contra-indicated in cancer of the liver, in acute attacks of hepatic colic, in cases of acute gastro-duodenitis, and in hepatic abscess.

The method of procedure is the following, the patient's **454** knees being well drawn up and the shoulders slightly raised, so as to completely relax the abdominal muscles:—

1. Deep breathing with arm raising, four to eight times.

2. Abdominal massage (**389**). Whatever aids the portal circulation will assist the liver.

3. Tapping (**313**) over the entire region of the liver (Fig. 31), best executed with the patient lying on the left side, which renders it possible to reach the liver behind as well as in front.

4. Fulling (**244**).

5. Kneading. Standing at the left side of the patient, place the left hand behind the liver, against the lowermost ribs of the right side, and with the other hand stroke and knead the liver by pressing up underneath the ribs on the right side. When in normal position, the liver lies half an inch above the lower border of the ribs. The direction of the strokes should be from the loin along and beneath the inferior border of the ribs to the epigastrium, and across to the opposite side.

6. Hacking (**316**) over the liver.

7. Spatting (**314**).

8. Deep vibration (jarring) (**302**).

9. Inspiratory compression. Have the patient take a deep breath, and then contract the abdominal muscles as firmly as possible while holding the breath. Compression with the hands may be made over the region of the liver at the same time.

10. Laughing exercise, consisting of the syllable "ha" uttered in an explosive way, and up and down the scale.

455   Massage in Diarrhœa.— Abdominal massage is of very great value in certain cases of chronic diarrhœa. Of these, two very distinct classes are benefited by massage, each requiring, however, a different mode of application. In cases in which undigested food substances are passed soon after eating, indicating excessive peristalsis, with deficient activity of the digestive fluids, abdominal massage should be applied for half an hour a short time before each meal. In cases in which the diarrhœa is due to intestinal catarrh, resulting from dilatation of the stomach, whereby the food is retained in the stomach for so long a time that fermentation takes place, causing irritation of the intestinal membrane when the fermenting food substances at last find their way out of the stomach, massage of the stomach (**451**) should be applied soon after eating, or within an hour after each meal.

456   General massage, especially massage of the shoulders and back, should be combined with abdominal massage in these cases, and massage should be employed at least once daily. Ordinarily, manipulation of the abdomen for ten or fifteen minutes is sufficient when the application is made after meals.

457   Pelvic Massage.— This form of massage, first introduced by Major Thure Brandt, a Swedish gymnast, in 1874, has been variously modified by different physicians who have taken up its employment since the favorable reports of Brandt, especially Norström, of Stockholm, Jackson, of Chicago, and Bunge, of Berlin. The method of Brandt and Norström consisted chiefly in supporting the uterus with one finger placed in the vagina and behind the cervix, then making intermittent pressure with the other hand placed externally over the fundus, the uterus being compressed between the two hands. Jackson added gentle manipulations of the abdominal walls, and Bunge extended the manipulations to the abdomen.

458   Pelvic massage concerns the following organs : —

1. The uterus.

2. The uterine appendages— ovaries, Fallopian tubes, broad, round, and other ligaments.

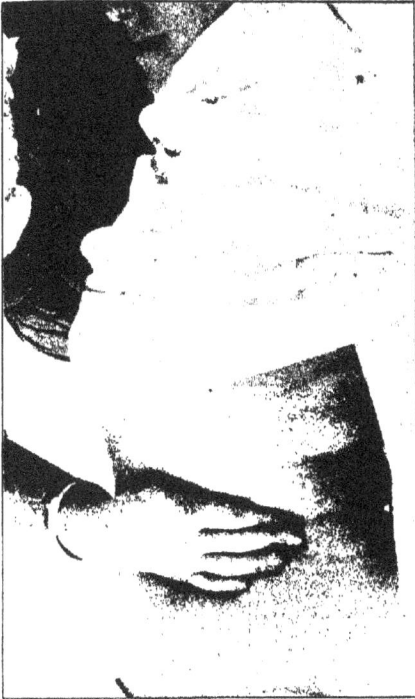

Fig. 96. Replacement of Stomach.

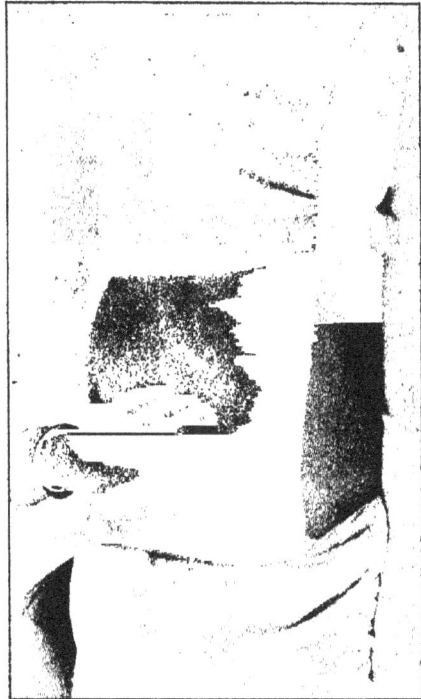

Fig. 98. Massage of Liver.

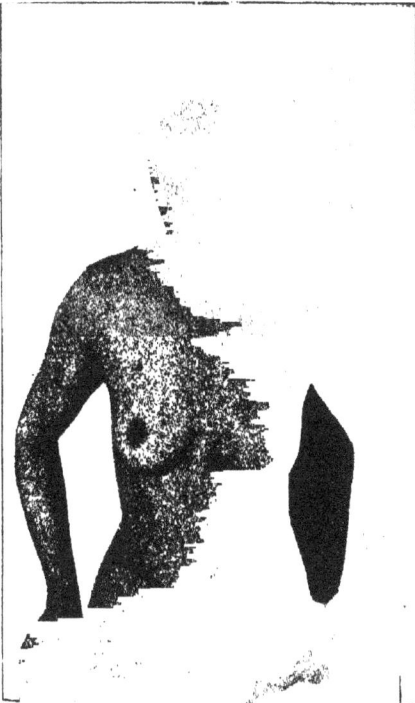

Fig. 95. Prolapse of Colon (Meinert).

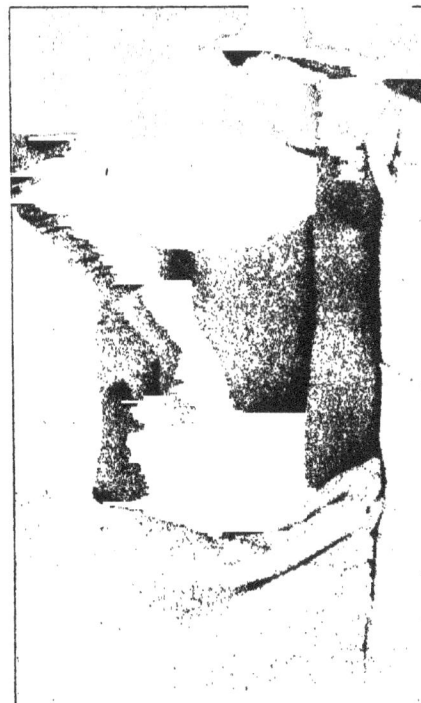

Fig. 97. Replacement of Right Kidney.

PLATE XXXV. — Replacement and Massage of Abdominal Viscera.

3. The vagina, in cases of rectocele and cystocele.

4. The rectum, in cases of prolapsed and relaxed rectum.

5. The prostate in men; sometimes, also, the bladder, in cases in which it is atonic.

6. The coccyx, in cases of coccygodynia, in both sexes.

Pelvic massage should never be undertaken by any person **459** who is not a qualified and experienced physician. The success of this procedure depends, first, upon a correct diagnosis; and secondly, upon special aptitude on the part of the masseur.

It is scarcely possible for a person to become proficient in **460** this special application of massage without personal instruction from some one who has by long experience become skilled in its employment and in the selection of cases to which it is adapted.

It is hoped, however, that the student may obtain an intelligent idea of pelvic massage by the following description of the method which some twelve years' experience has led the writer to adopt:—

Position.—The patient lies upon the back, with the heels well drawn up, the knees separated, the hips slightly elevated, arms by the side, and the head (not the shoulders) supported by a thin pillow.

1. Preliminary movements (**461-467**).
2. Intermittent compression of the uterus (**468-470**).
3. Digital kneading of the uterus (**471**).
4. Lifting movements (**472, 473**).
5. Vibration of the uterus (**474**).
6. Kneading of the appendages (**475**).
7. Digital kneading of the round ligaments (**476**).
8. Stretching of adhesions and kneading of exudates (**477**).
9. Nerve compression (**478**).
10. Massage of the abdominal muscles (**480**).
11. Finishing movements (**481-483**).

1. *Preliminary Procedures.*— The manipulations practiced **461** in pelvic massage are rendered very much more efficient by the application of a few preliminary movements for the purpose of placing the abdominal and pelvic contents in the most favor-

able condition possible in any given case. It should be remembered that in pelvic displacement there will always be found, also, displacement of the abdominal contents. When the uterus falls backward, the folds of intestines which have formerly been behind it, aiding and supporting it in its position, change their position, overlying it above and in front. Replacement of the uterus requires, first of all, a replacement of the intestines; in other words, room must be made for it in its old position before it can be restored to its normal place.

462   It should also be borne in mind that in most cases, displacement of the pelvic viscera is accompanied by a serious disturbance in the positions of the various abdominal organs. There will be found in nearly every case of this sort, displacement of the colon and stomach, and not infrequently displacement of one or both kidneys, and occasionally downward displacement of the liver. It is consequently evident that pelvic massage should always be preceded by such manipulations as will, so far as possible, aid in the restoration of the abdominal viscera to a normal position and condition.

463   The preliminary movements which I have found most effective, are : (1) Deep breathing ; (2) Lifting abdominal contents ; (3) Inspiratory lifting.

464   (1) *Breathing Movements.*—The patient is made to execute a few full breaths (Fig. 73), in which the lower part of the chest and the abdomen are well expanded with inspiration, and drawn in as far as possible with expiration.

465   (2) *Lifting the Viscera.*—After the patient has taken three or four deep breaths, the physician stands at the patient's left, and, with his back to the patient, places the ulnar edge of the two hands, with the fingers extended, just over Poupart's ligament, and parallel with the ligament, the fingers pointing toward the pubes. From this position the hands are moved slightly upward, the edge of the hands being made to sink as deep into the abdomen as possible without severe pain, the arms being slightly rotated at the same time, and the hands drawn upward in such a way as to grasp the contents of the

abdomen and drag them upward.   This movement is repeatedly
executed during the act of inspiration, the patient continuing
to take deep and full breaths, expanding the lower chest and
abdomen as previously described.   See that all displaced
viscera are in perfect position.

Essentially the same movement may be executed with the **466**
patient in the knee-chest position.   The masseur stands with
his back to the patient's head, and reaching around the patient
with one arm, drags the bowels upward during inspiration.

(3) *Inspiratory Lifting* (Fig. 74).— A number of years **467**
ago, when engaged in a series of experimental studies of intra-
abdominal pressure, and while one day administering pelvic
massage to a patient in whom the uterine supports were greatly
relaxed, I observed that with each forcible inhalation the
uterus was lifted upward a distance of half an inch or more.
I noticed also that the patient was breathing almost wholly
with the upper chest.   In order to intensify the effect of the
inspiratory lifting, I caused the patient to exhale completely,
and then to make the movement of inspiration by lifting the
upper chest forcibly while keeping the glottis closed, so that
the air could not enter the lungs.   The effect of this procedure
was very remarkable, the uterus being lifted in an upward direction more than an inch.

2. *Intermittent Compression of the Uterus.*— The prelimi- **468**
nary movements being completed, one, or, when possible, two,
fingers (index and middle fingers) of the left hand are introduced into the vagina and crowded upward behind the cervix,
the uterus being first placed in perfect position, then lifted
upward and forward as far as possible without giving too much
pain.   The extended fingers of the right hand are at the same
time pressed upon the abdominal wall just above the pubes, so
as to impinge upon the fundus, covering as large an area of the
uterus as possible.   Firm, intermittent pressure is then made,
continuing for two or three seconds, with intervals of one or
two seconds, this being repeated six to twelve times.   In this
procedure the pressure of the external hand will fall chiefly
upon the top of the fundus.

In many cases it is difficult to tilt the uterus forward, even after the previous lifting of the abdominal contents which has been described. In the effort to restore the uterus to its normal place, much assistance may be obtained from manipulations with the hand employed externally. The extended palm may be used in lifting the abdominal contents, working from the pubes upward ; or the closed fist may be pressed backward just above Poupart's ligament and the pubes, and crowded upward while the patient makes breathing movements. By this means the way may be cleared so that the tips of the fingers can finally be gotten down behind the uterus, even in cases of retroversion.

Sometimes the cervix must be grasped between the two internal fingers and used as a lever to pry the fundus up, when the organ has sufficient firmness to admit of such a procedure. It is often necessary to work the fingers of the external hand down upon one side at the same time that the internal fingers are crowded up as high as possible. In this way a fundus lying in the hollow of the sacrum may be slid up over the promontory of the sacrum, when the fingers of the external hand, working down beneath it, will quickly bring it into position.

469 When the vaginal orifice is too small to admit of two fingers, a useful application of massage may be made by the aid of one finger introduced into the vagina, or even a single finger operating through the rectum. A single finger, however, has less perfect control of the uterus, and in cases of extreme backward displacement it is often impossible to completely replace the uterus by means of one finger only working internally. A better method, in cases in which the vagina will admit of but one finger, is to introduce the forefinger into the vagina and the middle finger into the rectum. The remaining fingers of the hand should not be flexed, but extended and separated from the middle finger, and slid over the coccyx. A special advantage in the last-named method is that it facilitates palpation of the ovaries and tubes, the movements of the middle finger not being restricted by the vaginal walls.

Without allowing the uterus to drop down in the pelvis, **470** the two fingers of the left hand are now transferred to the front of the cervix, the uterus being supported by the external hand, the fingers of which are made to pass down deep behind the fundus. The intermittent pressure previously described is now renewed, the uterus being pressed from before backward. This procedure should be repeated six to twelve times.

These procedures must be executed with the greatest care to avoid giving the patient pain, thereby exciting contraction of the abdominal muscles, which necessarily interferes with the manipulation.

3. *Digital Kneading of the Uterus.*—The fingers of the left **471** hand being returned to the first position behind the cervix, thus supporting the organ, the fingers of the right hand execute a circular digital kneading movement, beginning at the top of the fundus, and enlarging the circle until the fingers are made to press down the sides of the uterus and all about it. A slight change in the direction of the pressure made by the fingers of the left hand enables them to antagonize constantly the movements of the right hand, so that the uterus may be by this means very thoroughly manipulated in nearly all cases, and except in patients who are very fleshy. This procedure is continued from one to five minutes.

4. *Lifting Movements.*—The preceding manipulations will **472** have completely freed the uterus from the overlying intestines, so that the top of the fundus will be lying in immediate contact with the peritoneal surface of the anterior wall of the abdomen. By the combined action of the internal and external hands, the uterus can now be freely lifted forward so that its form may be easily outlined by the fingers of the right hand. The action should be intermittent.

After lifting it forward as far as possible without inconven- **473** iencing the patient, the uterus is released, and allowed to drop down, then again lifted, the action being repeated six to twelve times, at intervals of two to three seconds, the uterus being held forward for a like period. The purpose of the lifting is to bring the blood vessels under tension, thus emptying the venous sinuses, which are filled with fresh blood as the uterus returns to its former position.

474   5. *Vibration of the Uterus.*—While supporting the organ with the fingers of the left hand behind the cervix, the thumb or one or more fingers of the right hand, is applied to the top of the uterus, and fine vibratory movements are communicated to it. This is a powerful means of stimulating the uterine circulation.

475   6. *Digital Kneading of the Appendages.*—In pelvic massage the manipulations should not be confined to the uterus alone. The ovaries, tubes, and the broad and round ligaments may be masséed thus: After lifting the uterus well forward, freeing it from the overlying intestines, the fingers of the left hand are directed toward an ovary. Starting as low down as possible, firm pressure is made in an upward direction, while the fingers of the external hand are made to coöperate in an effort to grasp beneath the ovary and tube and lift them forward. At the same time, gentle digital kneading movements are executed, the pressure of the external (right) hand being directed toward the fingers placed internally.

476   7. *Digital Kneading of the Round Ligaments.*—The fingers in the vagina should be directed toward the inguinal canal while digital massage is executed by the fingers of the right hand traveling in a curved line from the external ring along the side of Poupart's ligament and toward the fundus. The internal fingers will, to some extent, follow the movements of the right hand, so as to compress the tissues between the fingers of the two hands.

477   8. *Stretching of Adhesions and Kneading of Exudates.*—When adhesions and exudates are present, firm pressure should be made directly upon the bands of adhesion or the masses of exudate with the tips of the fingers which operate internally, counter-pressure being made externally ; and, so far as possible, the morbid parts should be grasped between the fingers of the two hands, and thus subjected to digital massage. Adhesions are also stretched by the lifting movements of the uterus previously described.

9. *Nerve Compression.*—The sacral plexus of the spinal **478** nerves and several of the lowermost pairs of ganglia of the sympathetic are accessible to digital pressure through the vagina; and in appropriate cases these, as well as other nerve structures, may be stimulated by gentle compression in connection with other procedures. One of the largest nerve masses accessible to compression through the vagina is the hypogastric plexus, which is located on the anterior surface of the sacrum, just below the promontory. A row of four or five sympathetic ganglia lies on either side of the median line just over the junction of the sacrum and the ilium, the anterior aspect of the sacro-iliac synchondrosis. A single ganglion (*coccygeal ganglion*, or *ganglion impar*) lies in front of the coccyx. Pressure made upon these points stimulates the ganglia and their branches, and by this means excites the circulation in the pelvic vessels.

Nerve compression in this region, as in other parts of the body, must be applied with very great discretion. This procedure should never be employed in cases in which inflammation, active congestion, or excessive hyperæsthesia exists. It is only appropriate in cases of passive congestion, atony, subinvolution, and general relaxation of the parts.

It is generally well to alternate some of the above-described **479** procedures, especially the lifting and kneading movements, instead of adhering closely to the order in which they have been given for the purpose of precise description.

Upward deep kneading movements executed with the closed fist may be advantageously alternated with the other movements mentioned.

10. *Massage of the Abdominal Muscles.*—After the internal **480** manipulations, the muscles of the lower abdomen and inner thighs should be gently masséed. The procedures most useful are the following, employed in the order named: Tapping, hacking, spatting, centripetal friction, and finally, stroking.

11. Finishing movements : —

481   (1) Knees separating, breathing. The patient should inspire while separating the knees, and expire while closing them. The vigor of the exercise may be increased by making a slight resistance to the movements of both adduction and abduction (Fig. 71). The movements should be made at the rate of ten to twelve per minute.

482   (2) Hips raising (Fig. 82), breathing in as the hips rise, and breathing out as they sink. This movement should be repeated from four to eight times. The movements of knees separating, hips raising, and breathing may be executed simultaneously.

483   (3) The treatment should be concluded by having the patient turn upon the face, and administering percussion — tapping, hacking, spatting, beating, and clapping over the sacrum and fleshy portions of the hips.

484   The following points should be carefully observed in the administration of pelvic massage : —

1. Never administer pelvic massage to erotic patients, nor in cases of vaginismus, acute pyosalpinx, pelvic abscess, growing tumors of the uterus or ovaries, rectal ulcer, acute vaginitis, irritable urethra, or inflammation of Skene's glands, until after these conditions have been removed. The best results are obtained in cases of subinvolution of the uterus, relaxed ligaments, recent exudates, and passive congestions with little sensitiveness. Kesch recommends that uterine massage should be applied especially during menstruation, but does not give what seem to the writer to be valid reasons for the recommendation. My opinion is very positive that massage should be discontinued during this period.

2. Before treatment, have the patient thoroughly empty the bladder and bowels, employing an enema, if necessary, or a coloclyster (large enema in right Sims's or in knee-chest position). A hot vaginal douche should also be administered.

3. No movements should be made with the hand used internally except with the ends of the fingers.

4. The force employed should generally be sufficient to produce slight pain.

5. In cases of flexion, the flexion should, if possible, be straightened during the manipulation. In all cases of displacement, the uterus must be restored to proper position.

6. Care must be taken to have the patient breathe deeply and regularly during treatment.

Massage of the Prostate.— In cases of enlarged prostate due to thickening from inflammation, especially in recent cases, much can be accomplished by massage properly administered. Massage of the prostate should be preceded by abdominal massage, and followed by inspiratory lifting, deep breathing, and percussing the sacrum (**313-317**). **485**

1. Introduce one, or better two, fingers, well oiled, into the rectum, making firm pressure against the prostate, but taking care not to press so hard as to bruise the membranous urethra. With the right hand, make pressure just above the pubes. After pressing the parts for two or three seconds, allow a rest for an equal period, repeating the pressure from six to twelve times.

2. Make gentle friction over the prostate in a downward direction for the purpose of pressing out of the ducts the stagnant secretions.

3. Make gentle friction over the prostate by pressure of the fingers, moving from below upward, covering the posterior surface of the organ, to empty the blood-vessels.

Care should be taken to have the patient empty the bowels and bladder thoroughly before the treatment is applied. Sometimes the patient is unable to completely empty the bladder ; in such cases a catheter should be passed.

Massage of the Coccyx.— This procedure is useful in cases of coccygodynia accompanied by painful points adjacent to the coccyx or its ligaments. The bowels and bladder should be first emptied, as in all forms of pelvic massage. Proceed as follows ; — **486**

1. With the patient in the right Sims's position, pass one finger, or better two fingers, of the left hand into the rectum, applying them to the anterior surface of the coccyx. With the fingers of the other hand applied externally, make a suitable degree of pressure, and knead the affected parts between the fingers, giving special attention to points of induration or pain. In cases in which the parts are extremely tender, begin the movements at a little distance from the most painful points, gradually encroaching upon the more sensitive tissues. The manipulation may be continued for three to ten minutes.

2. Apply to the sacrum, tapping (**313**) and hacking (**316**) movements; to the more fleshy parts, clapping (**315**), spatting (**314**), and beating (**317**).

3. Employ deep vibration, placing the hand over the lower end of the spine (**302**).

4. Apply stroking with the palm of the hand from the coccyx upward, outward, and downward along the inner surfaces of the thighs.

487   **Massage of the Rectum.**—This procedure is useful in cases in which the sphincter muscle is relaxed, and applicable to many cases in which the muscle has been over-stretched by officious and unnecessary dilatations applied by so-called "orificial surgeons." The most important movements are the following:—

1. Percussion with the finger tips, tapping (**313**).

2. Fulling (**244**) about the verge of the anus, care being taken to avoid bruising the parts, which should be well lubricated. The manipulations should be very delicate, the tissues being carefully picked up with the ends of the fingers and thumbs.

3. Thumb kneading of the anus and the tissues immediately adjacent, care being taken to roll the parts in when they are everted.

4. Hacking (**316**).

5. Beating (**317**).

6. Pressure (**154**) and vibration (**302**). Firm pressure with the palmar surface of the fingers or with the closed fist in an upward direction, accompanied by a vibratory movement.

7. Percussion of the sacrum and hips, as in massage of the prostate and coccyx (**485, 486**).

8. Inspiratory lifting (**467**).

Massage of the rectum should be preceded by abdominal massage. This procedure, as well as the following, is seldom required.

Massage of the Vagina.—This procedure is useful in **488** cases of rectocele, cystocele, and relaxed vagina, and is applicable to cases in which for any reason a suitable surgical operation cannot be performed. It is also valuable in cases of rigidity of the perineum, as a preparation for confinement, for which it may be employed daily during the last six or eight weeks of pregnancy. It should be resorted to in all cases of pregnancy in which there has previously been an operation for repair of the perineum. Proceed as follows:—

1. Lifting abdominal contents (**465**).

2. Lifting uterus and appendages (**472**), two fingers of the left hand being placed internally, the other hand coöperating externally, as in massage of the uterus.

3. With patient in knee-chest position, lift the bowels (**466**).

4. With knee-chest or Sims's position, fingers placed upon thighs, tips of thumbs at the mouth of the vagina, roll the tissues in as much as possible, lift upward, and manipulate the perineum with the thumbs.

5. With the index finger of the left hand in the rectum and the thumb in the vagina, compress and knead the posterior wall of the vagina.

6. With the closed fist firmly placed upon the perineum, make strong vibratory movements (**302**).

7. Apply percussion to the sacrum and the buttocks (**483**).

8. With patient lying upon the back, the heels well drawn up, raising of hips and full breathing (**482**).

9. Knees separating and breathing, with resistance (**481**),
10. Inspiratory lifting (**467**).

489   **Massage of the Face.**—This procedure is useful for developing the muscles of the fleshy portion of the face, improving the circulation (hence the complexion), removing wrinkles, especially about the eyes and the corners of the mouth, and also relieving facial neuralgia and muscular twitching.

490   For persons with fleshy faces, about all that can be done by general facial massage is to knead the tissues by compressing them with the thumb and fingers against the underlying bony surfaces, working outward from the mouth, the nasal openings, and the eyes. Care should be taken to work toward the points at which the blood vessels emerge.

491   In persons with thinner faces, the tissues of the cheek may be grasped between the thumb and finger. When indurations are present, the protected finger may be introduced into the mouth and placed against the cheek, while massage is applied with the tip of the thumb or with the fingers of the other hand. The little finger, covered with soft cotton, may be introduced into the nose and ears, although this procedure is very seldom required. Make use of the following manipulations:—

492   1. Digital kneading, working outward from the eyes, nose, and mouth, at which points many muscles find their insertion.

2. Petrissage, or grasping-kneading of the muscles of the face.

3. Massage of the orbit (Fig. 101), care being taken to avoid the eyeballs. Place one thumb upon the lower lid and the other just beneath the eyebrow, within the margin of the orbit. Make traction outward, drawing upon the inner corner of the eye; then change the position of the thumbs so as to massér all the muscles about the eye. Massage about the eye improves both the nerve and the muscular tone of the eye, and in this way often relieves muscular asthenopia, frequently due to general weakening of the eye, which renders annoying or injurious slight muscular inequalities which are not noticeable

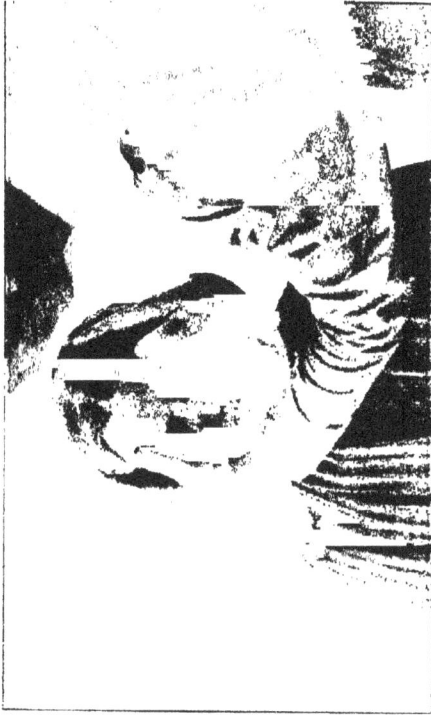

Fig. 100. Massage of Face for Removal of Wrinkles.

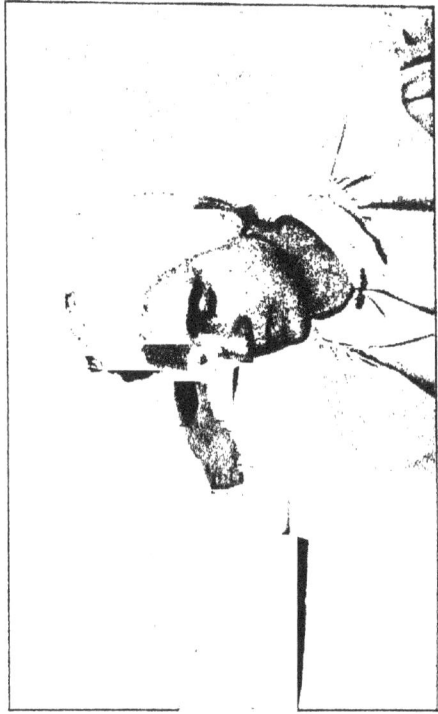

Fig. 102. Massage of Eye.

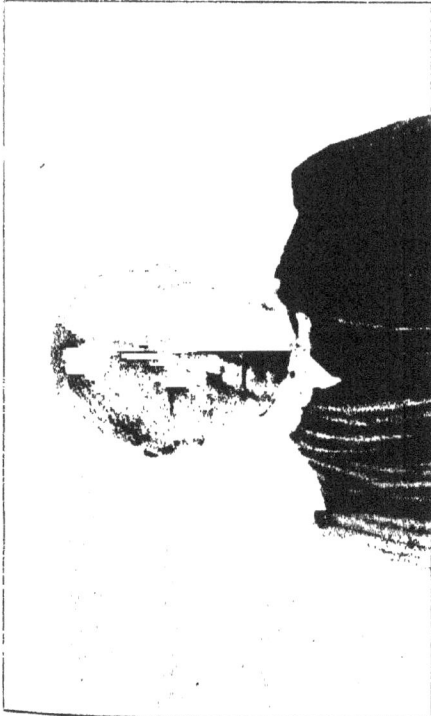

Fig. 99. Wrinkled Face before Massage.

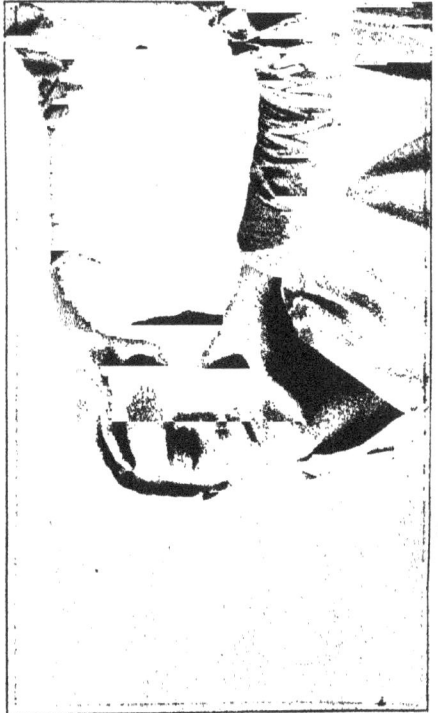

Fig. 101. Massage of Orbit.

PLATE XXXVI. — Massage of the Face.

when the muscles are well developed. The attention of those neurologists and oculists who think it necessary to operate upon every case of muscular asthenopia is especially called to this statement. The habit of rubbing the eye for relief, which prevails almost universally among persons thus suffering, is a strong suggestion of the utility of massage administered systematically and in a skillful manner.

Special attention should be given to the nose, working from **493** the root of the nose downward and outward. Relief is often afforded in cases of nasal obstruction from catarrh by facial massage, which is due to the fact that the lymphatics of the face arise from the mucous membrane of the nose.

Massage for Wrinkles.— Facial massage may be made **494** useful in removing wrinkles (Figs. 99 and 100), which as often indicate unhealthy tissues as advancing age or a wearisome existence. Wrinkles are best relieved by making traction upon the skin in a direction at right angles with the wrinkles, the wrinkled part being thoroughly manipulated to restore the natural flexibility of the skin, which has been lost. The patient must also be taught how to smooth out the wrinkles by cultivating a suitable facial expression. For example, the vertical wrinkles of discontent or despondency may be made to disappear by smiling, which wrinkles the face in an opposite way.

In friction of the face, special care should be taken to avoid **495** making so great pressure as to cause irritation of the skin.

Compression of the nerve trunks which supply the face is **496** a valuable procedure in many cases. The chief points to which pressure should be applied are shown in Fig. 32.

The different useful procedures in general facial massage **497** may be applied in the following order : —

1. Digital kneading of the cheeks, nose, and orbit.

2. Petrissage.

3. Stroking, localized as may be indicated when wrinkles are present.

4. Ear rolling (**503** [3]).

5. Stroking along the inferior border of the lower jaw.

6. Friction of the neck (**433, 435**).

498 **Massage of the Eye** (Fig. 102).—Massage of the eye was first suggested by Donders. The writer first saw it applied by Landolt, of Paris. It has been found to be useful in ulceration and cloudiness of the cornea, hypopyon, and in the early stage of glaucoma. Massage of the eye increases the vascularity of the eye, and encourages drainage.

499 Reibmayr noted that when masseing one eye, the other eye became, during the first minute, dilated; second minute, contracted; while in the third minute, the pupil of the eye masséed became smaller than the other, showing that massage of the eye, through reflex action, affects the controlling nerve centers as well as the eye itself.

500 Massage of the eye must be applied with very great delicacy of touch. Proceed as follows: Have the patient close his eye; place the fingers of the hand upon the temple a short distance from the orbit, and the tip of the thumb upon the upper lid of the closed eye. Make gentle rotary movements, gradually increasing the pressure, but taking care that it be not so great as to cause pain. Patients whose eyesight is impaired often remark that they are able to see better after the application.

501 **Massage of the Ear** (Fig. 103).—This procedure is of great value in middle-ear disease, catarrhal disease of the Eustachian tubes, in chronic disease of the middle ear unaccompanied by suppuration, and in cases of perforated membrana tympani. It may also prove useful in cases of tinnitus aurium.

502 Politzer recommends derivative massage as a means of relieving the pain of otitis media and of furuncles. In case of acute inflammation, the manipulations should be confined to the tissues about the ear, avoiding the ear itself.

503 The following procedures are the most effective:—

1. Digital kneading, friction, and stroking about the ear,—in front, behind, and beneath. This procedure is especially useful as a derivative measure.

2. Intermittent pressure upon the tragus in such a manner as to close the external meatus. The pressure should be both applied and withdrawn suddenly, but without too great force. The rate should be sixty to one hundred per minute. Its purpose is to exercise the structures of the middle ear.

3. Ear rolling (Fig. 103), with the fleshy portion of the thumb applied to the ear in such a manner as to cause it to fit into the external ear, and close the orifice ; the right hand to the left ear of the patient, and the left hand to the right ear. By means of a rolling movement, the ear will be stretched in different directions, and the meatus may be opened and closed in such a manner as to secure alternate compression and rarefaction of the air in the external auditory canal, thus imparting movement to the membrana tympani and to the ossicles connected with it. This measure may often replace the mechanical means ordinarily used for treating the middle ear.

4. Stroking of the Eustachian tube, by pressing one or two fingers into the furrow behind the maxillary bone, starting close to the ear, and following the groove down beneath the jaw. By pressure thus applied to the Eustachian tube, it may be emptied of obstructing mucus ; and when in a state of chronic inflammation, useful reparative processes are set up. An itching in the throat from which many patients complain is frequently due to an irritation at the orifices of the Eustachian tubes, which may be readily relieved by this means.

Massage of the Larynx (Fig. 104).— This measure is **504** especially valuable in chronic disease of the larynx, particularly in cases in which the vocal cords are relaxed, or in which there is weakness of voice from insufficient development of the laryngeal muscles. The object aimed at in massage of the larynx is to relieve congestion, if it exists ; to improve the blood and lymph circulations, stimulate nutrition, and thus strengthen the muscles and the nerve supply of the part.

The following are the most useful procedures : — **505**

1. Derivative massage of the neck (**433, 435**).

2. Fulling (**244**) of the skin overlying the larynx.

3. Digital kneading (**268**), in which the fingers are worked into all the irregularities of the larynx, and between it and the surrounding tissues.

4. Lifting, in which the larynx is seized between the thumb and finger just below the *pomum Adami*, and crowded upward. The vigor of this procedure may be increased by holding the larynx up while the patient swallows.

5. Tapping (**313**).

6. Deep vibration (seize larynx and vibrate) (**302**).

Friction strokes are intermingled with the other measures mentioned.

506 **Massage of the Heart.**— The position of the heart would seem to render it inaccessible to the application of massage ; but Oertel, in 1889, contributed to the literature of massage, a paper upon "Massage of the Heart," in which he claims to have obtained great advantage from the use of massage in such a manner as to influence the heart directly. He employs massage of the heart especially in connection with his system of treatment by mountain climbing, and considers it indicated in the following conditions : —

1. When the heart muscle is weak, either as the result of anæmia, impaired nutrition, or obesity.

2. When the arteries are imperfectly filled, resulting in passive or venous congestion.

3. In cases in which there is mechanical obstruction in the circulation, resulting from valvular lesions, diminution of the respiratory field, pressure of tumors, or anything which increases the work of the heart.

4. In connection with gymnastics for strengthening the heart.

507 Massage of the heart is contra-indicated —

1. In acute or recurring endocarditis or pericarditis.

2. In myocarditis.

3. In sclerosis of the coronary arteries and in general arterio-sclerosis.

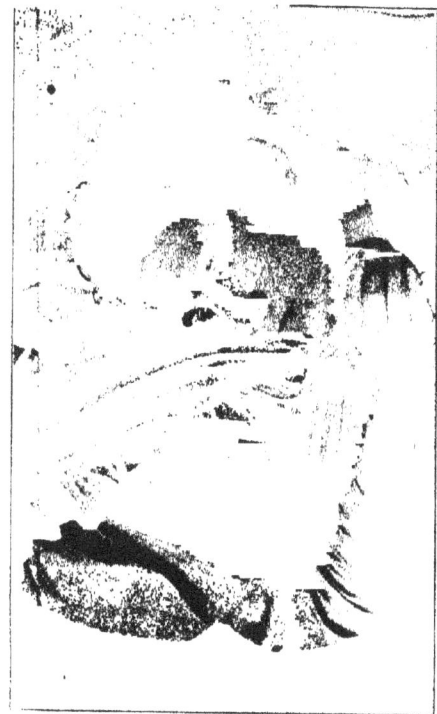

Fig. 104. Massage of Larynx.

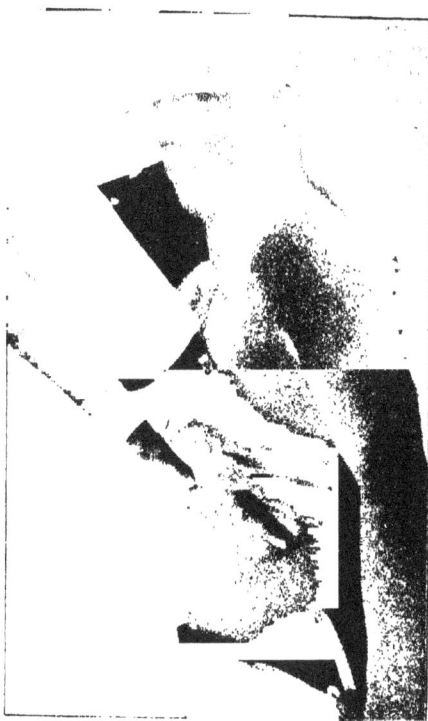

Fig. 106. Massage of Heart   finishing position

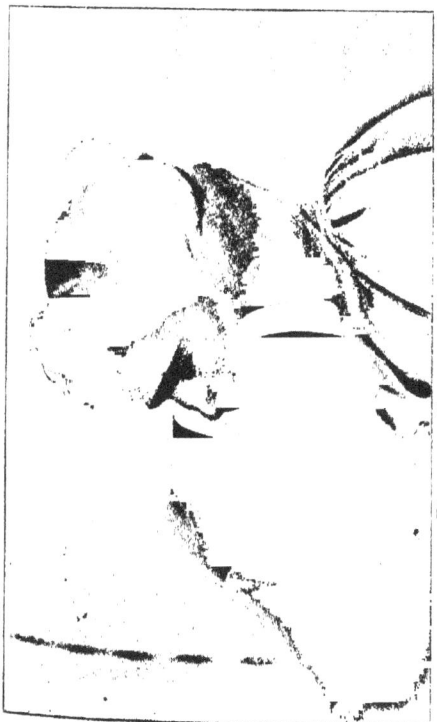

Fig. 103. Massage of Ears.

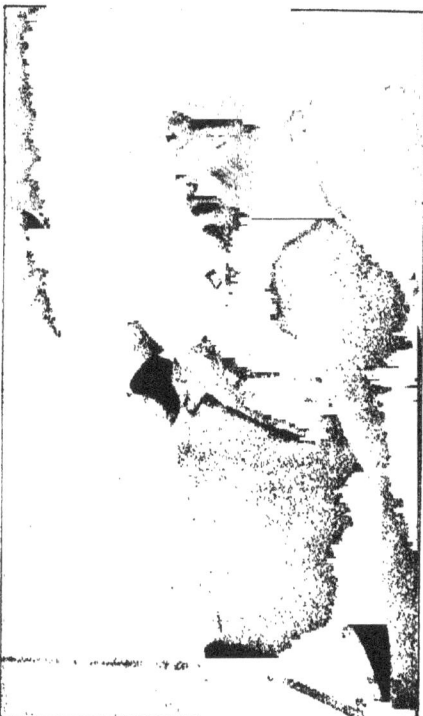

Fig. 105. Massage of Heart — beginning position.

PLATE XXXVII.—Special Applications of Massage.

Massage of the heart is applied during expiration only, and **508** in the following manner : With the patient reclining, the head supported upon a pillow, the masseur stands at his head, and, bending over the patient, applies his hands to the sides of the chest at its extreme upper part, the fingers touching the chest at the axilla, while the thumbs are directed toward the sternum (Fig. 105). The patient should be instructed to breathe deeply, slowly, and regularly. At the end of inspiration, and just as the act of expiration begins, pressure should be made with the hands, which at the same time should move gradually downward and forward until the thumbs fall upon the xiphoid cartilage (Fig. 106). The effort should be made to narrow the chest laterally, and at the same time to compress it antero-posteriorly. It is especially important to prevent increase in the antero-posterior diameter of the chest during expiration. The application of pressure should be gradual, increasing as expiration proceeds and as the hands glide downward. The greatest force should be applied between the fifth and eighth ribs, the maximum of pressure falling over the latter.

Massage of the heart is beneficial — **509**

1. In completing the act of expiration.

2. Through direct pressure made upon the heart, whereby its nutrition is favorably influenced, as in massage of other muscles.

Massage in Scoliosis.—Apply massage (**426**) only after **510** first putting the patient into a correct position. The following procedures are helpful in accomplishing this : In mild cases, patient lying on face, arms stretched upward ; in cases in which the patient has lost the power to correct the deformity by voluntary effort, side lying on quarter circle, concave side uppermost. Massage may also be applied with the patient suspended by head and shoulders, or hanging by the arms.

Untwisting the Patient.—The patient, sitting, passes the **511** arm of the high side in front, with the hand on the opposite

10

shoulder; while the hand of the low side is passed behind, and rests upon the back. Useful in cases of rotation.

512 Three degrees of deformity may be described : —

1. Deformity reducible by the patient's unaided, voluntary efforts.

2. Deformity readily reducible by manual assistance or such mechanical assistance as the patient can apply.

3. Deformity irreducible by manual assistance, and not easily reducible by mechanical aid.

513 The first class is curable ; the second class may be curable, and can certainly be benefited ; the third class is incurable, but may possibly be somewhat improved, and will require the permanent use of mechanical support.

514 *Method of Testing the Patient's Ability to Correct Deformity without Assistance.* —

1. Give usual directions for correct standing **(575)** (Figs. 108, 109, and 110).

2. Rest-standing position (hands at back of neck, arms in line).

3. Standing, arms stretched upward.

4. Rest-close-standing (heels and toes together).

515 *Exercises.* — The following exercises are valuable for patients of this class, to be used in connection with massage : —

1. The patient sitting untwisted **(511)**, leans forward, then raises the body backward against resistance applied to the head.

2. The patient sitting untwisted, operates a pulley weight with each hand.

3. Rowing, sitting on an inclined plane, high side of body on high side of seat.

4. Sitting on an inclined seat, untwisted, use pulley weights in opposite directions, high side pulling down, low side pulling up ; high side pulling from behind, low side from in front ; both sides simultaneously pulling from opposite sides toward the body.

5. Hanging from swinging rings or "ladder-wall," the low side grasping higher than the high side.

Method of Correcting Curvature by Manual Assistance. — **516**

1. For posterior curvature, patient should bend forward at hips, holding hips back. As the patient rises, press upon the convexity of the curve; and tell him to raise the chest, and draw the head back and the chin in.

2. Patient should take downward-bend position; one side of back higher than the other indicates rotation (see accompanying cut). Masseur, placing one hand upon highest part, and having the patient rise, should at the same time make gentle resistance.

3. Patient s h o u l d stand facing the table, thighs t o u c h i n g the table, and bend forward at the hips; head erect, chin well d r a w n in. Masseur should place his hands upon the con- vexity of the curve, and have the patient raise the trunk backward.

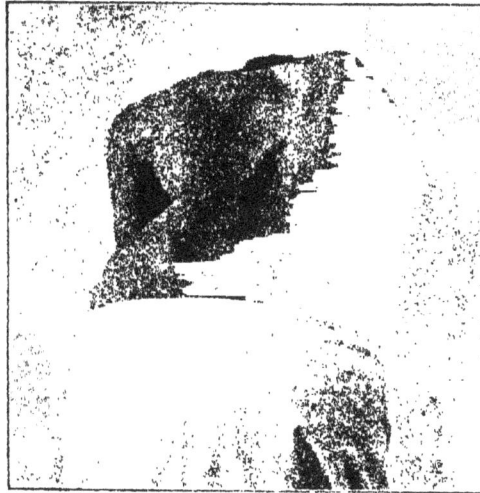

SPINAL CURVATURE WITH ROTATION.

4. Patient standing, the masseur should place one hand on the convexity in front, the other on the convexity behind, and stroke with firm press- ure from before backward. If necessary, repeat with the patient in rest-standing position, or rest-forward-bend standing. *

In applying massage to the back in scoliosis, particular at- **517** tention should be given to percussion, especially of the concave side. Use all the different kinds of percussion movements. Make pressure upon the prominent surfaces. Endeavor to work the spines into position by pressure and manipulation with the thumbs. A daily hot and cold douche or sponging of the back is of great importance in these cases, as a means of stimulating the nutrition of the tissues.

---

* These and other gymnastic positions are fully explained in another work by the author, now nearly ready for publication.

518 **Massage of the Joints.**— There is no single class of cases in which the benefits derived from massage are more evident than in those of chronic joint disease or of recent injury to the joint; at the same time there is no one class of cases in which large discretion and experience are of greater importance. Excessive manipulation of an irritable joint or of a joint the ligaments of which have recently been injured, as in case of a bad sprain, may do almost irreparable injury, and will certainly subject the patient to a great degree of unnecessary suffering, and may discourage him altogether, thus depriving him of the great benefits to be derived from massage skillfully administered. It may be laid down as a principle, that massage of the joints should never be applied in such a manner as to produce any considerable degree of pain. Slight pain is often produced by the first manipulations, especially in cases in which there has been much loss of motion, but the pain thus induced should be of a transient character, subsiding within a short time after the manipulation. When the pain increases for some days afterward, the manipulation has been applied in a violent or bungling manner, or the application should have been derivative rather than made directly to the joint.

519 A matter which requires the most careful discrimination is that of determining when manipulations should be applied directly to the joint, and when above or below it. Briefly, the best advice upon this point is this: When a joint is very sensitive, derivative massage only should be employed for a week or ten days at the beginning, the manipulations being gradually brought nearer the joint from day to day.

520 A careful examination of the tissues in a case of chronic rheumatism of a joint will show rheumatic nodules lying along the course of the lymphatics above the joint. In a fleshy person it is not always easy to find these, but a delicate touch will generally discover them. The work should begin upon the tissues above the joint for the purpose of opening up these obstructed channels, and thus acting indirectly upon the lymphatics and blood vessels of the joint.

The derivative effects may be greatly increased by giving **521** special attention to the healthy joint next above the affected joint, in the employment of strong traction, pressure, and other joint movements. The lymph and blood channels are largest in the vicinity of the joints, and by acting upon these by means of joint movements, pressure, and manipulations, the vessels of the joint below may be drained, especially after the lymph channels connecting the two have been opened up.

It must not be forgotten that in cases of chronic joint disease **522** the muscles and other tissues about the joint are affected, as well as the joint itself. This is especially true of chronic rheumatism, and is evidenced by muscular atrophy, induration, or fatty degeneration, one or the other of which conditions is nearly always present in chronic joint disease.

It is useful to know that certain muscles or muscular groups **523** suffer more than others in connection with joint disease. For example, when the knee is involved, the *quadriceps* atrophies; in hip joint cases, the *glutei* muscles are chiefly affected; in cases of the elbow, the *biceps* and the *brachialis anticus;* in cases of the shoulder, the *deltoid* and *supra-* and *infra-spinatus.* **524**

In *derivative massage* (**238**), fulling, friction, and deep kneading are most effective. In the manipulation of a joint, begin with light friction and pressure. If these applications are tolerated, add digital massage, working between the ligaments, and following all the irregularities of the ends of the bones and the articulating surfaces so far as accessible. Later, add percussion, first tapping, afterward hacking.

Joint movements should be employed from as early a **525** period as possible in cases of joint disease, so as to prevent the limitation of movement, or to restore motion which has been lost. The application must at first be very gentle indeed, and should not be carried to such an extent as to produce continued pain. The derivative manipulations which are first employed should be continued in connection with applications to the joint, since the effect of kneading a joint is to increase the circulation through it; while the effect of derivative massage is not to carry the blood through the joint, but rather around it, thus relieving excessive local congestion, or hyperæmia, by diverting the blood into other channels.

526   By the combination of local and derivative massage applied in connection with compression of the joints and gentle joint movements (**342**), the vital activity of the part may be greatly increased.   In cases of extremely painful joints in which heat and congestion are marked symptoms, derivative massage may be employed upon the soft parts both above and below, and joint movements should be applied to the joint above, care being taken to avoid motion of the affected joints.

527   Centripetal friction applied to the tissues and next joint above, relieves painful joints by increasing the surface circulation, and so diverting the blood from the joint itself.   Downward stroking below the joint also affords relief by lessening the supply of blood to the joint.

528   The cautions which have been given respecting the manipulation of affected joints, apply, of course, only to those in which the disease is active, or to painful or congested joints. In many old cases of joint disease there is a decreased vascularity and also a morbid and decreased secretion, as is evidenced by a grating, snapping noise, and other sounds induced by motion of the joint.   When this condition exists, the massage should be applied directly to the joint itself.   Even though it should have the effect to slightly increase the pain at first, the ultimate result will be improved nutrition of the joint, and the restoration of the normal secretion.   I have seen some most remarkable results in cases in which improvement would certainly have been regarded as most improbable.

529   In rheumatic gout and in old cases of rheumatism, very persevering efforts are required.   The maximum amount of benefit to be derived from massage is not always obtainable except by its continuous employment for several months, and

sometimes even two or three years. In one case under the writer's care,— a lady who had suffered from rheumatic gout for many years,— the limbs were flexed to nearly a right angle, and the patient had despaired of again standing upright ; but at the end of two years she was able to walk erect without the aid of a cane.

In cases of chronic rheumatism and rheumatic gout, it **530** must be remembered that the patient is suffering from a diathesis, and that the disease is not a purely local malady ; consequently, general massage, hydrotherapy, proper regimen, and other measures must be combined with the local treatment.

It is of great advantage also, to employ local applications **531** of electricity as well as hydrotherapeutic measures, in these cases. The irritation occasioned by manipulations is usually promptly relieved by a hot fomentation, followed by a heating compress, which should be applied thus : Wring a linen towel out of water as cold as can be obtained. If the patient is feeble, it should be wrung dry ; in a more vigorous person, a larger amount of water may be retained. The towel is wrapped tightly about the joint, and is then covered with oiled muslin, and closely wrapped with several folds of flannel, which should be applied in such a manner as to prevent any air from reaching the moist surface. It is generally well to change these compresses three or four times a day. When there is considerable heat in the joint, they may be changed more frequently with advantage.

In old cases in which the tissues are much relaxed, or in **532** which secretion is deficient, the hot and cold douche is the most effective means of stimulating the vital activities of the joint. Massage and hydrotherapy combined are twice as beneficial in the treatment of chronic joint troubles as either used alone. Together they are capable of effecting a cure in every case in which a cure is possible.

Massage for Sprains.— The treatment of sprained joints **533** by massage is by no means a recent idea. Massage has been thus employed in Germany for more than thirty years, and was

used in England half a century ago ; but the method is so dia-
metrically opposed to that in common use by the profession,
that it has been but slowly adopted. It also requires special
skill, while the employment of the old method of immobilization is compatible with any degree of ignorance and stupidity.

The value of this method is now so well established that it
is not necessary to offer statistics in support of it. Any physician who has once had the satisfaction of seeing the victim of
a severe sprain walking about without inconvenience at the
end of a week or ten days, who under the old regimé would
have been crippled for months, and possibly have suffered the
loss of a limb, will require no further argument to convince
him of the efficacy of this mode of treatment. Much skill and
experience are needed, however, to enable a masseur to accomplish a rapid cure. The following is the method : —

534   Apply massage as soon after the injury as possible, beginning with derivative manipulations of the soft parts above the
affected joint and of the joint next above it. Centripetal friction, with quite firm pressure, applied very carefully, may be
advantageously employed upon the joint itself from the very
first, but other manipulations of the joint itself should be de-
ferred for a day or two. The derivative manipulations should
gradually approach the joint from above, until by the second or
third day the joint itself is reached.

535   Careful joint movements should be executed after the
second day, pains being taken not to carry flexion or extension
so far as to produce the feeling of resistance, as this will bring
a strain upon the bruised or lacerated ligaments or pressure
upon the injured articulating surface. If there is much swelling, the external tissues are probably the chief seat of injury.
Both external and internal parts may be injured.

536   At first, when the manipulations are very light in character, the massage should be applied twice daily ; later, when
more vigorous measures of treatment are employed, once a
day is sufficient. After each manipulation, apply a tight bandage, taking care to begin the bandage at the toes. If there is

much pain, apply a hot pack, followed by a cool compress, for an hour; or place the feet in hot water, and gradually increase the temperature until it is as hot as can be borne. Continue bath for fifteen minutes. This is an excellent means for relieving local congestion. It may be used once or twice a day, the bandage being applied immediately after the bath.

I think it very advantageous to employ these hydrotherapeu- **537** tic measures in connection with massage. Cold water has been much recommended in the treatment of sprains, and has certainly been highly successful, although less rapidly curative than massage. By the combination suggested, most rapid results may be obtained, and the patient may be saved from great and prolonged suffering.

Muscular Rheumatism.— In muscular rheumatism, **538** pain is occasioned by use of the affected muscles. There is often also considerable loss of both motion and elasticity in the muscle. Frequently, rheumatic nodules will be found along the course of the lymphatics. Muscular rheumatism may exist alone or in connection with a like affection of the joints, as in the last-named disease the rheumatic process not infrequently extends from the joint to adjacent muscles.

Daily manipulation is essential in the treatment of muscular **539** rheumatism. The most important procedures are friction, deep kneading, hacking, rolling, wringing, chucking, stretching, and such resistive movements as will act upon the affected muscles, together with movements of the joint acted upon by them.

Fomentations and heating compresses are of special value **540** in these cases. Rheumatism of the muscles, as well as of the joints, is connected with a systemic condition, or diathesis, which must also receive attention. Not infrequently — in the majority of cases, in fact — there is to be found dilatation of the stomach; and complete relief will only be obtained by a combination of local measures with such general treatment as will correct the constitutional condition, which includes careful adaptation of the diet to the state of the digestive organs, and an antiseptic regimen. Local treatment of the stomach is essential in many cases, also general tonic and eliminative measures.

541 **Massage of the Breast** (Figs. 111 and 112). — The procedures in massage of the breast consist of gentle grasping, compressing, rubbing, and fulling movements, beginning at the periphery of the breast and working toward the nipple. The manipulation is very similar to that usually employed in milking. The parts should be thoroughly lubricated, and care taken to avoid so great pressure as to bruise the tissues. The manipulations should not be employed when the breast does not contain milk, as harm will thus be done rather than good. The purpose is to remove the milk from the obstructed channels in the gentlest manner possible, and thereby relieve the over-distended ducts. When hardness of the breast exists in the puerperal or nursing woman, milk is almost always present, although the patient may feel very certain to the contrary.

542 It is, as a rule, improper to manipulate a breast when suppuration exists. It should not be taken for granted, however, that suppuration is present because the patient has had a chill, and shows a rise of temperature, as the application of massage, even under such circumstances, will often result in resolution. But the greatest utility of massage of the breast is as a means of preventing an over-accumulation of milk, with resulting chill, fever, and suppuration. Violent or bruising manipulations, however, may result in great damage, encouraging suppuration rather than preventing it.

543 Manipulation of the breast is sometimes employed as a means of encouraging development of the organ, especially in cases in which the nipple is unusually small or retracted. In applying massage for this purpose, the areola should be drawn back by pressure with the thumb and forefinger until the nipple becomes prominent. It should then be seized and drawn forward, as by the action of the child's lips when nursing (Fig. 112), a pinching and rolling movement being at the same time applied. The proper time for such applications is during the later months of pregnancy. It should be remembered, however, that manipulation of the breast sometimes has an exciting effect upon the pelvic organs, and any marked indication of such a result should be considered sufficient reason for discontinuing the applications. This treatment is also an excellent means of hardening the skin of the breast and the nipple, and hence is a useful precaution against soreness of the nipples from nursing.

Massage in Pregnancy.—Massage is a most valuable 544 means of preventing a variety of the most serious complications of pregnancy and parturition. A woman who is accustomed to active muscular employment during the period of gestation will not require the assistance of massage ; but for those women who lead sedentary lives or who are lacking in physical development, massage affords a most excellent measure of preparation for the parturient process. Both general and local massage are of value in these cases. General massage should consist of the ordinary procedures, with this exception : Special care must be taken to avoid violent manipulations of the abdomen and too vigorous percussion of the lower portion of the back, especially at the beginning of the treatment. The " deep " procedures in massage should not be undertaken unless the masseuse has had special experience in these cases, and knows how to reach the colon without disturbing the gravid uterus. The chief aim of the manipulations should be to develop the muscles, and hence they will principally consist of fulling movements and petrissage of all the muscular structures of the abdominal wall. Lifting of the abdominal contents will also be found extremely useful in many cases, relieving the strain upon the back, and aiding in the "rising" of the uterus, which is likely to be delayed in women of feeble muscular development, resulting in many distressing pelvic symptoms.

Massage of the Perineum.—This procedure is espe- 545 cially valuable in cases of rigid perineum, and cases in which a laceration has previously occurred and has been repaired by an operation. By suitable manipulations, the parts being thoroughly lubricated, the structures of the perineum may be rendered stronger and more elastic, so as to be able to bear a larger amount of stretching. The applications should be as follows: With the patient lying upon her side, in the left Sims's position, the operator stands facing the back, with the fingers resting upon the buttocks, and manipulates the perineum, using the thumbs in alternation, stretching the tissues away from the median line. Only one thumb should be used at once, stretching in opposite directions, as by the use of both, the stretching might be overdone and the skin irritated.

546 The patient should also be made to execute breathing movements, in which both the abdominal and the perineal muscles are vigorously contracted during the act of expiration. Under the instructions of a physician, the manipulations may be somewhat extended and varied by introducing the forefinger into the vagina or the rectum, the muscle being grasped between the forefinger and the thumb, and thoroughly pressed and stretched.

547 **Neuralgic Pain.**— Massage is one of the most effective means of relieving neuralgic pain. General massage acts by improving the blood and the general nutrition. Dr. Chapman has very well said that "pain is the cry of a hungry nerve for better blood." With better blood and better nutrition, the cause of neuralgic pain is usually removed. Local massage may act both as a derivative measure and as a means of directly stimulating the nutrition of the nerve itself, according as the applications are made in a derivative manner or applied directly to the nerve.

548 All the various procedures of massage may be used in the treatment of neuralgia. The most effective measures for direct application are nerve compression and vibration. Vibration may be employed either by manual or mechanical means. Mechanical vibration may be simply ordinary shaking, or what may be termed musical vibration. Musical vibrations were first employed and brought to the attention of the profession by Mortimer Granville, of London, whose "nerve percuter" the writer has had in use for some twelve years. Dr. Granville believes that pain is due to disharmony, or morbid vibration, in a nerve, and has found in his experience that acute, sharp pain is best relieved by musical vibration of a low tone, while dull, heavy pain is best relieved by high-keyed vibrations. He thinks that relief is obtained by interruption of the discordant nerve vibrations, which he considers the cause of the pain.

Charcot claims to have obtained good results with the **549** vibrating helmet for relief of painful head symptoms. I have not found Mortimer Granville's nerve percuter entirely satisfactory, as it is very prone to get out of order, but have obtained good results from the use of a percuter constructed by modifying Bonwell's dental engine. The writer has recently had constructed an electrical device by which vibrations may be applied directly to a nerve trunk, or to any desired point accessible from the surface of the body. (See Fig. 121.)

Writer's Cramp.—This disease, which appears under **550** various forms, and to which different terms are applied as it occurs in writers, telegraph operators, piano players, or persons engaged in other occupations which chiefly employ the muscles of the forearm, is more amenable to massage than to any other mode of treatment. Three distinct phases are described, characterized respectively by trembling, spastic contraction of the muscles, and paralysis. All three phases of the disease are sometimes found present in a single case. This condition is largely the result of unbalanced muscular and nerve action.

The following procedures are the most effective in reliev- **551** ing it : —

1. Thorough kneading of the fingers and dorsal interossei (**213, 274**).

2. Kneading of the palm (**275**), especial attention being given to the fleshy masses of the palm of the hand ; and rolling of the hand (Fig. 47).

3. Kneading of the forearm with very firm pressure (**277**).

4. Hacking (**316**) of forearm and arm.

5. Stretching of the finger, wrist, elbow, and shoulder joints (**342, 372-376**).

6. Vibration — shaking (**303**).

Centripetal friction, with firm pressure, should be used in alternation with the various procedures named.

552　In addition to the passive movements of massage, the patient should be directed to take special exercises. These exercises should be so directed as to bring into action the muscles which antagonize the affected muscles or those which are most employed in the exercise which has given rise to the disease. In writing, the interossei are used in such a way as to fix and steady the fingers, holding the metacarpal bones tightly together; hence these muscles should be exercised in the opposite direction, which will be accomplished by causing the patient to separate the fingers, at the same time making resistance, which may be offered by grasping the extended fingers between the thumb and forefinger, then directing the patient to spread his fingers, the pressure being carefully graduated to the condition of the muscles, and increased from time to time.

553　The patient may take the exercise by himself, making resistance with the opposite hand, or applying it by means of a rubber band slipped over the fingers. As the muscles gain in strength, a stronger band may be used, or another may be added, the number of bands being increased as the muscles gain in strength. These exercises should be taken four to eight times daily.

554　Writing exercises are also useful. These exercises should be at first chiefly confined to such letters as give the patient the greatest amount of trouble. They should begin with blackboard work, or writing with a pencil in a very large hand. The purpose of this exercise is a double one ; first, to gradually train the muscles to execute proper movements ; and, second, to train the motor centers in the brain, which acquire a perverted habit through the long-continued morbid action of the muscles. As the muscular balance is improved, the letters are gradually decreased in size. Such letters as *l* and *n* are good ones for practice. To these, other letters may be added later, such as *f*, *t*, *g*, and combinations of letters, as *li*, *lim*, *lo*, *log*, *fog*, *fit*, etc.

The writer has succeeded in curing some extraordinarily **555** bad cases of this kind which had previously resisted all measures of treatment, including operative procedures.

Massage in Heart Disease.— There is no condition in **556** which massage is of greater value than in the treatment of disorders of the heart. Space is lacking for a consideration here of the pathology of cardiac disease, nor is it necessary that the masseur should possess this knowledge. It is important, however, that the trained masseur should know that different forms of cardiac disease require very different, indeed actually opposite, applications of massage, so that it is quite possible to do much harm by inappropriate measures, as well as incalculable good by the skillful employment of judicious procedures. For practical purposes, the various forms of cardiac disease may be classified in relation to the indications for the application of massage, as follows : —

1. *Overaction of the heart*, due to overcompensation from **557** valvular disease, to disease of the lungs in which the respiratory field is lessened, or to hypertrophy, the result of overtraining. Excessive action of the heart is indicated by its heavy beating (not palpitation, but excessive force of beat), strong, full, and sustained pulse, and congestion of the head, often accompanied by insomnia.

2. *Weakness of the heart*, a condition resulting from dila- **558** tation from advanced valvular disease, from fatty degeneration, or from hemorrhage or long existing and exhausting disease, as a prolonged attack of fever accompanied by high temperature. Heart weakness may be recognized by the feeble, frequent pulse, easily extinguished by pressure with the finger ; by the bluish, or cyanotic, appearance of the face or lips ; and by the inability of the patient to exercise to any extent without quickly getting out of breath.

3. *Functional disorders of the heart*, such as palpitation **559**

and intermittent or irregular beating. These troubles are, in the great majority of cases, connected with disturbances of digestion.

The treatment indicated for these conditions is as follows :—

560 *Massage for Overactive Heart.* — This condition requires, first of all, rest in bed. Massage is essential in these cases : (1) To obviate the evils which arise from long-continued rest in bed ; (2) to aid in quieting the overactive heart. For the accomplishment of the first purpose, abdominal massage should be administered daily. Moderate breathing exercises should be employed for five minutes before and after each meal, and on first awaking in the morning. The only general procedures which should be employed are stroking (**169, 175**) and centrifugal friction (**194**), the purpose being not to accelerate the circulation of the blood in the vessels, but rather to retard it. Care should be taken, even in the application of the measures named, to avoid the employment of too great a degree of force in the friction movements, as the reflex action occasioned thereby may result in giving the treatment an exciting, rather than a sedative, effect.

561 *Massage for Weak Heart.* — In cases of extreme weakness of the heart ; that is, cases in which even so small an amount of exercise as that involved in walking slowly for a short distance, cannot be taken without producing shortness of breath, the patient must first of all be put to bed. He must not be allowed to stand upon his feet at all, nor even to sit up, but must be kept in a horizontal position either in bed or on a cot, or in a reclining chair. In a case of this kind, nearly all the procedures of massage are beneficial, with the exception of centrifugal friction, which should be avoided. The measures of greatest value are centripetal friction (**193**), respiratory exercises (**381-384**), joint movements (**342-376**), and massage of the heart (**506-509**), all of which should be employed from two to four times daily. Abdominal massage (**389-424**) should also be applied, care being taken, however, to avoid the use of too much force, as it is not desirable to draw too large a quantity of blood to the abdomen.   In joint movements, great care must be taken not to overdo in exercising.   The force employed should not be so great as to cause the patient to breathe rapidly.   The slightest evidence of breathlessness or quickened respiration on the part of the patient, as shown by increased movements of the anterior nares, is an indication that the treatment has been too severe.

In order to avoid the possibility of injury from joint move- **562** ments, care should be taken not to apply a movement to the same joint twice in immediate succession.   Beginning with one arm, apply gentle flexion and extension, first to the wrist, then to the elbow, then rotate the shoulder joint, describing the circle but once ; next proceed to the other arm, then take the opposite leg, then the other leg.   Now return to the arm first treated, and so continue until each of the extremities has been gone over from two to six times.   Centripetal friction should be applied to each limb immediately after the application of the movements, and before proceeding to the exercise of another part.

In employing the flexion and extension, care should be **563** taken that the movement is carried to the extent of quite decided resistance, otherwise the circulation will not be excited. Flexion and extension thus applied to a joint constitute an invaluable pumping process, in which the lymphatics and vessels of first one side and then the other are alternately stretched or compressed and emptied, then relaxed and filled.

When the patient becomes able to bear a considerable **564** amount of purely passive flexion and extension without excitement of the heart, the movements should be made at first slightly, and later more strongly, resistive.   Resistive movements are most safely and effectively executed in these cases by having the patient first flex the joint to be operated upon, and then attempt to hold it in a flexed position while the masseur extends it ; the movement is then reversed ; that is, the patient extends the limb and holds it rigid while the masseur overcomes the rigidity in flexing it.   Very little force should be used at first.

11

565 When sufficiently recovered to allow some exercise upon the feet, the patient may be taught to operate upon his own joints by executing flexion and extension movements without the aid of the masseur. This may be accomplished thus : Extending the limb (an arm, for example), the patient renders it rigid by contracting both the flexor and extensor muscles as forcibly as possible. Flexing the joint to the fullest extent, the flexor and extensor muscles are again brought into a state of firm rigidity by voluntary contraction. The movements should be applied in a rotating series, passing rapidly from one joint to another until all the joints of both the upper and the lower extremities have been exercised, and then repeated as directed for passive movements administered by the masseur.

566 A patient suffering from cardiac insufficiency, as is the case with other patients for whom the "rest-cure" is employed, cannot be cured in bed. The purpose of rest in bed is to restore the balance of the circulation. When this has been accomplished, as indicated by improved aëration of the blood, outwardly manifested by the disappearance of the blue color of the lips or skin, and of œdema of the face or extremities, or of dropsical accumulations in the abdomen and chest or the pericardial sac, the patient may begin to take exercise upon the feet.

The exercise must not be carried so far, however, as to cause an increase of the dropsical accumulation in the feet or the abdomen. Great care must be taken that the patient does not take such violent or long-continued exercise as to cause breathlessness, or even a decided increase in the rate of breathing. When this precaution is disregarded, the breathlessness will increase from day to day, even though the exercise be not increased, and the patient's former condition will gradually return, necessitating his again being put to bed, and the employment of the same measures as before.

567 Walking and other voluntary exercises should stop just short of a decided increase of respiratory activity, so that the heart shall not be to any degree excited. The greatest care will be required at the beginning of exercise to avoid going beyond the safe limit.

Passive, active-passive, and voluntary exercise of the joints, **568** with the patient in a horizontal position, should be employed for half an hour after each effort of the patient to become accustomed to exercise in a vertical position, and will be found a very excellent means of quieting the heart. Among the most useful exercises in which the patient may at first engage, is the use of the treadle, which has the motion of the velocipede without the incitement to overexercise which accompanies the use of this admirable means of exercise.

By degrees the patient may be accustomed to more and **569** more severe effort, until such exercises as slowly climbing a hill of moderate grade, or a flight of stairs not too steep nor too long, may be attempted. It is only by voluntary exercise, gradually and systematically increased, that a patient suffering from cardiac insufficiency can be brought to a state in which he may be said to enjoy health, and in which he is comparatively safe from the extension of the pathological condition under which he is laboring.

That exercise is the only means by which a muscle can be strengthened is a principle which applies to the heart as well as to every other muscle of the body.

Massage for Palpitation of the Heart.— As palpitation and **570** other forms of functional disease of the heart are, in the majority of cases, due to a disturbance of the sympathetic nerve arising from some disorder of the abdominal viscera, special attention should be given to abdominal massage in this class of cases. Palpitation may arise from dilatation of the stomach and resulting indigestion, or from the dragging upon the abdominal sympathetic, due to prolapse of the stomach and bowels, a floating kidney, a prolapsed liver, or a dislocated spleen. Care should be taken to see that each viscus is in its proper position, replacement being performed by the methods previously described, when necessary. Lifting the abdominal contents is especially important, and in cases of dilatation of the stomach, massage of the stomach must be applied in such a manner as to empty the organ of its fermenting and decomposing contents. In some instances, lavage of the stomach is essential as a preliminary measure whereby the disturbing poisonous substances may be removed. Massage of the heart (**506-509**) is also useful as a means of assisting the heart to acquire its normal rhythm. Massage of the stomach (**451, 452**) and replacement of the viscera (**439-450**) should be employed at least twice a day. In case the viscera are prolapsed, an abdominal bandage must be worn, being carefully applied after the viscera have been replaced. General massage is required daily.

571   **Special Exercises to be Employed with Massage.** —Every masseur or masseuse ought to be skilled in gymnastics, as some of the morbid conditions which most urgently require the employment of massage are the result of deficient exercise and incorrect positions in standing and sitting. Weakness of the muscles of the trunk is the principal cause of prolapse of the abdominal and pelvic organs and of deformities of the spine, and is either directly or indirectly the cause of a great variety of functional disorders of the abdominal and pelvic organs, as well as local and general nervous maladies for which massage is frequently prescribed.

572   Massage alone is not sufficient to effect a permanent cure in these cases, for the reason that it does not remove the original cause. It is only capable of palliating or temporarily removing the consequences, and not the cause. It is necessarily of great importance that gymnastics should be combined with massage. I constantly employ manual Swedish movements, gymnastics with apparatus, Swedish educational gymnastics, and various outdoor exercises, such as bicycle riding, horseback riding, rowing, etc., as necessary complements of massage.

573   The limits of this work are too narrow to permit the consideration of the subject of physical culture and exercise. This I have considered at length in another work, but will present the following brief suggestions with reference to the best manner of strengthening the muscles required in assuming a correct poise in standing and sitting, feeling sure they will be found helpful, if intelligently employed : —

Correct Poise.—A correct sitting or standing poise is a **574** forcible position. In *standing*, the position should be such that a line drawn just in front of the ear will fall over the point of the shoulder, and strike the foot at the root of the toes. The position of a person when standing correctly is such that he can immediately rise upon the toes without swaying the body forward. In standing or walking, the weight of the body should fall upon the ball of the foot.

The proper standing poise may be obtained by the follow- **575** ing simple means (Figs. 108, 109, and 110) : Stand with the back against the wall. Place the body in such a position that the hips, heels, shoulders, and back of the head are in contact with the wall. The arms should be held straight, and close to the sides. Now flex the neck backward until the top of the head is in contact with the wall, allowing the shoulders to move forward, keeping the arms straight, and the heels and hips still in contact with the wall. After bending the head backward as far as possible, and thereby pushing the shoulders forward, raise the head, holding the shoulders in the exact position assumed when the head was flexed backward, and draw the chin well in ; the position will now be found to be correct. Care must be observed to hold the chest well forward, the shoulders back, and the arms extended downward at the sides.

In *sitting*, the seat of the chair should be at such a **576** height that the soles of the feet can rest squarely upon the floor, and it should also be of the proper width so that the hips can touch the back. The shoulders should rest against the upper part of the chair, but the center of the back should not touch the chair, unless the chair-back has a strong forward curve. The chest should be held well forward, with the chin drawn in, and the legs should not be crossed. A bad sitting position is responsible for more maladies of the chest, abdomen, and pelvis than is generally supposed.

577 **Exercises in Correct Poise, to be Taken in Connection with Massage.**— The author has found the following series of exercises of special service : —

Series A.— With the patient lying upon the face, the forehead resting upon the hands, placed one above the other, take the following exercises: —

1. Head raising backward four times.

2. Leg raising, leg and foot extended, each four times.

3. Leg raising, both together, four times.

4. Head and leg raising (Fig. 113), each leg two to four times.

5. Head and legs raising, both legs together, two to four times.

578 *Series B.*— Repeat the above exercises, with arms in rest position, patient lying upon back (Fig. 114).

579 *Series C.*— Patient lying upon back, with the heels drawn up to the body.

1. Hips raising (Fig. 82), two to eight times. The hips should be raised until the trunk and thighs are in line from shoulders to knees.

2. Knees separating (Fig. 71). The knees should be separated as widely as possible. Repeat four to eight times.

3. Hips-raising and knees-separating movements, thus : Separate the knees well, raise the hips, hold a few seconds, then bring the knees together while lowering the hips.

580 In assuming a correct position for the first time, a person may have a somewhat stiff and awkward appearance, but this will disappear as the ability to assume a correct poise easily and readily is acquired by practice.

The exercises of this series are especially designed to develop those muscles which tilt the pelvis backward, thus increasing the obliquity of the pelvis, a matter of much consequence in relation to correct standing, and also with reference to uterine displacements.

MECHANICAL MASSAGE.

Inventive genius has devised a considerable number of appliances by means of which a more or less perfect imitation of the action of the hands in the application of massage may be obtained. Zander, of Stockholm, and Taylor, of New York, as well as the writer, have invented machines for this purpose. For nearly twenty years the author has made use of various forms of apparatus designed to administer mechanical massage, or what is more commonly termed mechanical Swedish movements, with most excellent results in appropriate cases.

Mechanical massage may be advantageously used as a substitute for a number of the procedures of manual massage. I have, however, found no device quite equal to the human hand, for the administration of kneading movements. Shaking and vibratory movements, on the other hand, may be applied more efficiently by apparatus than by hand in cases requiring vigorous and prolonged application, for the reason that much more vigorous, rapid, and uniform movements can be executed by machinery than by the hand, and the movement may be continued as long as necessary ; whereas these movements are exceedingly trying to the masseur, and cannot be maintained, at best, for more than a few minutes continuously.

Several other procedures may be given by mechanical appliances quite as well as by the hand, and with even greater efficiency. A brief description of some of the more important means and methods employed in mechanical massage, or Swedish movements, will not be out of place in a work which undertakes, as does this, to cover the whole ground of the subject from a practical standpoint. The following is a brief description of the apparatus and modes of application which the author has had in use in the Battle Creek Sanitarium during the last fifteen to twenty years, and which have stood the test of practical use in some thousands of cases, not as an exclusive mode of treatment, but as an auxiliary means employed in connection with manual massage, exercise, hydrotherapy, electricity, and other rational methods.

The meager knowledge which has heretofore existed in regard to the functions of the sympathetic nerve and its relations to the activities of the viscera, has rendered difficult an explanation of the remarkable therapeutic results which have been constantly witnessed from the employment of mechanical massage, especially in the treatment of hepatic and digestive disorders. Now that the functions of the great sympathetic nerve and of the abdominal ganglia and solar plexus are coming to be better understood, it is very clear that the application of strong vibratory or shaking movements to the abdomen may produce powerful physiological and therapeutic effects through the stimulation of the sympathetic. When it is recollected that the great abdominal brain controls the nutrition of the entire body through its influence upon the circulation and its universal control of glandular action, it must be clearly seen that therapeutic applications capable of affecting this portion of the nervous system cannot be made without marked results.

The observations of the late eminent Professor Charcot have called the attention of the profession to the powerful physiological and therapeutic effects of vibration in the treatment of organic disease of the spine, one of the most intractable classes of maladies. The confidence in mechanical massage as a therapeutic measure inspired by the great prestige of this renowned Parisian physician, has encouraged the writer to give publicity to some of the observations which he has made upon this subject during the last twenty years, and to describe some of the various means employed by him. Among the several devices made use of are a number which were invented by Zander and Taylor, who have also been working in this line ; but the majority of those which the author con-

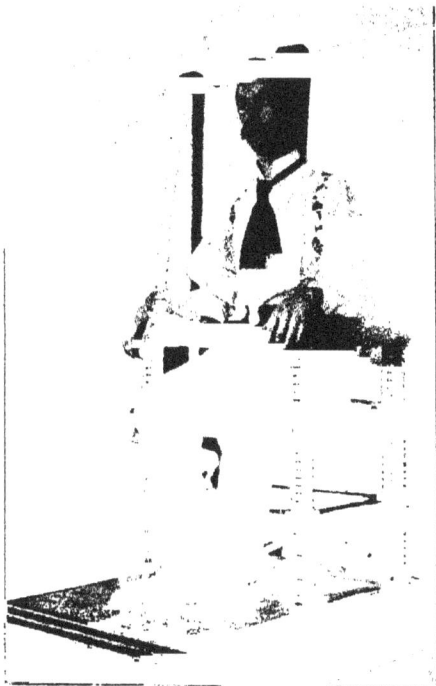

Fig. 115. Vibrating Chair.

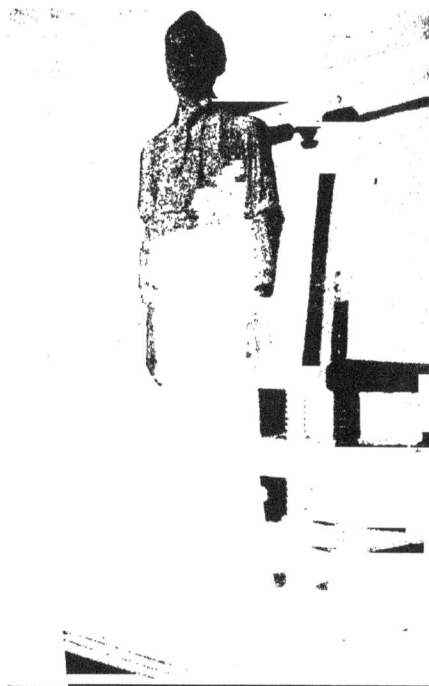

Fig. 116. Vibrating Platform.

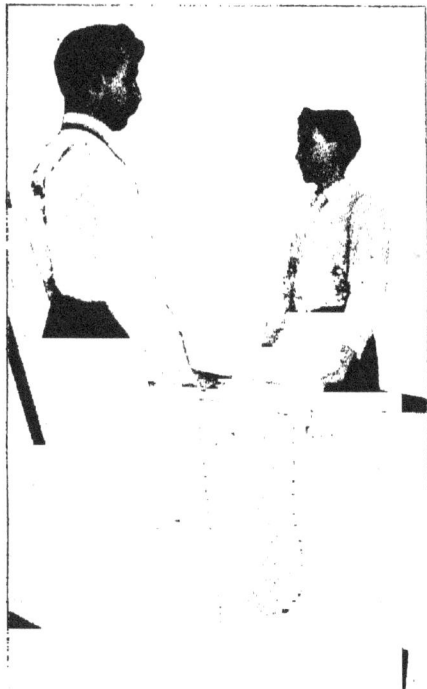

Fig. 117. Vibrating Bar.

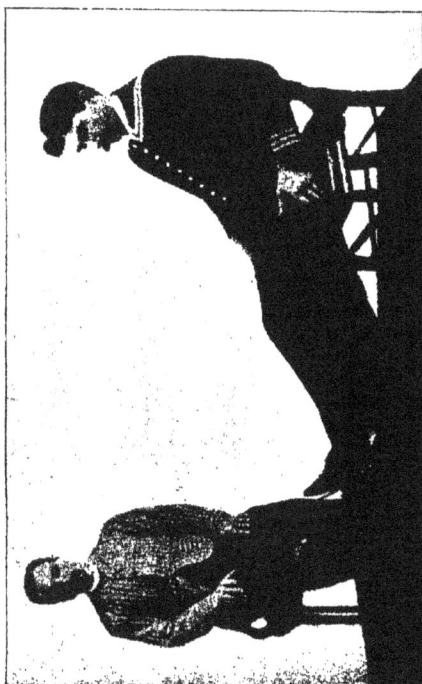

Fig. 118. Endwise and Lateral Vibration of
the Feet and Legs.

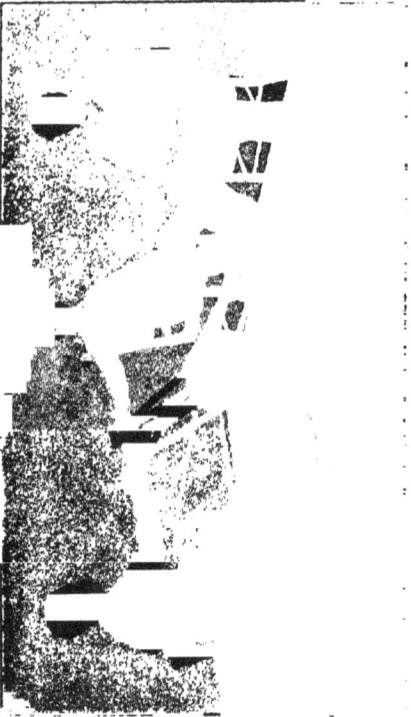

Fig. 119. Rotary Vibration of the Legs and Arms.

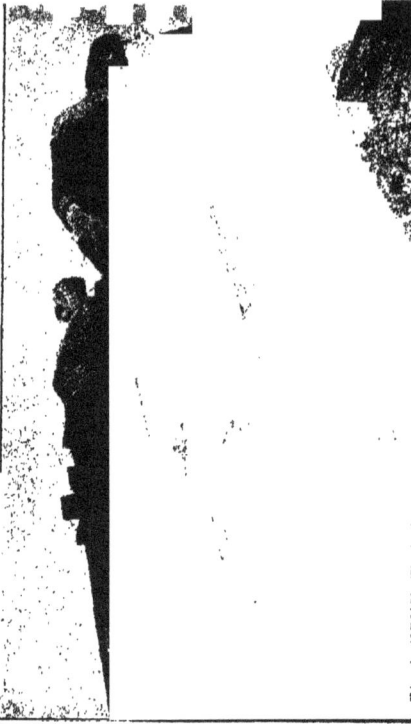

Fig. 120. Vibration of the Trunk.

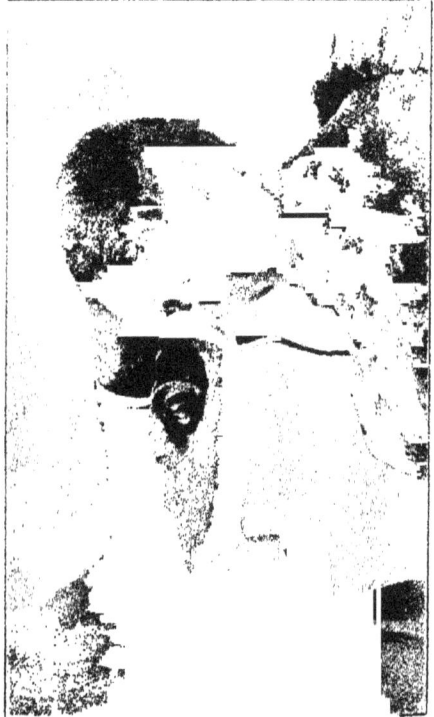

Fig. 121. Nerve Percuter.

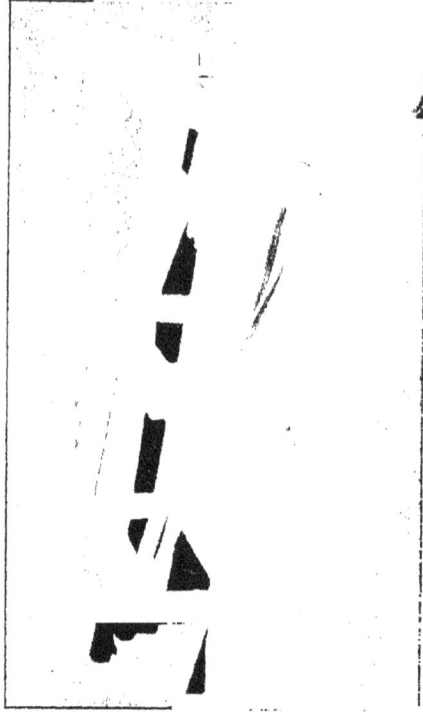

Fig. 122. Apparatus for Kneading the Abdomen.

siders the most effective are the outgrowth of his own personal experience, and have been constructed after designs furnished by him. Several devices other than those described have been made and utilized, and have been found not without merit, but are not described here for lack of space.

Mechanical Vibration.— One of the most useful of all the several forms of mechanical massage is mechanical vibration. The highest rate of movement which can be attained by the hand is ten to twelve to-and-fro movements per second ; whereas, by the use of mechanical, electrical, or acoustic devices, effective vibratory movements may be produced at any rate desired between forty or fifty per second to ten times that number. Vibratory movements forcibly communicated to the body at the rate of six per minute, have been shown to produce at first a distinct muscular contraction with each oscillation ; but if the vibration is long continued, the individual contractions become gradually less distinct, and after a time merge one into another, so that the contractions become continuous, or tetanic. From this fact it is apparent that mechanical vibration is capable of producing very decided physiological results as a mode of exercise ; and that it exercises a powerful influence upon the circulation is a frequent observation. My patients constantly report that vibratory movements make them warm, and restore the balance of the circulation when disturbed by morbid reflex action, so that, while the feet are warmed, the head is cooled.

Carefully conducted experiments which I have made, show that the temperature of a part subjected to mechanical vibration is actually increased, the amount of the increase depending upon the length of the application, and the degree of depression below the normal temperature at the start.

Vibration is also one of the most efficient means with which the writer is acquainted for relieving the great variety of paræsthesias from which neurasthenic patients suffer, such as numbness, formication, tingling, etc.

The Vibrating Chair. — Figs. 115 and 116 represent a vibrating chair which I devised in 1883, and have since had in

constant use at the Battle Creek Sanitarium. The usual rate
of vibration which I employ is twenty per second. A person
needs to experience but a single application to become convinced of the powerful physiological effects which may be
produced by mechanical vibration. When seated in the chair,
strong vibratory movements are experienced, in which the
whole body takes part. The greatest amount of force is applied
to the lower portion of the trunk. The vibratory impulses
communicated are felt powerfully in the lower bowel, and
have a decided stimulating effect upon the rectum.

By placing the hands upon the arms of the chair, and
inclining the trunk either forward or backward, the impulses
may be transmitted more or less forcibly, as desired, from the
lower to the upper portions of the spinal column. The application should continue from three to ten minutes, to secure
decided physiological effects.

Vibrating Platform.— In standing erect upon the moving platform on which the chair rests, the muscles of the legs
are brought into powerful action. Not only the muscles of the
lower leg, but the muscles of the thigh, are thrown into tetanic
contraction by the strong vibratory movements transmitted
through the legs (Fig. 116). The application usually lasts
about five minutes. A separate platform may also be used.

The Vibrating Bar.— Fig. 117 is a very imperfect representation of an apparatus I had constructed several years ago,
in which a suitable mechanism drives a pair of horizontal bars
at a high rate of speed. In using the vibrating bar, the hands
are first placed upon it with the fingers spread and held rigid,
but with the wrists flexible. This throws the hands into violent
vibration without communicating the vibratory impulses to any
other portion of the body. The bar is then seized by the
hands, which grasp it tightly while the arm is partly flexed at
the elbow, the shoulder joint being relaxed. Then, straighten-
ing the arms and holding them rigid, the muscles of the
shoulders being fixed and the bar held firmly, the vibratory
movements may be communicated to the upper spine and head

with very great vigor, producing a powerfully stimulating effect upon the upper spine.

The vibratory impulses may also be communicated to the stomach, liver, loins, sacrum, rectum, and other parts, by bringing these portions of the body into direct contact with the bar.

Powerful endwise vibratory movements are given to the legs by placing the patient in a chair facing the apparatus, with the feet against the uprights which support the end of the bar opposite the driving mechanism. The vibratory movements obtained from this apparatus are applied to each part from half a minute to one minute.

Vibration of the Arms and Legs.—The legs are vibrated in three ways: (1) By means of an endwise movement; (2) by means of a lateral movement; (3) by means of a rotary movement. The effects of these three modes of vibration are similar, yet in some respects different. The time of application is usually from three to five minutes.

Endwise vibration is by far the most vigorous of the three modes. It is administered by means of a horizontal vibrating bar against the end of which the feet are placed, supported in suitable rests (Fig. 118).

Lateral vibration is administered by means of the same apparatus, the feet being placed against the side of the bar instead of the end (Fig. 118).

Rotary vibration is produced by means of a rotating bar against the end of which the feet are supported (Fig. 119). The leg is held straight, not flexed as in the cut. The same apparatus is used for the arms.

Nerve-percuter, or Vibrator.—This instrument, which I have recently had constructed, and to which reference has previously been made, consists of a metallic chamber in which a mass of soft iron is made to play to and fro with considerable force by means of an alternating electrical current passing through a coil of wire which constitutes a part of the chamber. The blows struck by the oscillating mass of iron are communicated to the portion of the body under treatment by a brass rod terminating in a knob. By means of this simple device, very vigorous vibratory movements may be applied to the head, to a nerve trunk, or to any part of the body to which it is desirable to make vibratory applications (Fig. 121).

Vibration of the Trunk.— In Fig. 120 is shown a method of applying vigorous vibratory movements to the trunk. The apparatus consists of a mechanism by means of which a strong horizontal bar is made to oscillate at the rate of 1200 to 1500 per minute. By means of suitable padded rests placed upon the bar, vibratory movements may be communicated to the back, the abdomen, or to either side, as may be desired. The special purpose of this apparatus is to communicate mechanical motion to the liver, stomach, bowels, and other abdominal viscera. It is a vigorous means of stimulating peristaltic activity, and of quickening the circulation in the large viscera of the abdomen. This apparatus the writer has had in use at the Battle Creek Sanitarium for twenty years, and has found it an exceedingly effective device. It is not simply a means of amusing the patient, but is capable of producing powerful physiological and therapeutic effects. The time of application to each part is usually from three to five minutes.

Mechanical Kneading.— By means of suitable apparatus, mechanical kneading may be applied in a very efficient manner to the bowels, the arms, the legs, and even to the whole trunk.

Mechanical kneading of the abdomen is one of the most useful of the several forms of kneading ; it may perhaps with justice be said to be the most useful of all. It is best administered by means of the apparatus shown in the cut (Fig. 122). The writer had this apparatus specially constructed for the purpose some twelve years ago, and has had it in constant use since. The apparatus consists of a table with a large aperture near the center of its top. In this opening plays a series of six vertically-placed bars, each surmounted by a suitable pad. Each bar is separately actuated by a cam, or eccentric, so that it has its own independent motion. These six eccentrics are so arranged as to give a wave-like form to the combined movement of the six kneading pads. Simultaneously with the vertical movement of this kneading device, the table top, with the patient which it bears, is made to move back and forth, thus changing the relation of the pads to the abdominal surface, and causing them to knead the entire abdomen. The two sets of movements are so timed that the wave-like kneading movement is made to follow very closely the course of the colon, thus bringing this part of the intestine especially under control. Zander has a similar machine.

I have found this apparatus of very great service in the treatment of constipation. It is not, of course, a panacea for this disease, which arises from many different causes; but it is a most efficient auxiliary to other measures, and not a few cases have been observed in which the patient traced the greater part of the benefit received from a systematic course of treatment to this apparatus alone.

Mechanical kneading of the abdomen is useful not only in constipation, but also in cases of dilatation of the stomach in which there is, as a result of the dilatation, a considerable degree of motor insufficiency, in consequence of which the stomach does not empty itself with normal promptness. This treatment is of value in all cases of slow digestion so-called, and should be used within an hour or two after each meal. The kneading is usually continued from five to fifteen minutes.

Mechanical kneading of the arms is executed by means of the apparatus shown in Fig. 123. When the pressure is made sufficient to prevent the rubbers from slipping over the surface, the movement is that of rolling, a form of deep kneading; with lighter pressure, it is that of friction. This is a valuable mode of utilizing mechanical massage. The time of application is from three to five minutes.

The legs may receive mechanical massage by means of a similar apparatus, shown in Fig. 124. This is an excellent means of aiding the circulation in cases in which the legs and feet are habitually cold. The application should be continued from five to eight minutes, or until the extremities are thoroughly warmed.

Mechanical kneading of various parts may also be employed, as shown in Fig. 123. The apparatus utilized is similar to that used for rotary vibration of the feet. A suitable pad is secured at the end of a bar, which is made to rotate while it rests against any portion of the trunk to which it can be conveniently applied. It is especially useful in making applications to the back, stomach, bowels, shoulders, and the region of the liver. In cases of gall-stones, it is a most excellent means of jostling imbedded calculi down into the bile duct, thereby hastening the emptying of the gall-bladder. It also facilitates the discharge of the fluid contents of the gall-bladder, and is thus a valuable aid to digestion. It will be apparent from these observations that this particular form of apparatus is a very efficient form of vibration, as well as a thorough kneading procedure. The time of application should be from one to three minutes to each part.

Trunk Rolling.—The apparatus represented in use in Fig. 125 consists of a pair of pulleys moving in alternation and in opposite directions, a fraction of a revolution in each direction. To each pulley is attached one end of a broad strap, which is passed around the trunk in such a manner that, as the strap is pulled first in one direction and then in the opposite, the tissues are acted upon very much as in certain forms of palm kneading. When applied about the waist, it is a very excellent means of administering a rolling movement to the muscles of the trunk, and a shaking movement to the viscera; when applied across the shoulders, the effect is that of deep kneading. This is a favorite apparatus with patients who are under treatment by mechanical massage. It was devised by the author about ten years ago. This application is so vigorous that it is not usually continued longer than from two to four minutes.

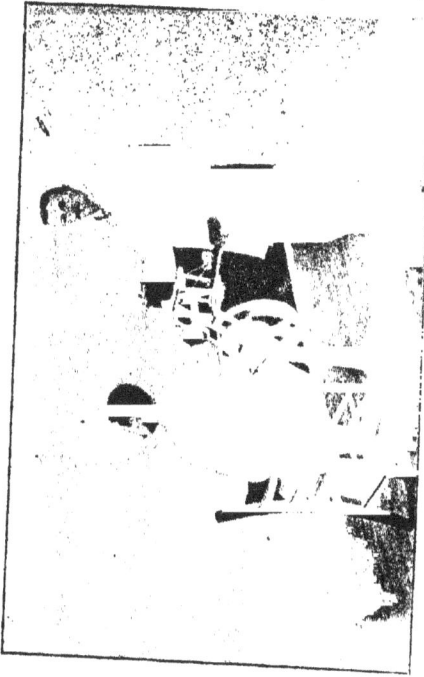

Fig. 123. Apparatus for Kneading the Arms.

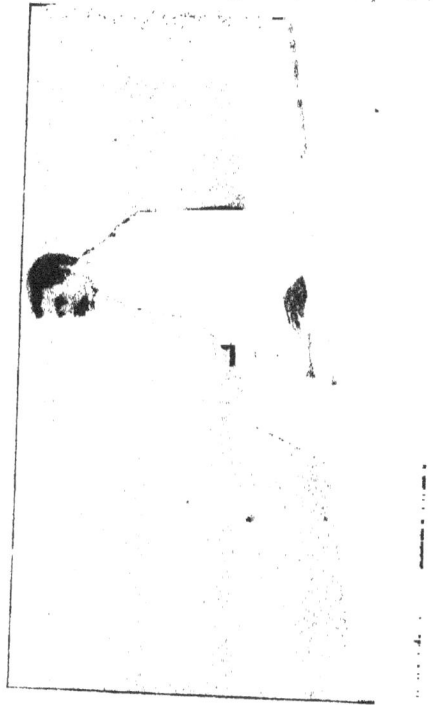

Fig. 124. Apparatus for Kneading the Legs.

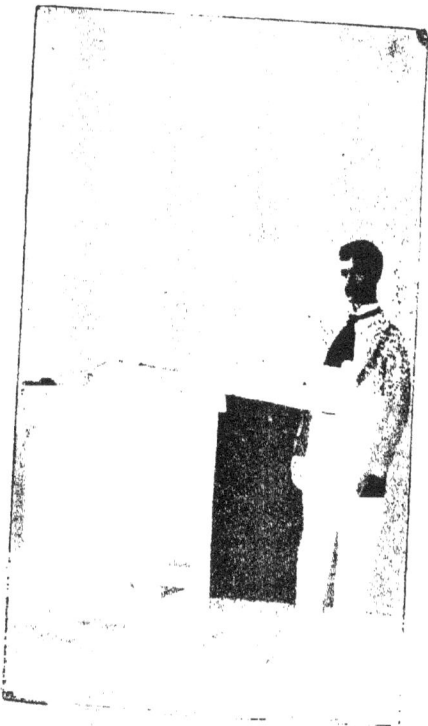

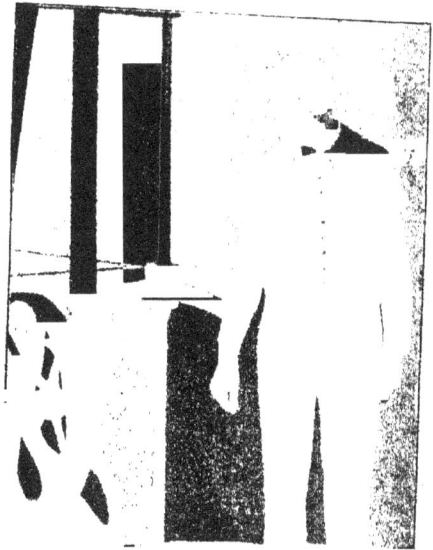

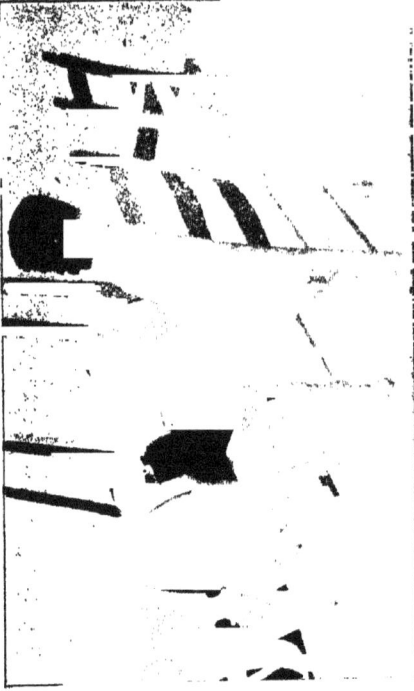

Fig. 128. Mechanical Friction of the Feet.

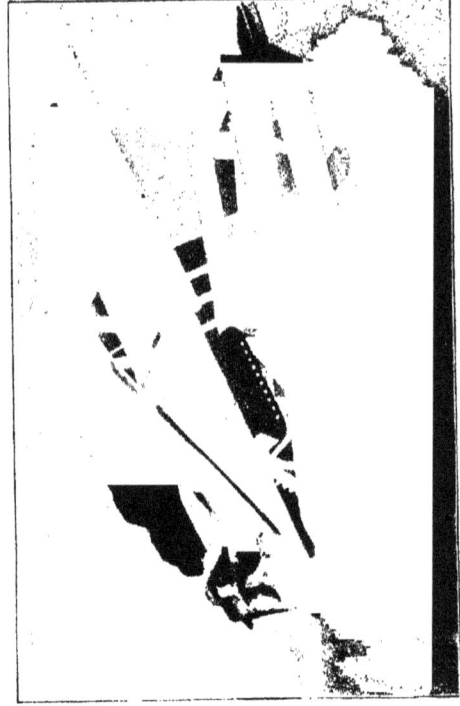

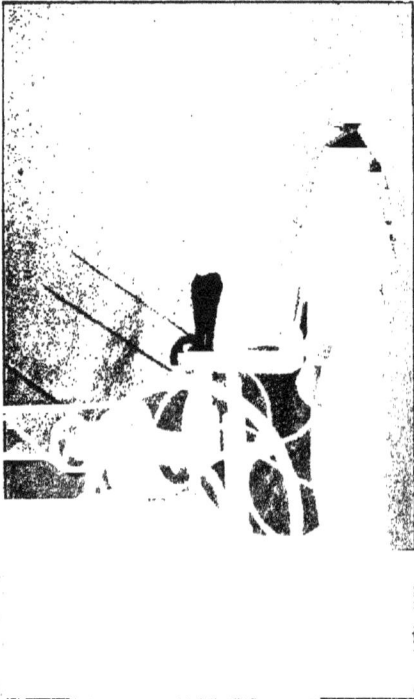

Fig. 127. Beating Apparatus.

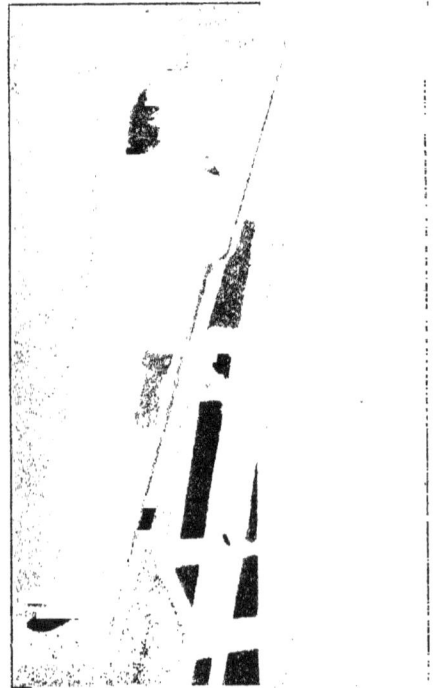

PLATE XLIII.— Mechanical Massage and Movements.

Mechanical Percussion.—There are two forms of percussion which may be administered mechanically, viz.: (1) Slapping ; (2) Beating.

Slapping is administered mechanically by means of a vertical revolving bar, to which is attached a broad strap about sixteen inches in length (Fig. 126). The strap is fastened to the bar at its middle, the two ends being free ; and thus two blows are struck at each revolution. Different degrees of force are secured by modifications of the speed with which the bar is made to revolve, the thickness of the strap, and the position of the patient in relation to the bar and the strap. The time of application, is from one to three minutes.

Mechanical slapping is a most effective measure for stimulating the surface circulation. In this respect it is not excelled by any procedure which can be administered by the hand. It is most usefully applied to the shoulders and back, the legs and thighs, and the soles of the feet.

Mechanical beating (Fig. 127) is an efficient mode of percussion, though less valuable in comparison with beating administered by the hand than is mechanical percussion in comparison with manual percussion. It is most effectively applied to the spine and chest, and over the abdomen. The apparatus shown was devised simultaneously by the writer and by Zander, of Stockholm. The usual time of application is from two to four minutes.

Mechanical Friction.— Friction may be applied to the soles of the feet by a revolving ribbed cylinder (Fig. 128), which was first used by Zander. The writer has added a number of features which have proved serviceable. One of these is the employment of an apron to cover the ribs of the revolving cylinder, thus preventing the wearing upon the patient's stockings or slippers ; another improvement is the insulation of the chair in which the patient sits, which I was led to make by noticing that sparks could often be drawn from different parts of the patient's body while receiving treatment from the apparatus. It is not an uncommon thing to see the hair of a patient sitting in the insulated seat, erected by the electric charge generated by the friction of the machine. It is possible that a certain portion of the static electricity may be generated by the driving belt. This phenomenon is of course chiefly confined to the colder months, when the atmosphere is dry.

The apparatus is a very valuable one, as it performs its work efficiently, and does something which cannot be so well accomplished in any other way. It is a favorite machine with our patients. The application is a very agreeable one, and may be continued almost *ad libitum* without injury. The usual time is from five to ten minutes.

Tilting-table.— In Fig. 129 is represented a tilting-table, which the writer devised nearly twelve years ago, and has had in use since. The patient lies upon his back while one end of the table top is lifted by means of a large cam operating beneath it. The patient lies with his head at the stationary end of the table.

The purpose of this apparatus is to secure what I have termed "vasomotor gymnastics." When the hand is raised above the head, a strong contraction of its blood vessels occurs, the effect being rendered visible to the eye by blanching of the skin. At the same time that the blood vessels of the arm are thus made to contract by a vasomotor reflex, the vessels of the corresponding portion of the brain also contract. By a repetition of the movement, real gymnastics of the muscular walls of the vessels may be executed, and thus relaxed vessels be contracted and strengthened, and local congestion relieved, if so situated as to come within the sphere of the reflex action set up by the change in the position of the arm.

This same principle applies with equal force to the lower extremities, which have a relation to the organs of the pelvis similar to that which the arms sustain to the brain. Leg raising, with the patient lying in a horizontal position, is one of the recognized and most valuable movements in the medical gymnastics of the Swedes. There is, however, a certain disadvantage in this mode of exciting vascular contraction. It is impossible to raise a limb by voluntary effort without a certain degree of strain, which involves holding the breath, and producing, as a result, an increase of pelvic and portal congestion, so that the exercise must to some degree defeat its own purpose. In this exercise, also, but one leg is raised at once. When the lower part of the body is elevated mechanically, there is no exertion on the part of the patient, consequently no strain, and both limbs are elevated at the same time ; thus the maximum effect is obtained.

This apparatus is of great service in all forms of pelvic congestion, in ovarian disease, uterine catarrh, displacements of the pelvic viscera, and in rectal disease of various forms. After spending a few minutes upon the tilting-table, rising and falling with its oscillations at the rate of about eight times a minute, patients suffering from the maladies named and others similar, almost invariably express themselves as experiencing a marked sense of relief. The effects of this mode of passive exercise of the blood vessels are so agreeable that patients are inclined to continue the application as long as they are allowed to do so. As a rule, ten to fifteen minutes is sufficient to secure decided physiological effects.

Pelvis Tilting. — Nearly all forms of pelvic disease give indications for the use of the tilting-table above described. In displacement of the womb or ovaries, however, as well as of the stomach, liver, kidneys, bowels, and other abdominal organs, it is important to combine with the vasomotor gymnastics described, the employment of position as an aid to restoration of the displaced viscera. This is accomplished by adding to the tilting-table above described a device by means of which the pelvis is lifted free from the table while the patient lies upon the face, thus causing the abdominal wall to sag downward (Fig. 130). As the table is tilted, the patient is lifted into such a position as to cause gravity to make an upward (in relation to the normal position) pull upon the viscera of the trunk. The device consists simply of an attachment placed

12

in the center of the table, which is made to rise more rapidly than the table itself, thus lifting the pelvis before the rest of the body, and holding it in this relation until the table returns to a state of rest. The effect of this apparatus is increased, if, while the patient is elevated, the attendant applies percussion or beating to the sacral region.

The use of this apparatus alone is not sufficient to restore displaced organs to position, but it aids greatly in relieving congestion, and is certainly a help toward a cure of visceral prolapse. The application should be made daily, or twice daily, and continued from eight to ten minutes each time.

Trunk-exercising Apparatus. — Figs. 131 and 132 represent forms of apparatus which are of substantial service in exercising the muscles of the trunk. Although the results obtained are different, the principle of both machines is the same, and is based upon the fact that the body involuntarily seeks to maintain its equilibrium.

Active-passive Rotation of the Hips. — Fig. 131 is an apparatus so constructed as to cause a seat to revolve in such a manner that its plane shall continually change, thus inducing the patient, when seated upon the apparatus, to contract the muscles of the trunk in maintaining his equilibrium, the body being steadied by the hands. There is thus secured a complete and perfect rotation of the hips. This is a most excellent form of exercise for persons with weak trunk muscles, which is the condition of most women who come under the care of the gynæcologist, as well as of a large share of the cases of nervous dyspepsia in both men and women. This apparatus has the advantage over other forms of gymnastic apparatus in that it brings the muscles into action automatically, as in walking, and thus secures a more complete and natural movement of the muscles of the trunk. The first applications with this apparatus should be brief, — not more than one or two minutes, — as the muscles of the trunk are brought into such vigorous action that they are likely to be overtaxed, especially in

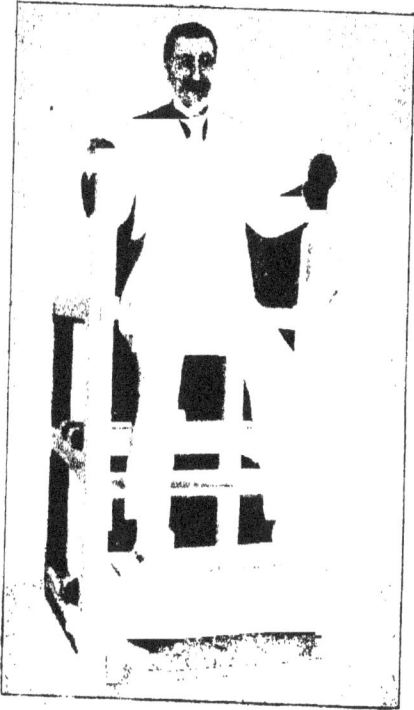

Fig. 131. Revolving Seat.

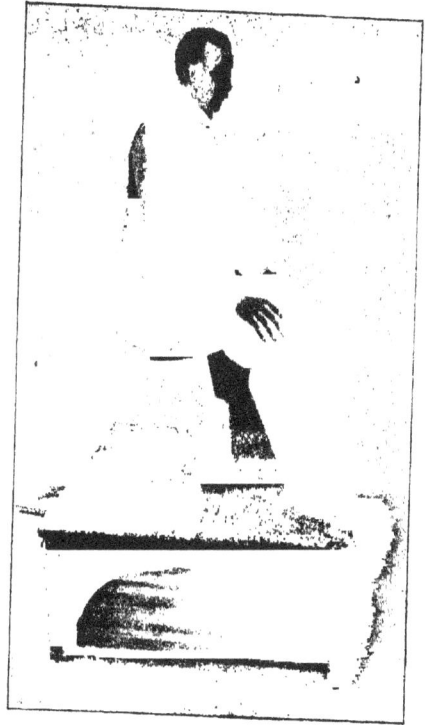

Fig. 132. Tilting-Seat.

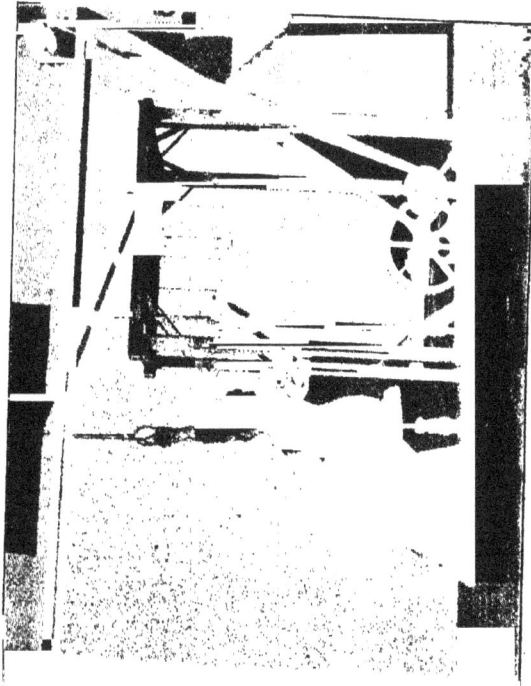

Fig. 133. Apparatus for Artificial Respiration.

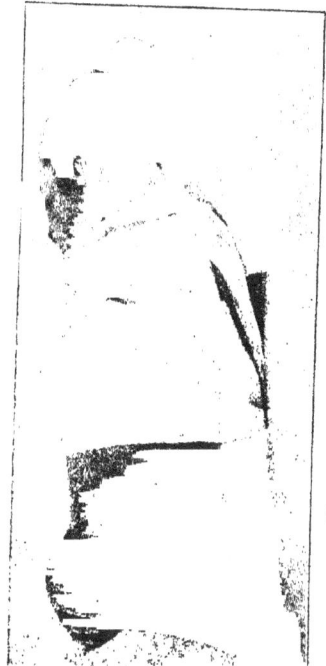

Fig. 134. Cannon-ball Massage.

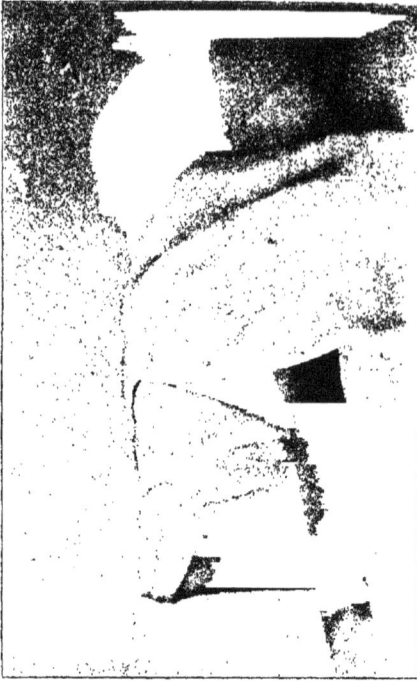

Fig. 135. Weighted Compress.

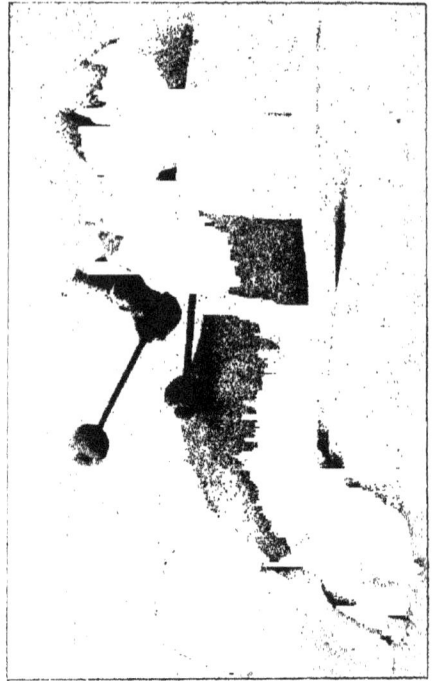

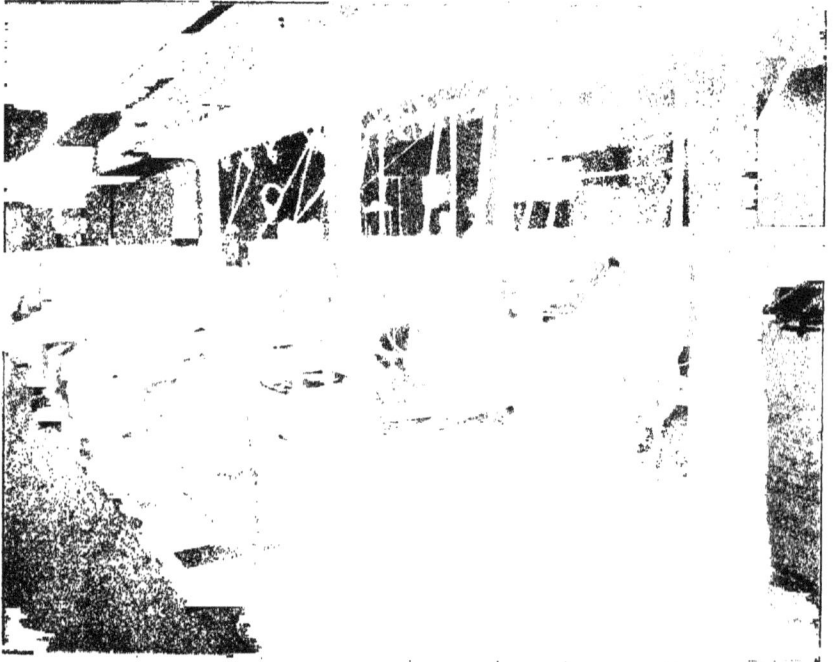

Fig. 137. Mechanical Swedish Movement Department of the Battle Creek Sanitarium.

PLATE XLV.

feeble persons. The apparatus may be used either with or without power attachment, but is usually employed without.

Trunk Flexion. — In the apparatus shown in Fig. 132 the movement is a tilting of the seat from side to side. It is used in two positions : (1) With the patient sitting parallel with the line of movement ; (2) with the patient sitting at right angles to the line of movement. In the first position, the patient is induced to make alternate flexion of the trunk forward and backward; in the second position, the patient flexes the trunk from side to side.

The use of this apparatus is indicated in the same class of cases as the preceding. Its action is less powerful, and consequently it is especially adapted to feeble patients at the beginning of a course of treatment, and as an introduction to the more vigorous movements. The action of this apparatus being less energetic than the preceding, the applications may be somewhat longer — two or three minutes at first, and longer after the patient becomes accustomed to them.

Mechanical Respiration. — In Fig. 133 is shown an apparatus by means of which artificial respiration may be mechanically administered. In its use the patient is seated upon a stool, the arms being placed over movable rests, which fall in the axillæ. The back is supported by a padded rest placed between the shoulders. When the machine is set in motion, the shoulders are lifted upward and backward in such a way as to expand the chest in an efficient manner, producing a strong inspiratory movement quite independent of any effort on the part of the patient. The effect is to correct the condition known as flat, or hollow, chest, and to give flexibility to the chest walls when they have become rigid in consequence of insufficient use. This apparatus is in part modeled after a similar arrangement by Zander, but several improvements have been added ; among others, is a device by means of which the arms, as well as the shoulders, are raised, thus increasing the vigor of the inspiratory movement.

In the use of this machine, the shoulders are alternately elevated and lowered, thus imitating exactly the movements executed in artificial respiration. The action of this apparatus being purely passive, the application may be somewhat extended—five to ten minutes or longer.

Cannon-ball Massage.— A cannon-ball (Fig. 134) covered with leather is a valuable mechanical accessory in the application of abdominal massage. The ball is simply rolled upon the abdomen, following the course of the colon from right to left. A ball weighing from four to six pounds is usually employed. I have found the cannon-ball very useful when employed in connection with other measures of treatment. It has an advantage in that it may be employed by the patient himself. It should be used for fifteen minutes morning and evening. In the morning it may be employed just before rising, or half an hour after breakfast.

The Shot-bag.— This is simply a bag containing a quantity of fine shot. The weight should be three or four pounds. It is used in a manner similar to the cannon-ball, being slowly rolled along the colon from right to left. In the writer's experience the shot-bag is less convenient for use in most cases than the cannon-ball. It is, however, better suited to cases in which there is a considerable degree of abdominal tenderness.

The Weighted Compress.— A quilted compress (Fig. 135) containing several pounds of fine shot, large enough to cover the anterior portion of the abdomen with the patient lying down, has been recommended and successfully used as an aid in inducing intestinal activity. The weighted compress acts simply by increasing the intra-abdominal tension, thus compelling the patient to breathe with greater vigor, and thereby administering to himself a sort of automatic massage to the abdominal contents, through the descent of the diaphragm, and compression of the organs between the diaphragm and the weighted abdominal wall. The cannon-ball may sometimes be advantageously employed in connection with the weighted compress.

The chief advantage of the cannon-ball, shot-bag, and weighted compress is that they may be used by the patient himself, without the assistance of the masseur. In the majority of chronic cases requiring abdominal massage, they are, however, scarcely sufficient in themselves to accomplish the results desired, but may be employed as useful adjuvants.

Muscle Beaters.—Some twelve or fourteen years ago, Klemm, a German empiric, introduced his so-called "muscle beater," consisting of elastic rubber tubes attached to a handle, which were used as a sort of cat-o'-nine-tails in whipping and flagellating various parts of the body. The inventor created quite an impression for a time by the cures effected by this simple means alone ; but the muscle beater is certainly a very imperfect substitute for massage, although it acts quite effectively in stimulating the surface circulation.

The muscle beater may be most advantageously employed upon thick and fleshy masses, and upon those portions of the body which are but slightly sensitive, as the back. The mode of application by a masseur is shown in Fig. 136. When the muscle beater is used by the patient in self-treatment, but one beater is ordinarily employed.

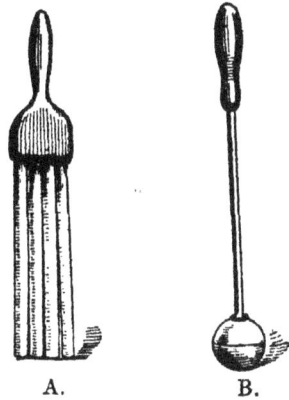

A.
Klemm's Muscle
Beater.

B.
Ball Muscle
Beater.

FIG. 138.

Various forms of muscle beaters have been devised. A form which I have found more convenient than that invented by Klemm (Fig. 138, A) consists of one or more rubber balls attached to a flexible rattan or whalebone handle (Fig. 138, B). One, two, or more balls may be employed, and of any size desired. The last-described form is an American invention.

Electric Massage.—Various appliances have been proposed for administering massage by means of a specially constructed electrode, thus applying massage and electricity at

the same time. A much better mode is the application of
electricity through the hand, by connecting the patient with
one pole, while the masseur connects himself with the other
pole by grasping the electrode with his other hand or fasten-
ing it about his arm. The application of electricity through
the hand is often useful, and sometimes even necessary;
but I have never been able to see any special advantage in
the simultaneous application of massage and electricity otherwise than in the employment of the electrical current by the
hand either held upon a fixed point, as in passive touch, or
with gentle stroking. My experience with various forms of
massage electrodes has led me to discard them as worthless.

SCIENTIFIC PHYSICAL TRAINING.

A difficulty which has been experienced by every intelligent physician who has undertaken to prescribe calisthenics, gymnastics, or any other form of exercise for his patients, is the lack of precise knowledge as to the strength of the patient, and the kind and amount of exercise appropriate in any given case. In a paper[1] which, with the apparatus to be presently described, was by request presented before the International Statistical Congress held in connection with the World's Fair at Chicago, I endeavored to show how this difficulty may be met; and, believing that at least some of those into whose hands this book may fall will be interested in this subject, I herewith present the substance of the paper referred to : —

Some twenty years ago I began the employment of calisthenics and Swedish movements, manual and mechanical, in the treatment of chronic invalids. A few years later I visited Stockholm, Sweden, and spent a short time under the tutelage of Professor Hartelius, in order to become better acquainted with the Ling system. For the past fifteen or more years I have made gymnastics a very prominent feature in the treatment of invalids of all classes coming under my care at the Battle Creek Sanitarium, and in this time have subjected to various forms of exercise, as a curative means, more than ten thousand invalids.

Early in my experience I became convinced that we have in voluntary muscular exercise one of the most powerful means of modifying nutrition. A more mature experience has fully established me in the belief that muscular exercise is one of the most valuable of all therapeutic agents. From the outset of my use of exercise as a means of cure, I appreciated a difficulty doubtless experienced by every person who has undertaken to make a definite prescription for exercise which should be

[1] "A New Dynamometer for Use in Anthropometry."

closely adapted to the needs of the individual for whom the prescription was made. This difficulty is found to be much greater in the employment of exercise for invalids than for that class of persons who usually come under the care of the physical director, owing to the greater degree of muscular asymmetry which is commonly encountered in invalid adults. In fact, it is a very rare exception to find among adults a person whose habits of life have not been such as to allow important muscular groups to fall into a state of idleness. This is well attested by the fact that such deformities as hollow chest, round shoulders, prominent abdomen, curvature of the spine, forward carriage of the head, and similar abnormalities are so prevalent that the majority of men and women who have reached the age of forty years or over, furnish illustrations of one or more of these defects. Among chronic invalids especially, it is exceptional to find a person who does not present asymmetry in some of the forms which I have shown in a series of outline studies of the human figure, presented elsewhere.[1]

In dealing with this class of patients, I experienced very great difficulty in adapting my prescriptions for exercise. to individual cases. In fact, I found myself constantly at a loss to know exactly what my patient needed, and was frequently embarrassed by the fact that, notwithstanding the exercise of the greatest possible care in making a prescription which I thought to be suited to my patient's needs, I had done harm rather than good, owing to the failure to recognize weaknesses which were quite as serious, though less manifest, than those which my prescription was intended to relieve, and which required a very different sort of treatment. I made use of the usual methods of anthropometry, exercising the greatest care in taking my measurements, only to be disconcerted by the fact that patients not infrequently decreased in measurement

[1] "Outline Studies of the Human Figure, Comprising 118 Figures, which Embody the Results of Several Thousand Observations, Embracing Studies of a Number of Different Civilized and Uncivilized Races."

while gaining in strength, or were discouraged by making little or no change in their dimensions, notwithstanding hard and persevering efforts in the gymnasium.

I soon discovered that measurements are of very little value indeed in dealing with adult invalids, however useful they may be in the management of the physical training of growing boys and girls and undeveloped youths. I learned that quality, rather than quantity, of muscle was the important thing in dealing with adults — at least invalid adults. Through the assistance of Professor Sargent, I possessed myself of all the various forms of dynamometers which had been constructed for use in testing the strength of the muscles of the human body. I found, however, that these dynamometers had so little range of adaptability that only a few muscular groups could be studied by their aid ; and, finding myself daily embarrassed in consequence of my inability to meet the requirements of my patients, and being unable to avoid most unhappy blunders in my exercise prescriptions, in sheer despair I sought to devise some accurate means for testing the strength, which could be adapted to the principal muscular groups of the body.

Having become accustomed in the physiological laboratory, to the use of the mercurial column as a pressure indicator, I adopted this as a source of resistance, and arranged a simple apparatus consisting of a closed cistern containing about half an inch of mercury, which received the lower end of a long piece of barometer tubing. The space above the mercury in the cistern was completely filled with water ; and with the cistern was connected, by means of three or four feet of rubber tubing, a strong rubber bulb about the size of an ordinary atomizer bulb. This was also completely filled with water. By compression of the bulb, the water contained in it was forced through the tube into the cistern, displacing an equal quantity of mercury, which was forced up into the glass tube. I found that a tube nine feet in height was sufficient to provide for as much resistance as was needed to balance all the force that could be brought to bear by a strong man in pressing the bulb. By means of various accessories, I arranged to apply to this bulb the force exerted by each of the principal muscular groups of the body,—extensors as well as flexors,— including the muscles of the trunk.

I encountered various difficulties, however, the chief of which were the gradual deterioration of the rubber bulb by use, and the frequent admission of air into the cistern by a change in the level of the rubber bulb, causing the mercury column to disappear from the glass tube. Closure of the upper end of the glass tube enabled me to shorten the tube, and diminish some difficulties, but it increased others. After several years of experimentation with the various forms of apparatus, I finally substituted a steel cylinder and piston for the rubber bulb, and connected this with the cistern by a metal tube, placing the apparatus upon a carriage which was made to slide up and down a vertical rod, so that there should be at no time any change in the relative positions of the cylinder and the cistern. In this arrangement I substituted oil for water, as in using water the steel cylinder and piston would soon become useless from rust. To my dismay, however, I soon discovered that the oil entered into combination with the mercury, and in turn deposited an adhesive precipitate upon the sides of the cylinder, seriously interfering with the movements of the piston, which must necessarily be as sensitive and delicate as possible. I tried various kinds of liquids without any advantage. Finally, the thought occurred to me that the oil and mercury might be separated by means of water, the relative specific gravity of which would keep the oil above and the mercury below. This simple device enabled me to overcome the last serious difficulty in the construction of the machine; and some three years ago I had constructed the apparatus, of which a cut is shown on the next page (Fig. 139). This apparatus has since been in constant use in the physical culture department of the Sanitarium at Battle Creek, Mich.

The dynamometer shown by Professor Seaver in his work on anthropometry, and which he has had the kindness to commend,

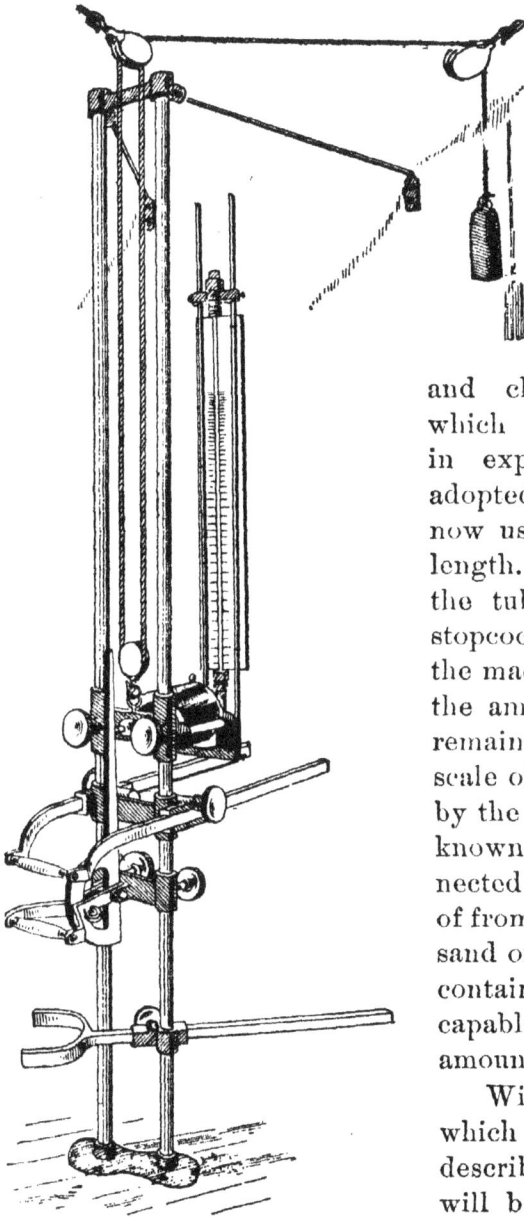

FIG. 139. DYNAMOMETER FOR TEST-
ING THE STRENGTH OF THE MUSCLES
(AUTHOR'S).

is my first instrument, which I discarded several years ago for the improved form which I have very briefly described. In order to dispense with the long tube, Professor Seaver suggested using a shorter tube, and closing the upper end, which I had previously done in experimentation. I have adopted this suggestion, and now use a tube one meter in length. At the upper end of the tube is placed a metallic stopcock, which is closed after the machine is adjusted, so that the amount of air in the tube remains always the same. The scale of the instrument is made by the application of weights of known value to the lever connected with it, and has a range of from one pound to one thousand or more pounds, as the air contained within the tube is capable of affording an infinite amount of resistance.

With this dynamometer, which I have very imperfectly described, but which I think will be clearly understood by reference to the accompanying cut, I have made, and had made by my assistants, careful tests of the strength of the principal groups of muscles in several thousand adults — both men and women. The muscular groups tested are as follows : For the upper extremities, hand flexors and extensors, forearm pronators and supinators, arm flexors and extensors, deltoid, latissimus dorsi, pectorals, and shoulder retractors ; for the lower extremities, foot flexors and extensors, leg flexors and extensors, thigh flexors and extensors, thigh abductors and adductors ; for the trunk, anterior, posterior, and right and left lateral muscular groups ; for the neck, anterior, posterior, and right and left lateral muscles ; for the thorax, the force of waist and chest expansion. Expiration and inspiration are also measured by means of Waldenburg's pneumatometer.

The accompanying physical charts (Charts I and II) are reduced copies of those which I use for recording the condition of the muscular system of my patients. These charts are constructed on a percental plan somewhat similar to that followed by Professor Seaver in his anthropometric chart. In making these charts, based upon the examination of six hundred men and a like number of women, the figures obtained for each group of muscles were arranged in a column in regular order, from the highest down to the lowest. The average of fifty per cent of those found in the middle column was obtained, and put down in the center of the corresponding column on my chart. Forty-five per cent, reaching five per cent above the upper level of the middle fifty per cent, were next added together, the average found, and the result placed in the same column, just above the previous result. Forty per cent, thirty-five per cent, and so on down to one per cent of the numbers above the middle, were cut out in like manner, the averages found, and the results properly placed. Proceeding in a similar manner, the figures were obtained for the lower half of the column. By treating the data obtained for each group of muscles in the body in this manner, I obtained a chart upon which I could make a graphic representation of the strength of the body, just as bodily dimensions have heretofore been

PHYSICAL CHART

Arranged from the results obtained in testing the strength of the individual groups of muscles in 500 WOMEN, by means of a Universal Mercurial Dynamometer, made and compiled under the direction of J. H. KELLOGG, M. D., Superintendent of the Sanitarium and Hospital, Battle Creek, Michigan.

Except when Otherwise Indicated, Quantities are Expressed in Pounds Avoirdupois.

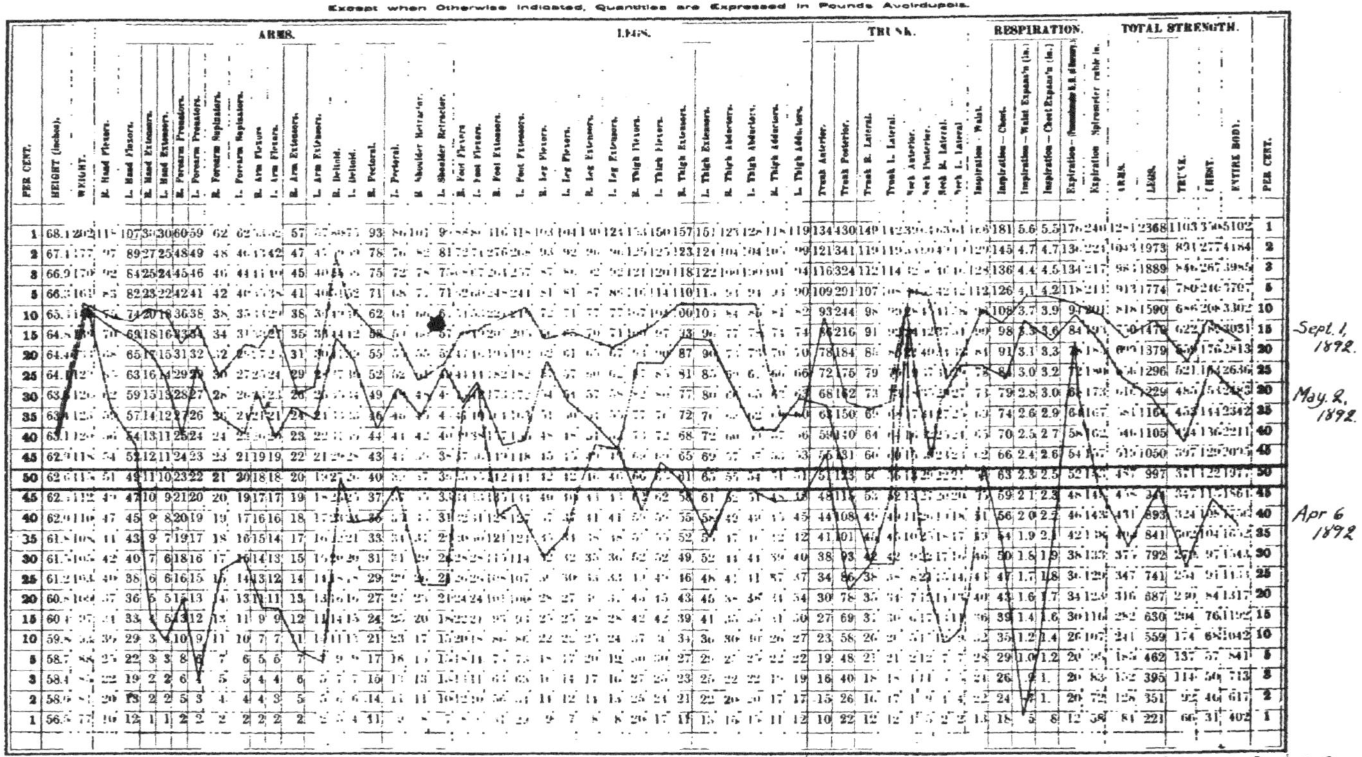

Label			
PER CENT.			
HEIGHT (inches).			
WEIGHT.			
R. Hand Flexors.			
L. Hand Flexors.			
R. Hand Extensors.			
L. Hand Extensors.			
R. Forearm Pronators.			
L. Forearm Pronators.			
R. Forearm Supinators.			
L. Forearm Supinators.			
R. Arm Flexors.			
L. Arm Flexors.			
R. Arm Extensors.			
L. Arm Extensors.			
R. Deltoid.			
L. Deltoid.			
R. Pectoral.			
L. Pectoral.			
R. Shoulder Retractor.			
L. Shoulder Retractor.			
R. Foot Flexors.			
L. Foot Flexors.			
R. Foot Extensors.			
L. Foot Extensors.			
R. Leg Flexors.			
L. Leg Flexors.			
R. Leg Extensors.			
L. Leg Extensors.			
R. Thigh Flexors.			
L. Thigh Flexors.			
R. Thigh Extensors.			
L. Thigh Extensors.			
R. Thigh Abductors.			
L. Thigh Abductors.			
R. Thigh Adductors.			
L. Thigh Adductors.			
Trunk Anterior.			
Trunk Posterior.			
Trunk R. Lateral.			
Trunk L. Lateral.			
Neck Anterior.			
Neck Posterior.			
Neck R. Lateral.			
Neck L. Lateral.			
Inspiration — Waist.			
Inspiration — Chest.			
Inspiration — Waist Expans'n (in.)			
Inspiration — Chest Expans'n (in.)			
Expiration — (Spirometer U.S. of Mercury.)			
Expiration Spirometer cubic in.			
ARMS.			
LEGS.			
TRUNK.			
CHEST.			
ENTIRE BODY.			
PER CENT.			

Section groupings: ARM. | LEG. | TRUSK. | RESPIRATION. | TOTAL STRENGTH.

Strength Measurements of _Miss D._

Taken Apr. 6, 1892. ___ May 2, 1892. ___ Sept. 4, 1892. ___ 189___ by ___

Apr. 6 1892
May 2, 1892.
Sept. 1, 1892.

CHART I.

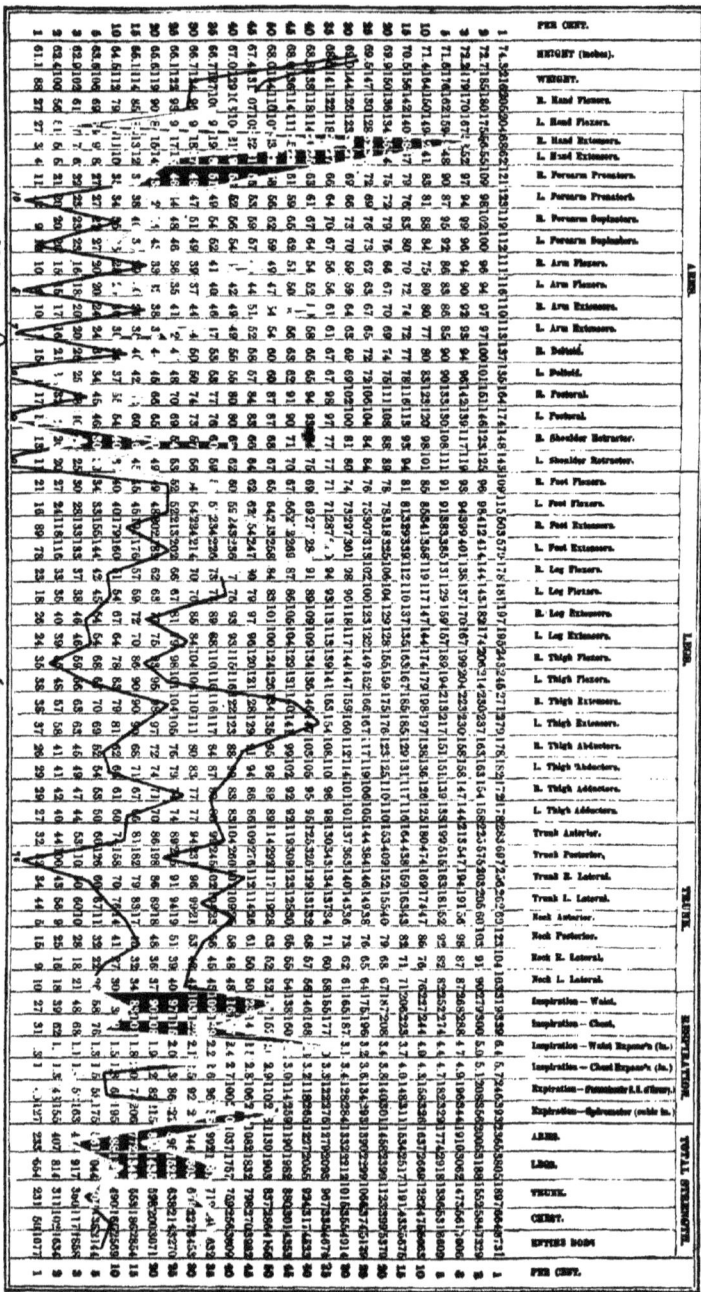

CHART II.

graphically represented upon anthropometric charts and tables.

At the right-hand side of the chart are arranged five columns for the totals of the arms, legs, trunk, chest, and the entire body, so as to bring under the eye at a single glance both the relative and the actual strength of the principal divisions of the body.

I have also prepared two other sets of tables, one based upon the examination of two hundred healthy men between twenty and thirty years of age, the other upon the data obtained from testing an equal number of women of the same age. This chart differs from the other chiefly in that the figures start at a higher level. In transferring the graphic representation of a person's muscular strength from one of these tables to another, I find that the characteristic features, although slightly modified, always remain the same.

As a further test of the value of the chart, I have platted the figures obtained for the various groups of muscles, and find that excellent curves are made. In the case of the left foot flexors, for example, an almost absolutely perfect binomial curve is obtained. The best test, however, for the value of this method of obtaining a basis for a prescription for exercise, is the fact that it meets in a most admirable manner the purposes for which it was designed.

The data afforded furnish exact information concerning the capacity of each of the principal groups of muscles in the body. Knowing the capacity of each muscle, it is easy to proportion the work in such a manner as to secure symmetry of development. My plan for accomplishing this is as follows : —

Taking 300,000 foot-pounds, one sixth of a full day's work, as the proper daily amount of exercise for a man whose total strength capacity is 10,000 pounds, corresponding very nearly to the greatest capacity shown upon my table prepared from two hundred young men in vigorous health, I have undertaken to establish a definite relation between the strength capacity and the total amount of work to be performed. This is accomplished by simply dividing the total amount of work done, by the total capacity of the muscles; that is, 1,800,000 is divided by 10,000, giving 180. In other words, for each pound of capacity, the muscles are capable of doing 180 foot-pounds of work daily, an interesting physiological fact thus for the first time determined. One sixth of 180 is 30. Hence it is clear that in a symmetrically developed man, with a total strength capacity of 10,000 pounds, each muscle, in order to do its proportion of the 300,000 foot-pounds prescribed, must do work to the amount of thirty times its lifting capacity represented in foot-pounds. It is only necessary, then, in order to ascertain the exact amount of work to be done by each group of muscles at each level, to multiply by thirty the figures of each column of the chart.

I have made a careful approximate calculation of the amount of work done in each exercise or set of exercises, with each apparatus in the gymnasium under my supervision. It is necessary to know the strength of the medicine as well as the needs of the patient. Knowing the amount of work required for each individual and for each set of muscles, and also the result obtained from each exercise, it is easy to construct tables of exercises exactly adapted to any capacity. I have arranged ten series of such tables, or day's orders, five for each of the two charts.

In making a prescription for exercise, I first note the total capacity of the individual, and then write down a number indicating the day's order which would secure for an individual of the given capacity the proper amount of work. Then, glancing over the chart, I note the low points, and check or underscore each of these, which indicates to the assistant who superintends the exercise in the gymnasium, that the work is to be doubled on all such points, so as to secure to the weak muscles such rapid development and growth as will enable them to overtake the rest of the muscles, and thus restore muscular symmetry. In practice, I find that this method never results in giving to a muscle more than a full day's work, and consequently there is no danger of injury resulting from this doubling of the amount of work to be done by the weak muscles. In case of complete paralysis of the muscle, it is of course necessary, at the beginning, to administer the exercise by electrical or mechanical means.

As a rule, I find it sufficient, for practical purposes, to divide the series of total capacities represented upon my table into five groups, instead of making a distinct schedule of work at each of the levels indicated by the several quantities representing total muscular capacity.

The ratio which I have established between the muscular capacity and the day's work is probably too small for those in vigorous health ; but I find it well suited to the class of persons coming under my observation, who are for the most part invalids or semi-invalids. The man who is in training, and desires to develop his whole body to its highest capacity, should be required to execute a full day's work, — 1,800,000 foot-pounds, or even more. In arranging a day's order of exercise, due account is of course taken of the work done in walking, running, and similar exercises which may be made a part of the program.

The patient does not undertake the first day to do all the exercises prescribed in the series, but gradually takes them up from day to day as he learns them, and becomes able to do them ; and by the end of two or three weeks, he is expected to have thoroughly mastered all the exercises given him, and to have become able to take each day all that is directed in his prescription. At the end of a month, another chart is made, the changes noted, and a new prescription prepared according to the requirements. It is a matter of frequent observation that the points which at the first examination are lowest on the chart, are so improved by the specific exercise directed to these particularly weak muscles that they become the highest ones upon the second chart.

The advantages of this mode of studying the condition of the muscular system, and the great change which may be effected by a precise and definite prescription for exercise, in combination with massage and manual and mechanical Swedish movements, is well shown in Chart I, which represents the muscular condition of a young woman at three different dates ; respectively, April 6, May 2, and September 1, 1892. The great irregularities of the first tracing, and the low levels reached by many of the arm groups of muscles, with the low level of the total strength, indicate a very weak and un-symmetrical development at the beginning. The young woman was stooped, round shouldered, hollow-chested, pale, anæmic, and possessed of very little vigor. Less than a month later, when the second tracing was taken, the patient had made a gain of nearly 800 pounds in total strength, the greater part of the gain having been made in the arms, which in the beginning were very much weaker than the legs, but which by special attention had become proportionately stronger than the legs. The chest had also gained even more than the arms, so that this portion of the muscular system was slightly in the ascendency. At this time another prescription was made, the effects of which appear in the further improvement shown by the test made September 1. By comparison of the totals, it will be seen that the asymmetry had largely disappeared.

No person is ever found whose chart gives a perfectly straight line ; but the nearer the approach to a straight line across the chart, the more perfect, of course, the symmetry.

At the time of the last test, September 1, this unsymmet-rical, feeble young woman would certainly have been pro-nounced one of more than average vigor and of excellent symmetry. She carried herself erect, her chest had become full and the respiratory movements deeper, and the whole body shared in the increase in physical vigor and stamina acquired by the muscular system.

By means of this method, it is possible to obtain exact knowledge respecting the requirements of each individual case. Possessed of this, it is not difficult to make a prescrip-tion which will be exactly adapted to the wants of the patient. It is possible to make, in less than a minute's time, a prescription which is more perfectly adapted to the needs of the individual examined, than could be made by the most elaborate study and the consumption of any amount of time, without the aid of the accurate data obtained by this method.

One of the charts herewith presented, that of Mr. A. (Chart II), shows the value of this mode of investigation in the diagnosis of morbid conditions affecting the motor system. The patient was suffering from paresis of the left arm. This would be apparent from the chart alone, without other evidence, as will be readily seen. The dynamometer picks out the particular groups of muscles which are affected by paresis or paralysis, and thus gives important indications respecting the location of the central lesion, of which the paralysis is merely a symptom. This chart also shows, in a most interesting manner, the value of the dynamometer as a means of indicating the progress made by a paretic patient under treatment.

Another advantage in this mode of studying the motor apparatus is the fact that the dynamometer tests not only the muscles, but the nerves and nerve centers as well, so that it is a precise measure of the condition of the individual's motor apparatus. It is a true measure of the dynamic energy of the body, and shows the actual ability of the individual to manifest energy through his muscular system as a whole, and through each particular part of it. The tape line merely gives the dimensions of a man,—it tells nothing as to whether he is alive or dead. The dynamometer gives us an accurate description of the living, active man. The chart obtained by means of a dynamometer enables the physical director to make a precise prescription for exercise without even seeing the subject, whereas the data furnished by the measurements of the tape line may relate to a man who is dead, or so completely paralyzed that all forms and degrees of exercise are alike impossible; so that without the aid of the dynamometer, anthropometry is a most unreliable guide and almost altogether useless, unless the subject is before the director, who, even then, is obliged to depend upon his intuitions and experience in arranging a pro-

13

gram for gymnastic work, rather than upon the indications of the tape line.

After several years' use of my dynamometer and the charts which it has enabled me to prepare, I am so thoroughly dependent upon these means of directing the gymnastic work of my patients that I should be quite at a loss to know how to prescribe for them without this or some other equally good means of exact diagnosis.

I ought, perhaps, to have said another word respecting the method of using the dynamometer. I have worked out an exact mode for testing each group of muscles. This method is followed with care in each test made. The general principle which I have followed is that the resistance of the dynamometer should be applied at the distal end of the bone which is operated upon by the group of muscles under examination, and in such a manner as to give the muscle an opportunity to act to the best advantage, at the same time isolating its action from that of other groups which might vitiate the results obtained.

I should not conclude this description of my dynamometer and the mode of using it without acknowledging my indebtedness to Dr. Jay W. Seaver, Professor Frank W. Howe, A. M., and Mr. M. W. Newton, who were acquainted with the instrument in the early stages of its development, for valuable suggestions which were utilized in its improvement; also to Dr. W. A. George, who compiled for me the first set of tables based upon the data obtained by the use of the dynamometer.

I am glad to be able to say at the present date (February, 1895), that the apparatus described has been adopted in the physical culture department of Yale, by the Government Military Training School at West Point, the Madison (Wis.) University, and by a number of other leading educational institutions and gymnasiums, as a basis for accurate work in physical training.

STUDIES OF INDIVIDUAL AND COMPARA-
TIVE MUSCULAR STRENGTH IN
MEN AND WOMEN.

A most interesting line of research which the dynamometer has enabled me to undertake, is a comparative study of
the muscular system in men and women. The studies of
this subject heretofore made have been chiefly based upon the
results obtained by the use of the tape line, which, as has
already been remarked, are practically valueless, and always
misleading. A few studies have been made by Quetelet and
others, based upon such incomplete tests as the strength of
the grasp of the hand, the weight which can be dragged over
a level surface, etc.; but the facts presented have been so
fragmentary as to be of little practical value.

In my personal studies by the aid of the dynamometer, the
principal comparisons which have been made are as follows,
the figures given (Table I, columns I-XIII) being based upon
the study of two hundred healthy men between the ages of
eighteen and thirty years, and an equal number of healthy
women of the same ages : —

1. A comparative table of the actual strength of each of
the several groups of muscles, and of all the muscles of each
of the principal divisions of the body, in the average man and
the average woman.

2. The relative strength of each group of muscles and of
the muscles of each division of the body, and also of the total
muscular strength, as compared with the average weight of
the body.

3. The strength of each group of muscles, of the muscles
of each of the principal divisions of the body, and of the total

strength of the body, compared with the average height in inches.

4. The strength of each group of muscles, and of the muscles of each of the principal divisions of the body, as compared with the total strength.

5. The strength of each group of muscles (right and left together) as compared with the strength of the corresponding division of the body.

6. The strength of the muscles of the left side of the body as compared with those of the right side of the body.

7. The strength of each group of muscles, of the muscles of each division of the body, and the total strength, in women, as compared with the same in men.

8. The strength of each group of muscles as compared with the antagonizing group.

9. The strength of the muscles of the arms as compared with the homologous, or corresponding, muscles of the legs.

10. A study of the muscular strength of men as compared with that of women of the same height.

11. A study of the muscular strength in short men and short women as compared respectively with that of tall men and tall women.

In a special paper the author will give an exhaustive statement of the results obtained by these various studies, only a few of which can be admitted to this work, for want of space.

In the accompanying table (Table I) will be found the figures indicating the principal of these relations, which are made more evident by a series of graphic diagrams presented in connection with the paper referred to.

The Relative Strength of the Various Groups of Muscles. — In Table II the figures which indicate the strength of each individual group of muscles for the average man and the average woman, are arranged in the order of their relative strength. It will be observed that the order in the two columns is not the same. Interesting differences and facts, a few only of which will be mentioned here, occur at many points: —

TABLE II.

TABULAR ARRANGEMENT OF THE SEVERAL GROUPS OF MUSCLES WITH REFERENCE TO THEIR RELATIVE STRENGTH.

MEN.		WOMEN.	
Muscles of Inspiration (pneumatometer)	.9	Muscles of Inspiration (pneumatometer)	.4
Muscles of Expiration (pneumatometer)	2.6	Muscles of Expiration (pneumatometer)	1.4
Neck Anterior	35	Neck Anterior	19
Hand Extensors	54	Hand Extensors	29
Neck Posterior	75	Neck Posterior	37
Arm Flexors	120	Arm Flexors	48
Neck Lateral	126	Arm Extensors	53
Arm Extensors	127	Forearm Supinators	57
Forearm Pronators	134	Forearm Pronators	57
Trunk Anterior	139	Neck Lateral	60
Deltoid	140	Deltoid	71
Forearm Supinators	143	Trunk Anterior	73
Foot Flexors	145	Inspiration (waist)	79
Shoulder Retractors	160	Inspiration (chest)	85
Inspiration (waist)	172	Foot Flexors	89
Latissimus Dorsi	185	Shoulder Retractors	95
Inspiration (chest)	190	Latissimus Dorsi	99
Leg Flexors	200	Pectoral	102
Thigh Abductors	206	Leg Flexors	116
Pectoral	209	Leg Extensors	123
Thigh Adductors	227	Hand Flexors	125
Leg Extensors	237	Thigh Abductors	135
Hand Flexors	249	Thigh Adductors	142
Trunk Lateral	287	Trunk Lateral	154
Thigh Flexors	303	Chest	166
Thigh Extensors	330	Trunk Posterior	173
Chest	365	Thigh Extensors	174
Trunk Posterior	380	Thigh Flexors	179
Foot Extensors	614	Left Arm	363
Left Arm	751	Foot Extensors	364
Right Arm	770	Right Arm	373
Trunk	1042	Trunk	516
Right Leg	1131	Left Leg	659
Left Leg	1131	Right Leg	663
Chest and Trunk	1407	Chest and Trunk	682
Both Arms	1521	Both Arms	736
Both Legs	2262	Both Legs	1322
Entire Body	5190	Entire Body	2740

1. One of the most curious facts noted is that the foot extensors, or calf muscles, in the average woman, have a strength almost exactly equal to that of the left arm.

2. The anterior muscles of the neck, in both men and women, have about half the strength of the posterior.

3. The hand flexors in men have just twice the strength of the arm flexors; in women, the hand flexors are nearly three times as strong as the arm flexors.

4. The anterior muscles of the trunk, the deltoid, the forearm supinators, and the foot flexors have almost equal strength in man ; in woman, the forearm supinators, forearm pronators, and the lateral muscles of the neck may be similarly grouped.

5. In man, the forearm supinators are considerably stronger than the pronators, whereas in women they are of equal strength, although much weaker than in man, these muscles being, in the average man, 2 1-2 times as strong as in the average woman.

6. In man, again, the thigh abductors and the pectorals have almost the same strength capacity; in woman, a similar parallel exists between the leg extensors and the hand flexors, and another group is found in the muscles of the back, the thigh extensors, and the thigh flexors, which are in the average woman almost exactly equal in strength capacity.

7. In man, the latissimus dorsi and the muscles which move the upper chest in inspiration, are equal in strength ; while in woman a similar parallel exists between the latissimus dorsi, the pectorals, and the shoulder retractors.

8. The inspiratory powers of the waist and chest are practically equal in woman ; while in man the inspiratory power of the chest is perceptibly greater than that of the waist, although in each case the respiratory strength in man is double or more than double that of woman. This fact demonstrates the fallacy of the idea that restriction of the waist is a means of giving woman a superiority in upper chest development, and so acting as a preventive of pulmonary disease. Men, without waist constriction, have greater relative strength in the upper chest than have women.

9. The total strength of inspiration (chest) is, in women, just 1-8 that of the total for the chest and trunk.

10. The strength of one leg is almost exactly equal, in woman, to the strength of the chest and trunk ; in man, the total for the chest and trunk is considerably greater than that for either leg.

11. The waist-expanding capacity is almost exactly 1–2 that of the total for the two sides of the trunk, in woman.

12. The thigh extensors in man have a capacity more than six times that of the hand extensors ; while the foot extensors have a capacity almost exactly twelve times that of the hand extensors, and double that of the thigh flexors.

13. The strength of the arm extensors, in men, is almost exactly 1–12 that of the entire arm.

14. The strength of the deltoid is, in woman, almost exactly 1–2 that of the homologous muscles,—the thigh abductors.

15. The lateral muscles of the neck have half the strength of the hand flexors, in both men and women.

Many other interesting comparisons might be made, especially those which relate to the strength of each group of muscles as compared with the whole body. This is graphically shown in one of the diagrams referred to.

The Strength of Each Group of Muscles in the Average Woman as Compared with the Corresponding Group in the Average Man. — (Table I, column III.) By referring to Graphic I, in which is shown the actual strength of each group of muscles in the average woman as compared with the corresponding group in the average man, the strength of man being taken as unity, it will be seen at once that the strength of the average woman falls far below that of the average man. A few comparisons will be found interesting : —

1. The thigh abductors, the group which is relatively strongest in women, have less than 2–3 the strength of the corresponding group in the average man ; while the total strength of the average woman is but a trifle more than half that of the average man (53 per cent).

2. The following groups of muscles in woman possess a relative strength of more than 1–2 that in man : Latissimus

dorsi, shoulder retractors, foot flexors and extensors, leg and thigh flexors and extensors, thigh abductors, thigh adductors, anterior trunk muscles, lateral trunk muscles, anterior muscles of the neck, muscles of expiration, as measured by the pneumatometer, and the leg muscles as a whole.

3. The following groups of muscles have, in the average woman, a relative strength of less than 1–2 that in the average man: Forearm pronators, forearm supinators, arm flexors, arm extensors, pectorals, muscles of inspiration, and the total for the muscles of the arms. The muscles of the arm, especially those of the forearm and those which act upon the forearm, are relatively the weakest muscles in the average woman.

4. The reasons for the unusual weakness of certain groups of muscles in women, are, in some instances at least, quite apparent. The weakness of the arm muscles is explained by the fact that women engage less than do men in laborious employments.

5. The legs are relatively stronger than the arms in women, for the reason that the amount of exertion by the legs is more nearly equal in the two sexes than in the case of the arms. The greater strength of the thigh flexors is, perhaps, due to the fact that the bones of the legs are, in women, shorter than in men, so that the muscles acting upon the thigh have a better leverage than in men. The same reason will hold good for the thigh abductors and adductors, which are relatively the strongest muscles possessed by the average woman. The greater width of hips perhaps affords another anatomical advantage to the muscles of the thigh in women.

These observations are entirely in harmony with the interesting fact pointed out by Quetelet and Sargent that the thigh is not only proportionately, but actually, larger in women than in men. The thigh is found to be relatively larger even in girls of twelve, and in girls of fifteen it is two inches larger than in boys of the same age. Increase in the size of the thigh is, in fact, one of the very first of all the sexual characteristics of a physical nature which appears as the girl ap-

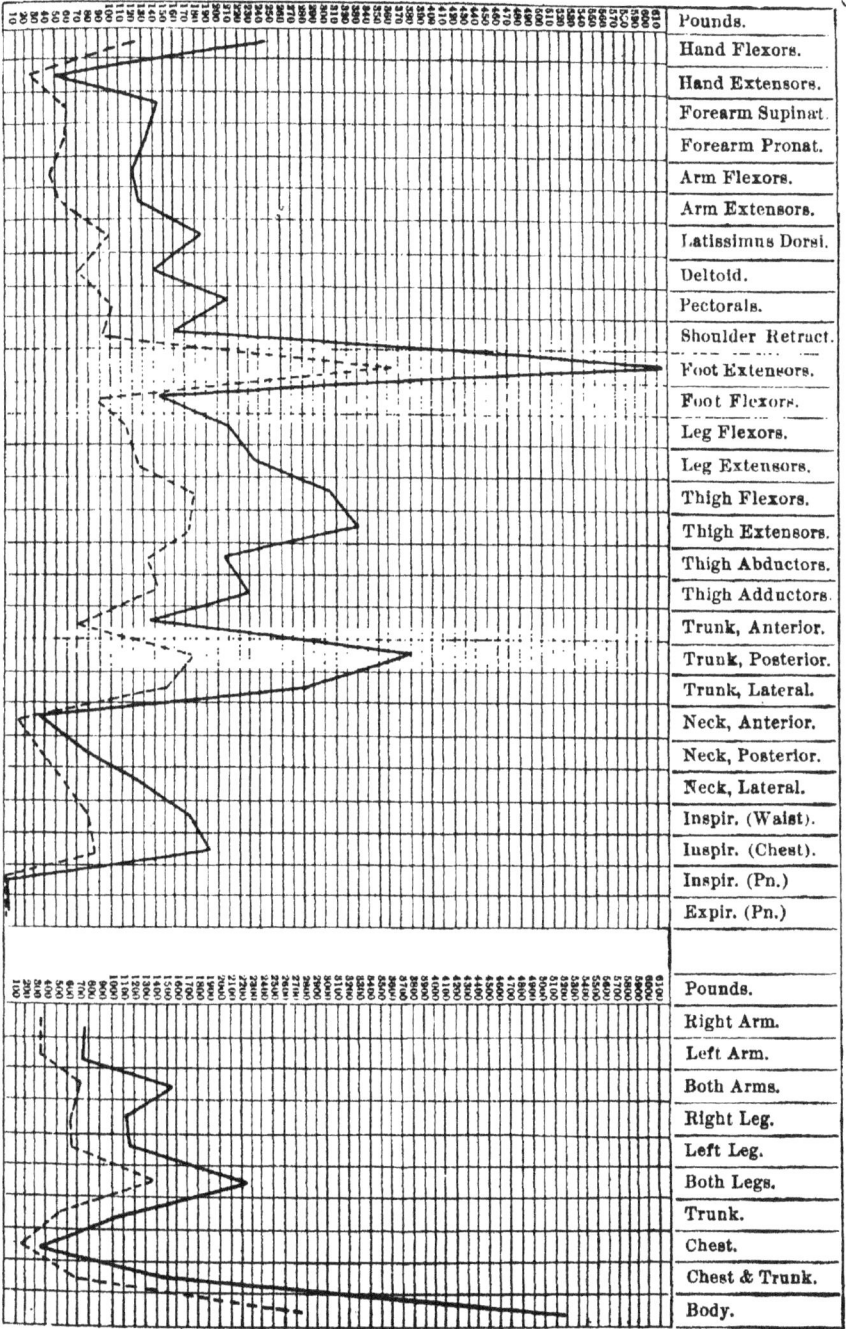

Pounds.

Hand Flexors.

Hand Extensors.

Forearm Supinat.

Forearm Pronat.

Arm Flexors.

Arm Extensors.

Latissimus Dorsi.

Deltoid.

Pectorals.

Shoulder Retract.

Foot Extensors.

Foot Flexors.

Leg Flexors.

Leg Extensors.

Thigh Flexors.

Thigh Extensors.

Thigh Abductors.

Thigh Adductors.

Trunk, Anterior.

Trunk, Posterior.

Trunk, Lateral.

Neck, Anterior.

Neck, Posterior.

Neck, Lateral.

Inspir. (Waist).

Inspir. (Chest).

Inspir. (Pn.)

Expir. (Pn.)

Pounds.

Right Arm.

Left Arm.

Both Arms.

Right Leg.

Left Leg.

Both Legs.

Trunk.

Chest.

Chest & Trunk.

Body.

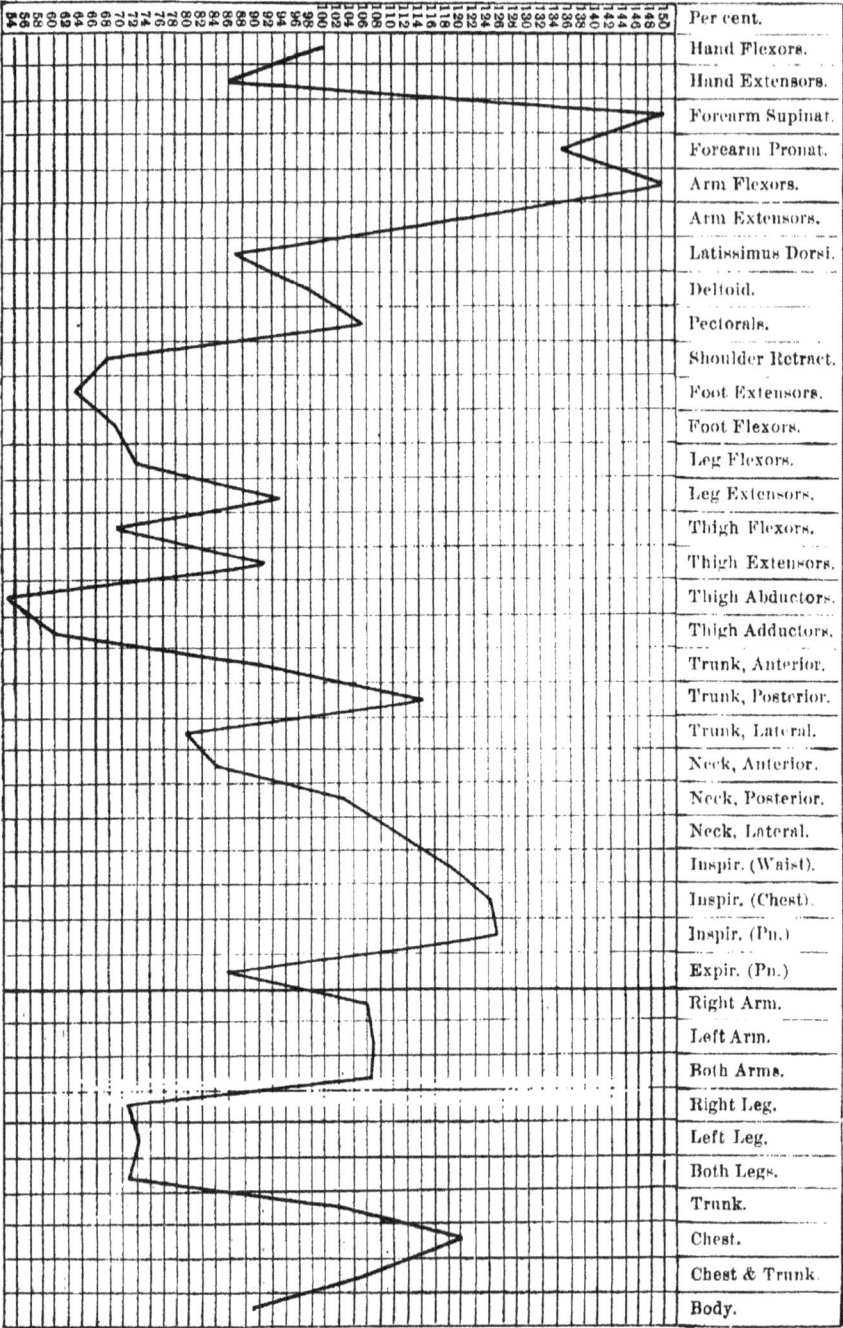

Per cent.

Hand Flexors.

Hand Extensors.

Forearm Supinat.

Forearm Pronat.

Arm Flexors.

Arm Extensors.

Latissimus Dorsi.

Deltoid.

Pectorals.

Shoulder Retract.

Foot Extensors.

Foot Flexors.

Leg Flexors.

Leg Extensors.

Thigh Flexors.

Thigh Extensors.

Thigh Abductors.

Thigh Adductors.

Trunk, Anterior.

Trunk, Posterior.

Trunk, Lateral.

Neck, Anterior.

Neck, Posterior.

Neck, Lateral.

Inspir. (Waist).

Inspir. (Chest).

Inspir. (Pn.)

Expir. (Pn.)

Right Arm.

Left Arm.

Both Arms.

Right Leg.

Left Leg.

Both Legs.

Trunk.

Chest.

Chest & Trunk.

Body.

proaches puberty. It is interesting to observe that the results obtained by the dynamometer entirely coincide in this particular with those noted by anthropometry.

Heretofore, there has been no means of knowing whether the larger thighs of women were the result of a greater pro. portionate development of the muscles, or simply a greater accumulation of adipose tissue. It is probable that both peculiarities in structure are present, but the dynamometer has clearly shown that the thighs in women are not only larger, but proportionately stronger, as compared with other muscles, than in men. As compared with men, the abductors are stronger in women of equal height, than in the average woman, the relation being 72 per cent for the former, as compared with 65 per cent for the latter.

Many of the facts already noted, and others, are made more clear by reference to Graphic II.

6. The muscles which are relatively weakest in women are the forearm pronators and supinators, and the arm flexors. The latter muscles are 2 1–2 times stronger in men.

7. A very marked superiority in favor of men is also noticeable in the muscles concerned in respiration.

The inspiratory strength of the waist and that of the chest, both as measured with the dynamometer and with the manometer, or pneumatometer, are relatively much weaker in women than in men, the disparity being : For waist inspiration, 1.18 ; chest inspiration, 1.24 ; and inspiration as measured by the pneumatometer, 1.25 ; or respectively, 2 1–5, 2 1–4, and 2 1–4 times greater strength for corresponding parts concerned in inspiration in man than in woman.

8. It is worthy of note, on the other hand, that the disparity in the case of expiratory strength, as measured by the manometer, is not so great, being only 86 per cent, or 1 6–7 times as great in man as in woman, the latter being unity. The explanation of this weakness of the inspiratory power in woman is clearly to be found in the impediment to inspiration afforded by the conventional mode of dress among

civilized nations, and the resulting deterioration in muscular structures. It is quite safe to predict that such a deficiency would not be found to exist in the case of savage women.

The obstacle existing in regard to inspiration does not exist in relation to expiration, since the constriction of the clothing would assist, rather than interfere with, expiration. If it be argued that the hindrance to inspiration presented by tight clothing ought to act as a sort of gymnastics and discipline of the respiratory muscles, whereby they would acquire greater strength, it is only necessary to say in reply that one of the best established principles in relation to muscular development is the fact that long-continued and unrelenting opposition to muscular movement finally results in the tiring out and disabling of a muscle, rather than in its superior development. This is clearly seen in various forms of spinal curvature, as well as in other acquired deformities.

9. The total for the chest falls at a point nearly as high as that for inspiration, the difference amounting to 1.20 in favor of the average man, indicating a total strength of the chest in the average man 2 1–5 times that of the average woman.

10. Another prominent point of weakness in women is found in the muscles of the back, which are in the average man 2 1–5 times stronger than in the average woman.

We have here one explanation of the constant complaint heard from women, of tired back. This undeveloped condition of the muscles of the trunk, particularly those of the back, may well be due to the constriction of corsets and tight skirt bands, and the consequent inability, as well as neglect, to make free use of the muscles of this portion of the body.

11. The pectoral muscles are also notably weak in women, which quite agrees with the weak inspiratory power of the chest previously referred to.

A number of other interesting facts will be learned by a careful study of Table I. These are more clearly shown in the graphic diagrams referred to, but which, for want of space, cannot be given here. A few points may be briefly mentioned, as follows : —

Relation of Strength to Height and Weight in Men and Women.— Without going into all the relations of strength to height and weight, which we have traced out, and which are based on the figures given in Table I, columns IV to VII, attention is called to the following as of especial interest : —

1. The strength of the average woman, in comparison with her weight, is less than 2–3 that of the average man, as compared with his weight.

2. The strength of the average woman, in comparison with her height, is only 4–7 that of the average man.

3. The total strength of the average woman as compared with the total strength of the average man is .53. The weight of the average woman as compared with that of the average man is .86. The height of the average woman as compared with that of the average man is .92. It thus appears that the average woman, while less than the average man in height, is still more inferior in weight, and presents a still higher degree of inferiority in strength. A comparative study of men and women between forty and fifty years of age would possibly show women to be somewhat less inferior in weight.

The full significance of these facts is recognized only when they are considered in connection with the law that weight increases with the cube of the height, whereas muscular strength increases only in the proportion of the square of the height. This principle gives the shorter individual an advantage over the taller, so that while, according to this law, we might expect to find women weaker than men, they should not be weaker than men in proportion to their height.

To make this point clearer, let us take an example : The average strength of 12 men, each 70 inches in height, was found to be 5483 lbs. The average strength of 14 men, each 65 inches in height, was found to be 4653 lbs. The calculated strength of the men, compared with that of the average man, is found to be exactly 5425 lbs.—only 58 lbs. less than the actual strength observed.

Applying the same rule in a comparison of men and women, the following result was obtained : The average strength of 25 men having an average height of 69 inches was found to be 4810 lbs.; the average strength of 34 women, 64 inches in height, was found to be 2652 lbs. The calculated strength of a woman 64 inches in height, obtained by the same rule, and taking the average strength of 25 men 69 inches in height as a basis, is 4130 lbs. By this we see that, applying the ratio of the square of the height as a means of determining the strength for a person of given height, women fall far short of the strength they should possess, the deficiency in the above case being 1478 lbs. In other words, the strength of woman is only 64 per cent of what it should be, as compared with man.

An actual comparison of men and women of the same height brought out the deficiency still more clearly. The average strength of 19 healthy women between the ages of eighteen and thirty years, 65 inches in height, was found to be 2660 lbs.; the average strength of 14 healthy men of the same age and the same height, was found to be 4653 lbs.

We find in these observations an interesting confirmation of the correctness of the principle that the strength of two persons of different height will be in direct ratio to the squares of their heights. It also appears that the actual facts, as observed by the comparison of the average strength of a large number of men and women of equal height, agree very closely with those shown by calculation, since the 19 women with an average strength of 2660 lbs. should have had an average strength equal to that of the 14 men, whereas they fell short 1993 lbs., or 43 per cent. According to this, the strength of the average woman is 57 per cent that of the average man of the same height.

4. The strongest single group of muscles in the body in relation to body weight is the foot extensor group, which, in men, lifts 4.4 times the weight of the body, and in women, 3.1 times the weight of the body.

5. The following groups of muscles in the average man (the muscles of both sides being included) are capable of lifting the entire weight of the body or more : Hand flexors, forearm supinators, deltoid, latissimus dorsi, pectoral, shoulder retractors, foot flexors, foot extensors, leg flexors, leg extensors, thigh flexors, thigh extensors, thigh abductors, thigh adductors, trunk anterior, trunk posterior, trunk lateral, inspiration (waist), inspiration (chest).

6. In women the hand flexors, foot extensors, leg extensors, thigh flexors, thigh extensors, thigh abductors, thigh adductors, trunk posterior, and trunk lateral are each able to sustain a weight equal to that of the body.

7. Those muscles which are able to lift a weight equal to that of the body in men but not in women, are the following : Forearm supinators, deltoid, latissimus dorsi, pectorals, shoulder retractors, foot flexors, leg flexors, trunk anterior, inspiration (waist), inspiration (chest).

8. It is interesting to note that the strength of each division of the body is more than sufficient to lift the entire body ; even the smallest total found — that for the chest in women — is able to lift 1 1-4 times the body weight. The highest total for a division of the body — that for the legs — indicates, in men, a strength 16 times that required to lift the body weight. The arms in men are able to lift 11 times the weight of the body, while the muscles of the chest and trunk combined are, in men, capable of lifting 10 times the body weight.

9. The foot extensors are, in men, a little less than fifty per cent stronger than in women, when compared with the body weight, although the flexors are but a little more than 1-3 stronger in men than in women.

10. The strength of the inspiratory muscles as compared with the body weight in men, is nearly twice that of women.

11. The lateral muscles of the neck have a strength, in relation to the weight of the body, nearly double that of the same muscles in women, a fact which is readily explained by the greater size of the head in men.

12. The back muscles are stronger in men, in proportion to total strength, doubtless in consequence of the heavier arms, shoulders, and head which these muscles are required to sustain.

Relation of Strength to Height.—In this relation, special interest attaches to the following figures, which express the number of pounds lifted for each inch in height:—

1. For men: arms, 22.5 ; legs, 33.4 ; trunk, 15.4 ; chest, 5.4 ; entire body, 76.7.

For women: arms, 11.7; legs, 21; trunk, 8.2; chest, 2.6; entire body, 43.6.

2. The strongest group of muscles in the body, in relation to height, is the foot extensors, which are able to lift a little more than 9 pounds for each inch in height, in men, and 5.78 pounds for each inch in height, in women.

Relative Strength of Flexor and Extensor Muscles.—(Table III.) It is evident that in order that bodily movements

TABLE III.

RELATIVE STRENGTH OF OPPOSING MUSCULAR GROUPS IN MEN AND WOMEN.

(The group first mentioned is taken as unity.)

MUSCULAR GROUPS.	MEN.	WOMEN.
Hand : Flexors — Extensors	4.61	4.31
Forearm : Supinators — Pronators	1.07	1.00
Arm : Flexors — Extensors	.94	.91
Latissimus Dorsi — Deltoid	1.32	1.39
Pectorals — Shoulder Retractors	1.31	1.07
Foot : Extensors — Flexors	4.23	4.09
Leg : Flexors — Extensors	.84	.94
Thigh : Flexors — Extensors	.92	1.03
Thigh : Abductors — Adductors	.91	.95
Trunk : Anterior — Posterior	.37	.42
Trunk : Right Lateral — Left Lateral	1.01	1.03
Neck : Anterior — Posterior	.47	.51
Neck : Right Lateral — Left Lateral	1.00	1.00
Inspiration — Expiration	.35	.29
Arms : Flexors — Extensors	1.47	1.41
Legs : Flexors — Extensors	1.41	1.50
Trunk : Flexors — Extensors	.58	.63
Entire Body : Flexors — Extensors	1.18	1.22

should be well balanced, the opposing muscles must be endowed with proportionate strength. With this fact in mind, the following comparisons are interesting : —

1. In the comparison of the relative strength of the flexor and extensor muscles, it is found that the greatest difference between the strength of the flexors and extensors exists in the case of the hand, in which, in men, the flexors have more than 4 1–2 times the strength of the extensors.

2. In the lower extremities, the foot extensors (corresponding anatomically to the hand flexors) are 4 times as strong as the opposing muscles.

3. The pronators and supinators of the arm are very closely balanced, as are also the arm flexors and extensors.

4. The latissimus dorsi is 1–3 stronger than the deltoid, and the pectorals are about 2–5 stronger than the shoulder retractors.

5. The leg flexors and extensors, thigh flexors and extensors, and thigh abductors and adductors, are very closely balanced.

6. The anterior trunk muscles are only 2–5 as strong as the posterior ; the muscles of the right and left side are of nearly equal strength.

7. The anterior neck muscles have a little less than 1–2 the strength of the posterior muscles ; while the lateral muscles of the neck, are of equal strength.

This relation of the anterior and posterior muscles of the trunk and neck is evidently the result of the greater work imposed upon the posterior muscles of the neck and trunk in sustaining the head and body.

8. The force of inspiration is but 1–3 that of expiration, as shown by the pneumatometer ; but with this statement must be considered the fact that the expiratory muscles have the assistance of the elasticity of the chest walls and of the lungs, which oppose inspiration, but aid expiration.

9. Coming to the totals, we find the muscles of the arms and legs standing upon a nearly equal footing. The flexors of the

arms are a little more than 50 per cent stronger than the extensors, while the flexors of the legs are slightly less than 1-2 stronger. In the trunk the extensors are stronger than the flexors, the flexors having a strength of only 60 per cent that of the extensors.

10. Considering the entire body, the flexors are in men 20 and in women 25 per cent stronger than the extensors.

These facts are interesting from a physiological standpoint, though the cause has not been fully determined. It is probable, however, that it is to be found in the greater amount of work which, as a rule, is imposed upon the flexors.

In comparing the figures for men and women, it is observed that they run remarkably close together, so that the above remarks, which are based chiefly upon the figures obtained for the average man, apply with almost equal exactness to the average woman. Practically, the only differences are the following : —

11. In men, the forearm supinators are a little stronger than the pronators.

The Strength of Each Group of Muscles, and of Each Division of the Body, as Compared with the Whole Body.—(Table I, columns VIII and IX.) The most prominent point brought out by this comparison is the fact that the strength of even the strongest group of muscles in the body — the foot extensors, the muscles of the calf — is small when compared with the total for the entire body.

1. The strength of the foot extensors is, in man, about 12 per cent, or 1-8 of the total strength.

2. Next in order are the muscles of the back, which have a capacity of .073 that of the body, or a little less than 1-14 of the total strength — about 1-2 the strength of the foot extensors.

3. The hand flexors have a strength of nearly 1-20 that of the body.

4. The lowest point, with the exception of expiration and inspiration, as measured by the pneumatometer, is reached by

the neck anterior, the capacity of which is only .7 per cent of the total for the entire body.

The Strength of Each Group of Muscles (right and left) as Compared with the Strength of the Corresponding Division.— (Table I, columns X and XI.) 1. The strength of the foot extensors is a little more than 1–4 the total for the legs.

2. The strength of the muscles of the back is more than 1–3 the strength of the entire trunk, exclusive of the chest.

3. The relative strength is found to be greater, in women, in the hand flexors, the hand extensors, the deltoid, the latissimus dorsi, the pectorals, and the shoulder retractors, as compared with the total for the arms. The foot extensors, the foot flexors, the thigh flexors, and the thigh abductors and adductors are also stronger in relation to the total for the legs, than in men. The anterior and lateral muscles of the trunk show a similar superiority; also the neck anterior muscles. It should be remembered, however, that in the total strength of the trunk muscles, the average woman is much inferior to the average man.

Strength of the Muscles of the Left Side of the Body as Compared with Those of the Right Side.— (Table I, columns XII and XIII.) In a symmetrically developed man, the muscles of the right and left sides should be found of equal strength, but the unequal training of the average man gives the right side of the body an advantage in the case of nearly every group.

1. In only three instances do the muscles of the left side exceed those of the right side, in the average man; viz., the thigh flexors, thigh extensors, and thigh adductors. Why the thigh flexors, extensors, and adductors should, in the average man, be stronger upon the left side than upon the right, is a question which I have not been able to settle. I have, however, for many years made this observation, and it is clearly shown in the average measurements made in more than one thousand men. It has occurred to me that, while we are right handed, we have a tendency to left-leggedness, and my

14

observations certainly seem to justify this idea , although the totals for the right and left leg are found to be exactly the same, a marked deficiency of the flexors and extensors of the left leg, as compared with the right, serving to counterbalance the excessive development of the thigh flexors, extensors, and adductors.

2. In the average woman, as in the average man, the left side is ahead of the right at three points. Curiously, however, none of these points coincide with the corresponding points in men. The points of left-side superiority in women are found in the shoulder retractors, foot flexors, and leg extensors.

3. In women, there is a greater degree of asymmetry, as regards bilateral development, than in men. The total strength of the left side of the body, in men, is 99 per cent that of the right side, so that the two sides of the body are very nearly balanced. In women, the total strength of the left side, as compared with the right, is a little less, or 98.6 per cent. This is what we should expect from the inferiority of woman, in relation to man, in muscular development.

Comparison of the Muscular Strength of Tall Men with That of Short Men.— (Table I, columns XIV to XVI.) The average heights of the groups compared were respectively: for tall men (15), 71.5 inches; for short men (39), 64 inches. No height in either group varied from the average more than one half inch.

In a comparative study of tall men and short men, it was found that tall men are at nearly every point stronger than short men. The total strength capacity for a short man was found to be 90 per cent that of a tall man. At four points only are short men superior to tall men; namely, the lateral and posterior muscles of the neck, the trunk laterals, and the deltoid.

The reasons for this difference are interesting. As has long been known, the difference between the height of short men and tall men is chiefly due to the difference in the length of the legs. The arms of the short man are longer in propor tion to his height than are the arms of the tall man. In view of this fact, we should expect to find the relative strength of the arms in short men greater than that of the legs. In the case of the muscles of the trunk and neck, the short man has an evident advantage over the tall man, in that his muscles have a better leverage. Both the neck and the trunk are shorter in the short man, thus giving an anatomical advantage which is apparent in the records made by the dynamometer.

Comparison of the Muscular Strength of Tall Women with That of Short Women.— (Table I, columns XVII to XIX.) The average heights of the two groups compared were respectively: for tall women (64), 66 inches; short women (88), 61 inches. No height in either group varied more than one half inch from the average.

In the comparison of tall women and short women, it is found that short women, while showing a total average strength of only 92 per cent that of tall women, are ahead at three points; viz., the pectorals, posterior trunk muscles, and the muscles of inspiration (waist).

The superiority of the pectorals is a characteristic which is not shown in short men, hence is probably accidental. The greater strength of the muscles of the trunk, and also of the waist-expanding muscles, is probably due to the anatomical advantage referred to in the case of short men.

It is interesting to notice that short women, as well as short men, show a superiority at this point over taller persons of the same sex. I think the fact is more than a coincidence, and is confirmatory of the explanation above given.

Comparison of the Muscular Strength in Men and Women of Equal Height.— (Table I, columns XX and XXII.) In the comparison of 45 men and 45 women of equal height, the average height being 65 inches, and no individual varying more than an inch from the average height, it was found that the average woman is slightly less inferior to the average man of the same height than is the average woman when compared with the average man considered without reference to height.

The figures are 57 per cent for the woman of equal height as compared with 53 per cent for the average woman. Two or three points are especially worthy of notice. The thigh adductors and thigh flexors of the woman of equal height have a relative strength slightly less than that of the average woman, the figures being respectively 60 and 62 for the adductors, and 52 and 59 for the thigh flexors.

Comparative and Relative Strength of Homologous Muscles in Men and Women. — (Table IV.) In this comparison the flexors of the hand are compared with the extensors of the foot, and *vice versa;* the deltoid with the thigh abductors; and the latissimus dorsi with the thigh adductors.

TABLE IV.

RELATIVE STRENGTH OF HOMOLOGOUS GROUPS OF MUSCLES IN MEN AND WOMEN.

MUSCULAR GROUPS.	MEN.	WOMEN.
Hand Flexors — Foot Extensors	.41	.34
Hand Extensors — Foot Flexors	.37	.33
Arm Flexors — Leg Flexors	60	.41
Arm Extensors — Leg Extensors	.54	.43
Deltoid — Thigh Abductors	.68	.53
Latissimus Dorsi — Thigh Adductors	.81	.70
Forearms — Legs	.76	.59
Arms and Shoulders — Thighs and Hips	.63	.54
Total Arms — Total Legs	.67	.56

This table presents the following interesting facts respecting the relative strength of homologous muscles : —

1. The hand flexors and hand extensors have each, in man, a strength about 2–5, and in women about 1–3, that of the corresponding muscles of the legs.

2. The arm flexors have, in men, 3–5, and in women, 2–5, the strength of the leg flexors.

3. The total for the arms is, in men, almost exactly 2–3 the total for the legs, and in women, a little more than 1–2.

4. The forearm has, in men, 3–4 the strength of the lower leg ; in women, 3–5.

5. The upper arm and shoulder have 3–5 the strength of the thigh and hip, in man ; a trifle more than 1–2 in women.

THE "REST-CURE."

The importance of rest as a therapeutic means in the treatment of certain forms of disease and morbid conditions, especially in surgical cases, has long been recognized by scientific physicians; but it is only within recent times that this most important of nature's various recuperative agents has been systematically studied, and a method of treatment organized to which the term "rest-cure" could be appropriately applied. Mitchell was not the first, however, to present the subject in a methodical form. John Hilton, president of the Royal College of Surgeons, of England, had, long before, dwelt with much emphasis upon the importance of rest in the treatment of disease, and devoted a volume of considerable size to its proper employment in painful maladies. It must be granted, however, that Dr. Mitchell was the first to conceive a systematic treatment by rest combined with massage and a regulated regimen, a fact which has received world-wide recognition by the medical profession.

As a therapeutic agent, rest belongs in the category of natural agents, with exercise, diet, baths, etc. It is perhaps for this reason that it was so long neglected, as were also dietetics and hydrotherapy, which have only recently begun to receive the attention that their importance demands. Sleep, nature's great restorative, is the most powerful of all recuperative measures, for the reason that during sound sleep the nearest possible approach to perfect physiological and mechanical rest is secured. Rest, even during sleep, is not absolute; otherwise the life processes would cease, and death ensue. The advantages of the rest afforded by sleep are illustrated by many facts.

Both plants and animals require physiological rest. During its waking hours, which usually correspond to those of daylight, the animal expends energy in muscular and nervous activity. It gathers its food at the cost of more or less exertion, and otherwise exercises its powers in providing for its individual comfort or that of others. During sleep these expenditures cease, and the energies of the body may be solely employed in the repair of the injuries and losses which have occurred during the hours of waking activity. It is during sleep, when the force of the vital powers is thus concentrated upon the organism itself, that both animals and plants make the principal part of their growth.

Physiological and mechanical rest has long been known to be the best means of promoting recovery in cases of injury, and it is equally valuable in recruiting depleted vital energies or in repairing a breach in the continuity of the tissues. In cold climates, trees and plants take physiological rest during the winter months; while in warm countries a similar rest is afforded by the dry season. The water-lily of Egypt flourishes in the canals during the wet season, when they are filled with water for irrigating purposes, but disappears utterly during the dry season, when the canals are empty, and their beds so dry and hard as to be used for roadways. When the floods come down the Nile, and the water flows into the canals, the lily, recuperated by its rest, blooms again. During the brief summer season of the Arctic regions, flowers and plants spring up after their long sleep, and attain maturity in a shorter period than in any other part of the world.

Another evidence of the universal necessity for rest is afforded by the fact that plants while in bloom, in many instances exhibit evidences of sleep very similar to those shown by animals, closing their leaves or their flowers when the sun approaches the western horizon.

Growth and exercise are in opposing relation to each other. It is true that exercise promotes growth, but the growth does not occur simultaneously with the exercise. On the contrary, during periods of vigorous exercise, growth is checked. Increased oxygenation and improved elimination resulting from exercise are means of systematic invigoration which promote growth, provided the exercise be not carried to an extreme. By too great exhaustion of the bodily forces, growth is lessened.

In the child, growth may be said to be chiefly confined to periods of rest and sleep. The full development of the body having been obtained, repair takes the place of growth. Incessant activity, which must necessarily be accompanied by the loss of sleep, produces a rapid waste of tissue, as well as anæmia from a diminution both in the number of corpuscles and in the hæmoglobin, or coloring matter, of the blood. Sleep promotes tissue production and repair.

Rest is necessary for the viscera as well as for the brain, the nerves, and the muscles. A viscus, as the liver or spleen, when at work, increases in size, from the unusual amount of blood circulating through its vessels. The diameter of the liver increases during digestion from half an inch to an inch. It is for this reason that the spongy viscera of the abdomen are each surrounded by an elastic capsule, which contains both muscular and yellow elastic fibers. The pressure of this elastic covering, constantly acting upon the organ, promotes its return to a state of physiological rest as soon as the demand for its activity has ceased.

Even the brain enlarges during activity. The thick skull does not permit an actual increase in the volume of the brain as a whole, but nature has provided an arrangement by which an enlargement of the active parts may occur. The large lateral ventricles which occupy the interior of the brain on each side are constantly filled with cerebro-spinal fluid. The optic thalami and the corpora striata, the most active portions of the brain, are so placed that they project into the ventricles. When distended with blood, and thus enlarged, as they are during activity, these bodies project farther into the ventricles, displacing a quantity of the cerebro-spinal fluid, which passes through the foramen of Monroe, the third ventricle, the aqueduct of Silvius, the fourth ventricle, the cerebro-spinal opening in the floor of the fourth ventricle, and the sub-cerebral spaces, into the vertebral canal. When the activity ceases, the pressure of the cerebro-spinal fluid causes it to return to the lateral ventricles, thus keeping them constantly filled, and providing suitable support for the blood vessels of the adjacent nerve structures. It has been shown that when the cerebro-spinal fluid is not present in the lateral ventricles, the brain cannot be injected without rupture of these vessels.

The rhythmical activity of the chest is another means of securing the return of the brain and the viscera to a state of rest after activity. The diminution in pressure which occurs during inspiration makes a strong draught upon the blood current in the direction of the heart, thus aiding especially the venous circulation of the brain and also that of the liver, as well as that of the other abdominal viscera.

Indications for Application of the " Rest-Cure." — More than twenty years' experience in the employment of the " rest-cure " in various forms has to the author amply demonstrated its value. It has been found especially successful in the treatment of the following conditions : —

Chronic Pain. — The rational treatment of painful maladies necessarily includes not only the recognition and treatment of the cause of the malady, but also mitigation of the pain itself, in consequence of the exhausting influence of long-continued pain, and the interference of this symptom with the normal processes of recuperation and repair. Rest and position are, in suitable cases, more effective in securing relief from pain than any of the ordinary sedative drugs, without rest. This is true of both local and general pains. The terrible pain of a felon may not infrequently be relieved to an astonishing degree by simply elevating the hand above the head. The pain of a rheumatic ankle sometimes disappears almost instantly upon the sufferer's assuming a horizontal position, with the foot elevated. The pain of an inflamed nerve, as in sciatica, yields to prolonged rest more certainly than to any other treatment. The neurotic young woman who in an erect position suffers

such intolerable spinal pain as to make existence almost un-
endurable, finds herself perfectly comfortable when in bed.
Pelvic and abdominal pains often disappear as if by magic
when the patient assumes a horizontal position. The relief thus
afforded is often brought about by the removal of the tension
upon the abdominal sympathetic nerve and its branches, which
is secured by a reclining position.

In a majority of cases of this kind, some of the abdominal
or pelvic viscera will be found displaced, or in a condition
termed by Glenard "enteroptosis." When the patient is in an
erect position, the stomach, liver, kidney, bowels,— one or all
of these organs,— being in a pendant or floating condition,
drag upon the sympathetic in a way which may set up pain
and morbid symptoms of the most varied character, and in
structures either near or remote. Pain attributable to irritation of the abdominal sympathetic from the cause mentioned,
may be locally expressed in any part of the body from the
heel to the top of the head. Rest in bed is a sovereign remedy
for cases of this kind.

Emaciation.— Progressive wasting of the tissues as indicated by a steady loss of flesh, is a morbid condition which
sometimes proves most refractory to therapeutic efforts, especially when the means employed are exclusively of a medic-
inal character. There is, in fact, no drug which can be relied
upon to secure a substantial and permanent increase in flesh.
Emaciation is an evidence of a serious disturbance of nutrition;
and when considerable in degree, or rapidly progressive, invariably demands a prompt and systematic application of the
"rest-cure." An improvement in weight can be expected only
as the result of an increase of residual tissue, or fat. This
requires, first of all, an improvement in digestive activity,
which may involve an increase in either the quantity or the
quality of the digestive work done. Not infrequently, patients
complain that, although they have a good appetite, and eat
large quantities of food, they nevertheless steadily lose in

flesh. In these cases, a thorough-going examination of the stomach fluid obtained after a test meal, shows the coefficient of digestive activity to be low,— in other words, the quality of the digestive products is so poor that they are, in large part, useless for the purposes of nutrition.

Successful treatment of these cases requires, next after an improvement in digestion by which a larger amount of tissue-building material can be taken in, a careful economizing of the vital resources. As far as possible, the activity of the bodily powers must be concentrated upon the building up of the individual. All external expenditures of energy must be cut off.

Food is consumed in the body in three ways only — for heat production, force production, and tissue building. The food elements consumed in heat and force production cannot be deposited as tissue, or, at least, cannot be retained ; consequently the amount of nutritive material used in this way should be limited to the smallest amount possible. In no way can the vital resources be thus economized so effectively as by the aid of the "rest-cure."

Fever.— In all cases in which there is any considerable rise of temperature or febrile activity, from whatever cause, rest is one of the most essential features of treatment. If the temperature rises daily three or four degrees above normal, the patient should be kept in bed. If the elevation of temperature is not more than one or two degrees, the patient may spend a part of the time only, in bed ; the balance of the time he may be dressed, if he desires, but should recline upon a cot, rolling-chair, or hammock. In this way the great waste of tissue which always accompanies fever may be very materially lessened, and the intensity of the febrile action greatly diminished. Rest in bed is one of the most valuable of all the means which can be utilized in the treatment of pulmonary tuberculosis, or consumption, during febrile paroxysms.

The necessity of rest is well recognized in the treatment of typhoid fever and other acute febrile maladies, but its impor-

tance in the treatment of pulmonary consumption is often overlooked. In the last-named disease the patient should be put to
bed whenever the temperature rises above 101°.

Neurasthenia.— This condition, commonly called nervous
exhaustion, is one in which the "rest-cure" has achieved
some of its most important and remarkable triumphs. The
value of the "rest-cure" in the treatment of neurasthenia
has come to be so thoroughly recognized that it is by some
considered almost a panacea. This view is an extreme one;
nevertheless, mechanical and, as far as possible, physiological rest of the brain and nerves is, for many cases of this
kind, most important as a requisite for recovery. This is especially true of those cases of nervous exhaustion sometimes
encountered in young men and women who have led aimless
and idle lives, and whose morbid condition is the result of a
mental and physical stagnation rather than excessive work.
In the case of overworked and worried persons, especially
those in whom the decline of health has been accompanied
by a loss in flesh, the "rest-cure" is indicated as a therapeutic measure of the first importance.

The Opium, Cocaine, Whisky, and Tobacco Habits.— In
the treatment of these poison habits I have found rest a
most valuable accessory means. The man or woman who has
long been addicted to such a habit will invariably be found in
a state of nerve exhaustion, and it is this condition of the
nervous system, and the veritable cyclone of nerve symptoms
which arises from it as soon as the toxic agent is withdrawn, so
that the patient becomes conscious of his real condition, which
renders the management of these cases so difficult. A person
habituated to the use of any poison cannot be considered cured
until the nervous system has been restored to a normal and
well-balanced state. If the drug is simply withdrawn, and the
patient left with a nervous system shattered by its pernicious influence, he will, in a majority of cases, find himself utterly unable
to resist the importunities of his worn-out and pain-racked nerves
for their accustomed solace. The morbid condition which con-

stitutes an ever-present incitement to the perpetuation of the habit must be removed before the patient can be regarded as cured. "Rest-cure" is as valuable in the treatment of this form of nervous exhaustion as any other.

Another very important reason for the employment of the "rest-cure" in these cases is the absolute control of the patient which it secures. The patient who has been long accustomed to the use of opium or cocaine, and even in some instances alcohol or tobacco habitués, require every possible assistance in getting through the first few days after the complete with-drawal of the accustomed drug, whether it is gradually taken away or suspended at once. In order to receive all the assist-ance possible from a rational system of treatment and by the aid of a trained nurse, the patient must remain in bed ; for during this period he will require an application of some sort not only every hour but almost every moment, to quiet his clamoring nerves, as well as to while away the weary hours and beguile his mind into a normal channel. I have found the "rest-cure" of great value in the treatment of a large number of cases of the opium habit and other forms of drug addiction.

Gastric Ulcer.—In this disease, there is not only marked wasting of the body in a majority of cases, in consequence of the disturbance of nutrition occasioned both by the ulcer itself and by the morbid condition of the stomach which precedes it, but there is also a local destruction of tissue, which is aggra-vated by exercise. The irritability of the stomach and the highly excited state of the solar plexus render exercise upon the feet, in many of these cases, extremely painful, such exercise often giving rise to most distressing paroxysms of pain and gastric crises. By rest in bed, the patient's forces are econo-mized ; nutrition is improved ; and more favorable conditions for recovery are secured.

Gastric ulcer is usually a consequence of long-continued hyperpepsia. Exercise upon the feet has a marked tendency to increase the hyperpepsia, and thus promote the development of the ulceration ; while mechanical rest has an opposite effect.

In most of these cases it is also necessary to give the stomach complete physiological rest by withholding altogether the administration of food by the mouth, and administering only specially prepared foods by means of the rectum. While the nutrition is thus restricted, absolute rest in bed is most important as a means of preserving the forces of the patient.

Hemorrhage.— After severe hemorrhage from any cause, as from the lungs in pulmonary disease ; from the uterus in cases of fibroid tumor or other diseases of that organ ; from the rectum, in consequence of ulceration or bleeding hemorrhoids ; or from any other cause whatever, a more or less prolonged rest in bed is of the utmost importance as a therapeutic measure, and is in the highest degree conducive to the replenishment of the blood. In a number of cases of this kind the writer has noticed, during rest, an astonishingly rapid restoration of the hæmoglobin and a return of the normal blood count.

Diseases Peculiar to Women.— While many diseases peculiar to women are the result of neglect to properly develop the muscles, especially those of the trunk, nevertheless, in a large number of the morbid conditions from which they suffer, a short course of "rest-cure" may be employed with very great advantage. This is especially true in all inflammatory diseases of the ovaries and uterus. Severe cases of uterine and vaginal catarrh are also greatly benefited by rest in a recumbent position. The effect of position upon the circulation of dependent parts is readily shown by noticing the change which occurs in the circulation of the hand when lifted above the head from the usual position by the side. If the veins are much swollen, as is likely to be the case when the arm swings by the side, it will be observed that instantly, when the hand is raised above the head, or even to the horizontal position, the fullness disappears, and the skin of the hand becomes blanched. This is not simply the result of gravity acting upon the blood, but is due chiefly to a decided contraction of the blood vessels in the hand. A like change occurs in the pelvic viscera. The swollen state of the blood vessels induced by the vertical position must greatly aggravate any pathological condition of the uterus or its appendages when congestion, either active or passive, is a prominent feature of the morbid state. The writer has frequently been told by patients that vaginal or uterine catarrh was always greatly increased during or after exercise upon the feet, and has seen such discharges disappear entirely during prolonged rest in bed, evidently as the result of the diminished circulation secured by the recumbent position.

Prostatic and Bladder Disease. — The remarks which have been made with reference to diseases peculiar to women are equally true with reference to acute disease of the bladder, urethra, prostate gland, or the genital glands, in men. An acute cystitis, urethritis, or prostatitis will be more readily benefited by rest in bed than by the employment of any other means. The same must also be said of orchitis, a disease which not infrequently resists treatment with great obstinacy, without the advantage of the recumbent position. In many cases of chronic disease of the bladder. in both men and women, "rest-cure" is of paramount importance as a therapeutic measure.

Bright's Disease of the Kidneys. — The various pathological conditions of the kidney included under the term "Bright's disease" not infrequently demand rest in bed as a necessary condition for a cure of the disease, or even an arrest of its progress. This is especially true of acute inflammation of the kidneys. In this disease there is a lessened ability of the kidney to eliminate poisons ; consequently, the disintegration of tissue which occurs as the result of exercise upon the feet necessitates increased eliminative work on the part of the kidney. Exercise on the feet, and even sitting or standing, also involves greater activity of the heart and a higher arterial tension. An abnormal increase in arterial tension may be, in itself, sufficient to cause the appearance of albumen in the urine. It is evident, then, that in cases of acute inflammation of the kidneys, whatever tends to increase the arterial tension must aggravate the disease ; and, on the other hand, the lessened arterial tension induced by rest in a horizontal position must favor recovery. In a somewhat extended experience in the treatment of this disease, the author has found rest an exceedingly valuable accessory.

Disease of the Heart.— In the history of a case of organic disease of the heart, the first morbid condition of grave character which requires the attention of the physician, is often over-compensation. The unusual amount of work required of the organ induces an excessive development of the heart muscle, and this excessive cardiac activity results in a variety of disturbing and often alarming symptoms. There is no way by which the heart's action can be so quickly and so safely quieted as by means of rest in the recumbent position. There is no drug which is, even in a small degree, a substitute for rest, in cases of this kind.

In cases of cardiac insufficiency, rest in bed is equally as valuable as in cardiac hypertrophy with overaction of the heart. When the heart has become so weak as to be unable to maintain the circulation, the relief from work afforded by rest in the horizontal position enables the heart to recover itself, so that, after a few days or weeks, as the case may require, the normal balance of the circulation is re-established ; the heart, no longer distended and embarrassed with blood from which it has lost the power to empty itself, recovers its tone ; the pulse becomes fuller and stronger ; the cyanosis disappears ; the swollen limbs return to their normal size; and the respiration is no longer embarrassed.

Nervous or Mental Irritability or Excitability.— For certain cases of extreme nervous or mental excitability bordering on acute mania, and especially in cases of acute mechanical excitement, rest in bed, accompanied by appropriate treatment, is a measure of such great advantage that I should feel very loth indeed to undertake the treatment of cases of this sort without its aid. Rest in the horizontal position not only lessens the waste of tissue resulting from abnormal nervous or mental excitement, but secures to the patient the isolation and quiet which may exercise in a high degree a calming influence upon his over-excited nerves.

The Significance of Pain.—In the selection of cases to which the "rest-cure" should be applied, it is necessary to understand clearly the significance of pain. Not infrequently the pain experienced is very remote from the part which is the real origin of the pain, and to which, accordingly, the therapeutic measures should be directed.

In the employment of the "rest-cure" as a means of relieving pain, it is very important to distinguish between pains which are purely local in character, and those which are of reflex origin. Local pains, or those originating in the parts· where they are felt, if involving but a small portion of the body, may require rest only of the part itself. But sympathetic, or reflex, pains generally require complete rest. This is true, for example, of the intercostal pains connected with pleurisy, either acute or chronic, or adhesions of the pleura resulting from inflammation. The pleura and the overlying tissues are supplied with branches from the same sensory nerves. This fact should always be kept in mind, and should lead to a careful examination of the lungs in cases in which thoracic pains are experienced.

Quite a large proportion of the external pains are connected with disease of the viscera. Pain between the shoulders or above the lower angles of the scapulæ, a very common chronic pain, indicates some disturbance of the fourth, fifth, and sixth spinal nerves. The nerve centers from which these nerves originate are those which chiefly give rise to the great splanchnic, or visceral, nerve, which is distributed to the stomach, liver, pancreas, and intestines. Its branches are also closely interwoven with the solar plexus and the lumbar ganglia of the sympathetic. It is consequently clear that the pain described may readily be produced by disease of the stomach, intestines, pancreas, liver, or some other viscus ; and a careful investigation will usually show a prolapsed stomach or liver, a floating kidney, sagging of the bowels, or several of these conditions

15

associated, whereby an abnormal and nerve-irritating condition is induced, affecting the branches of both the sympathetic and the splanchnics.

One-sided pain, is, as a rule, an indication of a one-sided disease, while bilateral pain indicates a morbid condition affecting both sides. Even in cases arising from disturbance of the viscera, this rule holds good more frequently than might be expected. Migraine affecting one side of the head is, in the experience of the author, frequently connected with extreme hyperæsthesia of the lumbar ganglion of the same side. If both ganglia are affected, the patient will say that the attacks occur simultaneously upon both sides, or extend from one side to the other. In these cases, the greatest tenderness will usually be found in the lumbar ganglion of the side upon which the pain first begins. In cases in which the attack begins in the back of the head, extending thence upward over the whole head, both ganglia are usually found equally affected. In cases of pain arising from visceral disease, rest in bed for a week or two at the beginning of the treatment is a measure of very great advantage. At the conclusion of the period of confinement in bed, care should be taken to keep the organs in position by a properly adjusted bandage and appropriate applications of abdominal massage.

Disadvantages of the "Rest-cure."—It should never be forgotten that rest in bed involves certain disadvantages, against which careful provision must be made. Man is naturally an active animal ; and habits of regular, systematic exercise are essential to the maintenance of the integrity of the vital functions. Absolute rest in bed, without the employment of proper preventive measures, is, in itself, sufficient in many cases to provoke grave morbid conditions. The muscles, of course, rapidly deteriorate under the influence of inaction, but this is a matter of small importance compared with the injury sustained by the liver and other viscera. It is a common observation in surgical wards and hospitals that a healthy man confined in bed from fracture of a limb, becomes bilious, sometimes even jaundiced, in consequence of interference with the functions of the stomach, liver, and bowels. The unpleasant effects of rest are readily understood when the important influence of exercise upon the viscera is recognized.

Exercise necessarily involves increased chest activity. The lungs constitute not only an air pump by which oxygen is supplied to the body, but, at the same time, exercise a most important influence in assisting the circulation and thus the functional activity of the stomach and liver.

The diaphragm not only acts as a great lymph pump, but by compression of the stomach and liver during the act of forcible inspiration, it exercises these important organs, and by promoting absorption, aids in emptying the stomach of its contents; while, by mechanical compression, it empties the liver of bile, and hastens the passage of the blood through its capillaries.

Perhaps more important still is the effect of exercise upon the general system in promoting the complete oxidation, or burning up, of the waste matters which are continually accumulating in the tissues through increased absorption of oxygen, and by draining off the poisonous waste substances prepared for removal from the body, and hastening their transportation to the liver, kidneys, lungs, bowels, and skin, through which they make their exit from the body. Diminished respiratory activity alone may be responsible for a congestion of the stomach and liver resulting in stomach and intestinal catarrh, infectious jaundice, and inactivity of the liver and bowels.

The horizontal position may also result in injury on account of the congestion due to the mechanical accumulation of blood in the dependent part. Pneumonia not infrequently results from lying continuously upon the back during a course of typhoid fever or some other disabling malady. Even cerebral congestion may result from the horizontal position.

These and other disorders, the nature of which may be inferred from what has been said in reference to the influence of rest in producing these morbid conditions, may be prevented by the adoption of proper measures, the most important of which are massage and manual Swedish movements. The utility of massage in these cases need not be argued, as it is apparent at once that it may be made, to a very large extent, a substitute for exercise, without expending the nervous energy of the patient, or making any large draughts upon his vital resources.

These facts give massage a value which cannot be overestimated. It is a means by which the patient may receive the benefit of exercise without effort on his part; and in most cases in which "rest-cure" is required, massage must also be employed as a complementary measure. A few exceptions only need be made. These are so important, however, that they must not be overlooked. First of all, it must be remembered that in febrile conditions, or at least in all cases in which any considerable degree of febrile activity exists, massage must not be applied, for the reason that it increases heat production. In most cases, bathing and rubbing must be employed to a greater or less extent; but care should be taken to avoid all manipulative measures except stroking and centrifugal friction, the tendency of which, as regards heat production, is the opposite of all the other processes of massage. In the employment of the "rest-cure" for the relief of pain due to visceral prolapse or other diseases of those organs, manipulation of the diseased viscera must be avoided except so far as may be necessary for replacement; but massage to the limbs and other parts of the body may very wisely be employed, since, when administered in this manner, it operates most efficiently as a derivative measure.

In acute Bright's disease of the kidneys, massage must be avoided, or at least should be confined to the gentlest measures, for the reason that the kidneys are crippled, and it is desirable that their work should be restricted as much as possible within safe limits. A vigorous application of massage may suddenly throw into the circulation so large a quantity of toxic and excrementitious substances as to overwhelm the kidneys and create an increase of irritation, the result of which might be disastrous. Stroking (**169-190**) and centrifugal friction are the only appropriate measures for cases of this kind until after there has been a marked diminution in the activity of the disease, as shown by a decrease in the production of albumen and an increase of urea, or a marked rise in the coefficient of toxicity.

In cases of excessive nervous and mental excitability, massage must be used only when great care is taken to select the right measures, and the treatment in such cases must be administered with unusual skill. The lighter measures of massage only are admissible in these cases. Percussion must generally be altogether interdicted. Gentle, deep kneading (**246**) and centrifugal friction (**194**) are most appropriate measures, and these should be employed derivatively.

Among the most valuable preventive measures to be employed in massage when administered in ordinary cases of "rest-cure," should be mentioned abdominal massage (**389-424**). Massage of the stomach (**451**), bowels, and liver aids greatly in counteracting the evil effects of rest upon these viscera, and in facilitating the processes of digestion and elimination, in fact promoting all the functions of the organs named, as well as those of the kidneys.

Another measure of greatest importance, in addition to general and abdominal massage, is to be found in lung gymnastics (**381-384**), which not only greatly aid the functions of the liver, stomach, and other viscera, but also relieve the brain of blood, thus preventing cerebral congestion, and promote elimination. Breathing exercises also promote the formation of blood, thus preventing anæmia, and greatly aiding the oxidation and elimination of waste matters. These exercises are valuable not only in ordinary cases, but in fevers, Bright's disease, and in fact in every case in which the "rest-cure" is employed, except acute pleurisy and pulmonary hemorrhage, in which, of course, it is important to secure as great a degree of quietude as possible.

The employment of lung gymnastics in fevers is a valuable means of combating the depressing tendency of the disease, and of preventing the pneumonia which frequently accompanies fevers of a low type. It also aids in lowering temperature, not only by cooling the blood, but also by assisting in oxidation and elimination of the toxic substances to which the rise of temperature is due.

Ewald measured the temperature of the stomach by a thermo-electric device, and found it to be, on an average, 1° F. higher than in the axilla. By making the patient breathe forcibly, even with the mouth closed, the temperature of the stomach was reduced to half a degree less than the axillary temperature. When the patient breathed steam at the temperature of the body, this lowering of the temperature of the stomach did not occur, showing that the internal temperature may be lowered by bringing the blood into contact with an increased quantity of cool air through forced respiration.

This measure has not been employed in febrile cases as much as it deserves to be. It is, of course, important that the patient should be entirely passive. The increased breathing activity should be secured by movements executed by the masseur, who, by raising the arms from the sides and drawing them upward, will aid inspiration; then, by returning them to the sides, and compressing the sides of the chest, may aid expiration. Cyanosis, which so frequently accompanies febrile action when the temperature rises to a dangerous point, may be made quickly to disappear by this means.

Position is a matter also worthy of mention as a means of combating some of the evil tendencies of rest. In cases with a tendency to cerebral hyperæmia, the head of the bed should be raised, thus utilizing gravity as a means of securing drainage of the brain. This is especially important in cases of apoplexy, and the same measure should be employed in pulmonary hemorrhage. In hemorrhage from other parts of the body, resulting in anæmia, the opposite plan should be followed, the foot of the bed being raised. This measure should also be adopted whenever it is desirable to antagonize congestion or inflammation in the lower extremities. Pelvic pain due to disease of the ovaries or of the bladder, prostate, or rectum, is often greatly relieved by raising the foot of the bed, in connection with rest in the recumbent position.

From what has been said, it is evident that massage is practically indispensable as a complementary measure of treatment in connection with the "rest-cure," and that it may be applied in some form in all cases requiring rest, and in such a manner as to greatly increase the advantages which may be derived from the "rest-cure."

After-rest Exercise.— A point of very great importance, to which attention should be called, is that rest alone seldom results in a radical cure. Rest secures a symptomatic cure, but does scarcely more than this, except to provide conditions favorable for recovery. Other recuperative measures must also be employed in connection with rest. Massage has been shown to be an invaluable remedy for this purpose. The "rest-cure" is only a preparation for exercise-cure. The patient who has been put to bed, and who has been relieved of his morbid symptoms by the rest thus obtained, must be made capable of enjoying good health upon his feet. To be cured in bed is not sufficient, as few sick people desire to spend their lives there. The patient must be gotten upon his feet, and enabled to endure at least an ordinary amount of exercise without injury, before he can be considered well. Neglect of this point has resulted in a failure to effect anything more than temporary relief by means of the "rest-cure" in perhaps a large proportion of all the cases in which this measure has been employed. But as this point has been considered quite fully elsewhere in this work, the reader is referred to what has already been said. The author would, however, emphasize the importance of supplementing, in every case, a course of "rest-cure" with a course of carefully graduated exercises, by which the patient may be safely introduced to life under ordinary conditions. The author expects to be able to place in press at an early date a work in which will be given many such series of exercises, adapted to different conditions.

RULES RELATING TO MASSAGE.

1. *Correct Use of Terms.*—In speaking of massage or its application, be careful to use correct terms (pp. 238, 239).

2. *Good Health Necessary.*—Of all persons, one who administers massage should have perfect health. The so-called magnetism which renders some persons so much more successful than others in massage, as well as in other callings, is largely the outgrowth of the vivacity, freshness, good cheer, and good nature which result from abounding health. A few things of special importance in this relation are proper diet; healthful, loose, and appropriate clothing; a daily cool morning sponge bath; and daily out-of-door exercise.

3. *Personal Cleanliness.*—Massage is hard work, equal to almost any form of manual labor. A masseur who does his duty will perspire vigorously; hence the necessity of due attention to personal cleanliness. Cleansing of the skin may be promoted by the addition of a little carbonate of ammonia to the water used for the morning bath. When one perspires freely, stockings and underclothing should be changed daily. After airing for a day or two, the same garment may be worn again for a day. Special attention must also be given to the hands, teeth, and also the nasal cavity, if a catarrhal condition is present, and to the hair and scalp.

4. *The Hands.*—Good hands are necessary for success in massage. The hands must be soft, warm, dry, strong, and elastic. A bony, sweaty, hard, or calloused hand is exceedingly objectionable. The hands should also be free from blemishes, such as warts, abrasions, chaps, etc. The nails should be trimmed close. Absolute cleanliness is the best means of promoting a healthy state of the skin of the hands,

as well as other parts. A perfectly clean hand is not likely to chap. Always wash the hands just before giving massage; doing so, if convenient, in the presence of the patient, or at least with his knowledge. Always wash the hands a second time just before manipulating the head, face, or neck, if the hands have been used upon other parts since washing. The following lotions are valuable for keeping the hands in a healthy state : —

(1) Comp. tr. benzoin.. dr. 4.
    Alcohol.. oz. ½.
    Glycerine.. oz. 1.
    Water... oz. 2.

(2) Borax.. dr. 1½.
    Carbonate of soda... dr. 1½.
    Carbonate of ammonia.. dr. 2.
    Aquae ammonia... dr. 4.
    Glycerine... oz. 1.
    Water to make... oz. 6.

5. *The Personal Appearance.* — Simplicity, neatness, and tidiness in dress are in the highest degree commendable. The personal appearance should be made attractive by extreme care and appropriateness in dress, without showiness, which always indicates vulgarity or ignorance. Nurses connected with a hospital in which a uniform is used should always wear it when on professional duty.

6. No person should undertake to practice massage who has not received a thorough practical training. Massage is both an art and a science, and only those who have had long practice can be thoroughly efficient.

7. Never countenance the belief that vitality, magnetism, or any other occult force is imparted by manipulation. Avoid flourishes.

8. Do not be hurried, flurried, nor out of breath from fast walking, in approaching a patient to administer massage.

9. Avoid a bustling, nervous manner.

10. Only in most extraordinary cases and under exceptionally justifying circumstances, and then only in the presence of

other persons, should a masseur or a masseuse administer massage to an adult person of the opposite sex.

11. The room in which massage is given should be well ventilated, temperature about 75° to 80° F.

12. As a rule, the patient should be undressed, or clad in a single loose gown. Care should be taken to keep the body well covered, with the exception of the part undergoing manipulation.

13. The patient should be placed in an easy, comfortable position.

14. The position of the operator varies with the part operated upon, but should always be such as is best suited for the part undergoing manipulation.

15. In bending over the patient, the body should be flexed at the hips, not at the waist or shoulders. By this precaution the masseur may avoid becoming round-shouldered. The height of the bed or couch should be such that the masseur will not need to bend to any great extent.

16. Movements of the hands should always be executed from the wrist.

17. Apply as much of the surface of the hands and fingers as possible to the part operated upon, thus distributing the pressure and saving time.

18. The body should be gone over systematically, for which purpose it should be divided into separate territories. Each part should be finished before going to another part.

19. Opposite sides of the body should be manipulated in succession, so as to intensify the effect upon the nerve centers.

20. The masseur should always keep in mind the anatomy of the body,— the outline of the bones, the location of the large nerves, arteries, and veins, and of the principal muscular groups,— and should take care to follow the bones, thinking of the bony framework as well as its covering of soft parts. Work down between the muscles and tendons, around the head of the bones, taking special care to work into all the

irregularities of the joints, where the blood vessels and lymph channels are the largest.

21. At the beginning, movements should be slow and gentle, being gradually increased in rapidity and force to the maximum, then gradually diminished to the termination.

22. As a rule, always employ the same rate of motion for the same movement. This indicates skill and good training.

23. It is well to run rapidly and lightly over a part before giving the more vigorous movements.

24. In the first application of massage to a patient not accustomed to treatment, great care should be taken not to produce soreness and black-and-blue spots. These unpleasant effects are especially likely to occur in fleshy and aged persons, owing to the feeble circulation in the adipose tissues of the first class, and the brittleness of the blood vessels of the second class. Fever convalescents and persons who have been long in bed are also liable to these effects, for similar reasons.

25. For relief of sensitive parts, employ only gentle stroking over the affected areas, and administer derivative massage to the muscles and other tissues of the vicinity, especially between the affected part and the heart. The painful part may be approached by degrees until applications can be made directly to it.

26. In many cases it is well to lubricate the hand with some unctuous substance, such as olive oil, fine vaseline, cocoanut oil, or cacao butter. The last-named substance is, perhaps, the best of all. It is solid at ordinary temperatures, melting, however, at the temperature of the body. A cake of cacao butter rubbed upon the hands occasionally during the administration of massage, keeps the hands well lubricated without smearing the body of the patient with a surplus of oil. In case oil is objectionable, talcum powder may be used.

27. Lubricants should always be used when much pressure is required, and where prolonged manipulation is necessary, also in the treatment of parts where the skin is extremely sensitive.

28. When it is desired to stimulate the skin to a high degree by friction, lubricants should be avoided. A part may be rubbed six to ten minutes when oil is employed; but the same surface should not be operated upon more than from two to five minutes when a lubricant is not used.

29. Some authorities recommend that the parts should be shaved before the application of massage, but this is rarely necessary; and when the treatment must be employed a long time, may become a source of serious inconvenience.

30. The amount of massage administered must be suited to each case and to the mode of application.

31. Do not recommend massage for everything.

32. General massage should never be given in cases of fever. Local applications should not be made to parts which are the seat of acute inflammation.

33. Fleshy persons do not bear massage well, for the reason that the manipulations set free a large amount of waste matter and imperfectly oxidized products which, absorbed into the system, produce the same effect as excessive exercise,—effects resembling those of consecutive or secondary fatigue, to which fleshy persons are very liable. Fleshy persons often complain of languor, lassitude, and lameness after massage, and the tissues are very easily bruised because of the weak circulation and on account of the excessive amount of adipose tissue. Another cause of this condition is probably the disproportion existing between the lymph spaces and the amount of waste matter set free, because so much space is occupied by fat and subcutaneous tissue.

34. Massage is contra-indicated in nearly all forms of skin disease, except in the thickened condition of the skin left behind by chronic eczema. It is also contra-indicated in cases of apoplexy and in the early stages of neuritis, when excessive irritability still exists, and should never be administered to abscesses, tumors, or tubercular joints.

35. *Order in General Massage.*—(1) Arms; (2) Chest; (3) Legs; (4) Abdomen; (5) Hips; (6) Back; (7) Head; (8) Neck.

36. *General Observations.*— Percussion is sometimes more effective in strengthening a weak muscle than either kneading or faradization.

37. Percussion and vibration should be avoided in hyperæsthesia. In such cases, deep kneading, stroking, and joint movements may be employed.

38. Deep kneading is especially suitable for excitable neurasthenics and patients suffering from chorea.

39. In infantile paralysis and other diseases accompanied by lowered vitality and diminished activity without increased sensibility, percussion is indicated.

40. In chorea and locomotor ataxia,— in fact, in most cases in which massage is valuable,— gymnastics should be added. In locomotor ataxia the patient should exercise by walking and standing with the eyes closed, to develop the coördinating centers.

41. In convalescence from fevers, massage must be applied with care, because of the disturbance of the heat-regulating function on the part of the body. The same is true in tuberculosis. Use chiefly friction in such cases.

42. Patients in whom the skin is rigid and inelastic, or in a "hidebound" condition, may be prepared for general massage by the administration of a warm bath.

43. In some patients the application of oil to the surface is objectionable through the irritating effect of oleaginous matters upon the susceptible skin, especially in persons subject to certain forms of skin disease. In such cases we have found a glycerine ointment compounded after the following formula, an excellent substitute: Glycerine, 15 oz.; boracic acid, 1 1–2 oz.; starch, 1 1–2 oz.; gum tragacanth, 1 1–2 oz.; oil of wintergreen, 1 dr.

After lubricating the surface with the ointment, a little moisture should be added by dipping the tips of the fingers in water. By means of a moist towel this lubricant can be completely removed after the treatment, leaving the skin delightfully smooth.

CORRECT USE OF TERMS.

So much ignorance and incorrect usage prevails in relation to the various terms employed in connection with massage and its administration, that it will be worth while to devote a few lines to this part of the subject, as no one thing is so suggestive of ignorance or proficiency as the misuse or correct use of terms.

Massage is a noun, the literal meaning of which is kneading, as a baker kneads bread. This word, like many other terms relating to massage, is derived directly from the French. It retains its French pronunciation, and is pronounced as though spelled *mas-sahzh*, and not as though spelled *massaj* or *massaje*, which is so frequently heard.

Masser is a verb, meaning the act of applying massage. It is pronounced as though spelled *mas-say*.— I masse; you masse; he massees (pronounced as though spelled *mas-sa-es*).

Masseing is the present participle, and is pronounced as though spelled *mas-sa-ing*.— I am *masseing*.

Masséed is the past participle, and is pronounced as though spelled *mas-sa-ed*.— I *masséed* a patient yesterday.

Masseur is pronounced very nearly as if spelled *mas-sur*. The term is applied to a man who administers massage.

Masseuse is pronounced very nearly as if spelled *mas-suse*. The term is applied to a woman who administers massage.

Pétrissage is pronounced as though spelled *pa-tris-sahzh*. It is a French term applied to deep kneading, as distinguished from superficial kneading.

Tapotement is pronounced nearly as though spelled *tah-pote mont*, and indicates the act of percussion.

[238]

Effleurage is pronounced as though spelled *ef-flur-ahzh*. It means light friction.

Centripetal,— toward the center. In relation to massage, the term is applied to movements made in the direction of the blood current in the veins.

Centrifugal,— from the center. This term is applied to movements made from the heart, or in the direction of the arterial blood current.

THE GENERAL PHYSIOLOGY, NAMES, NERVE SUPPLY, AND ACTIONS OF THE MUSCLES OF THE HUMAN BODY.

Physiology of the Muscles.— The following brief summary of the physiology of the muscles, while incomplete, will assist somewhat in understanding the relation of these structures, with which massage deals so directly, to other bodily organs : —

1. Muscular action is allied to ciliary and amœboid movements.

2. The source of muscular energy is the oxidation of glycogen stored in the muscles.

3. During work, the amount of oxygen absorbed and the amount of CO_2 given off by the muscles, is very greatly increased ; hence respiratory activity is increased.

4. Muscular activity is accompanied by the production of heat ; the muscles are the principal seat of heat production in the body. The thermic activities of the muscles are dependent, not only upon muscular activity, but also upon nerve control, through the heat-centers of the central nervous system.

5. Muscular activity is usually excited by nervous impulses received by the muscle at the rate of about ten per second.

6. The muscle has an independent excitability which induces contraction, as the result of the application of chemical substances, cold, electricity, and mechanical stimulus.

7. Acids and excessive heat produce stiffening of the muscles.

8. A single voluntary muscular movement may be made in one sixteenth of a second.

9. Contraction from electrical stimulation occurs more quickly than from voluntary effort.

10. With contraction of a muscle, contraction of the opposing muscle occurs simultaneously, beginning slightly later.

11. Voluntary contraction is allied to tetanus.

12. Tetanus is produced by electrical applications in which the current is interrupted at the rate of twenty or more per second.

13. Muscular contraction is propagated along the muscle at the rate of forty feet per second.

14. Muscles are most perfect machines. The best steam engine utilizes only one eighth of the force contained in the fuel as work, seven eighths appearing as heat. A muscle produces one fifth work and four fifths heat.

15. The amount of work a muscle can do is proportioned to its transverse section.

16. A human muscle is able to lift 125 pounds for each square inch in area of its transverse section.

17. Muscular strength varies at different periods of life. A new-born infant is able to sustain its own weight for 24 seconds by grasping a stick with its hands. The strength of adult men and women, in relation to the body weight, is shown in Table I.

18. The weight of the muscles in proportion to the body weight varies at different ages, being 23.40 per cent of the body weight of a new-born babe, and 43.10 per cent of the body weight in adults.

19. The amount of work done by a laboring man in eight hours is about two million foot-pounds.

20. Fatigue is the result of the accumulation, within the muscle, of the poisonous products of work; the muscle is rested when these products are removed.

THE MUSCLES, THEIR NERVE SUPPLY AND ACTION.

Name.	Nerve.	Action.
Head and Face.		
Occipito-frontalis	Posterior auricular, small occipital, facial.	Moves scalp and wrinkles forehead.
Attollens aurem	Occipitalis minor	Raises ear.
Attrahens aurem	Facial	Advances ear.
Retrahens aurem	Posterior auricular	Retracts ear.
Orbicularis palpebrarum	Facial	Closes eyelids.
Corrugator supercilii	Facial	Draws eyebrows down and in.
Tensor tarsi	Facial	Compresses puncta and lachrymal sac.
Levator palpebræ superior	Third	Raises upper lid.
Rectus superior (eye)	Third	Rotates eyeball upward.
Rectus inferior "	Third	Rotates eyeball downward.
Rectus internus "	Third	Rotates eyeball inward.
Rectus externus "	Sixth	Rotates eyeball outward.
Obliquus superior "	Fourth	Rotates eyeball down and out.
Obliquus inferior "	Third	Rotates eyeball up and out.
Pyramidalis nasi	Facial	Depresses eyebrow.
Levator labii superioris alæque nasi	Facial	Elevates upper lip, dilates nostril.
Dilator naris posterior	Facial	Dilates nostril.
Dilator naris anterior	Facial	Dilates nostril.
Compressor nasi	Facial	Contracts nostril.
Compressor narium minor	Facial	Contracts nostril.
Depressor alæ nasi	Facial	Contracts nostril.
Levator labii superioris	Facial	Elevates upper lip.
Levator anguli oris	Facial	Elevates angle of mouth.
Zygomaticus major	Facial	Draws upper lip backward and upward.
Zygomaticus minor	Facial	Draws upper lip backward and upward.

Levator labii inferioris.	Facial	Elevates lower lip.
Depressor labii inferioris.	Facial	Depresses lower lip.
Depressor anguli oris.	Facial	Depresses angle of mouth.
Buccinator.	Facial and inferior maxillary	Compresses cheeks.
Risorius.	Facial	Draws angle of mouth outward.
Orbicularis oris	Facial	Closes mouth.
Masseter.	Inferior maxillary	Mastication, molars.
Temporal.	Inferior maxillary	Mastication, incisors.
Pterygoideus externus.	Inferior maxillary	Moves lower jaw forward.
Pterygoideus internus.	Inferior maxillary	Raises and advances inferior maxillary.

Neck.

Platysma myoides.	Facial and superficial cervical	Wrinkles skin and depresses mouth.
Sterno-cleido-mastoid.	Spinal accessory and cervical plexus.	Depresses and rotates head.
Sterno-hyoid.	Descendens and communicans noni	Depresses hyoid.
Sterno-thyroid.	Descendens and communicans noni	Depresses larynx.
Thyro-hyoid.	Hypoglossal.	Elevates larynx.
Omo-hyoid.	Descendens and communicans noni	Depresses and retracts hyoid.
Digastric.	Inferior dental (facial)	Elevates hyoid and tongue.
Stylo-hyoid.	Facial	Elevates and retracts hyoid.
Mylo-hyoid.	Inferior dental	Elevates and advances hyoid; forms floor of mouth.
Genio-hyoid.	Hypoglossal.	Elevates and advances hyoid.
Genio-hyo-glossus.	Hypoglossal.	Retracts and protrudes tongue.
Hyo-glossus.	Hypoglossal.	Depresses side of tongue.
Lingualis.	Chorda tympani.	Elevates center of tongue.
Stylo-glossus.	Hypoglossal.	Elevates and retracts tongue.
Palato-glossus.	Meckel's ganglion.	Draws base of tongue upward.
Constrictor inferior.	Glosso-pharyngeal, pharyngeal plexus, and external and recurrent laryng'l.	Contracts fauces.
Constrictor medius.	Glosso-pharyngeal and glosso-pharyngeal plexus.	Contracts fauces.
Constrictor superior.	Glosso-pharyngeal and pharyngeal plexus.	Contracts pharynx.
Stylo-pharyngeus.	Glosso-pharyngeal and pharyngeal plexus.	Elevates pharynx.

NAME.	NERVE.	ACTION.
Palato-pharyngeus	Meckel's ganglion	Closes posterior nares.
Levator palati	Meckel's ganglion (facial)	Elevates soft palate.
Tensor palati	Otic ganglion	Renders palate tense.
Azygos uvulae	Meckel's ganglion (facial)	Raises uvula.
Rectus capitus anticus major	Cervical plexus	Flexes neck backward.
Rectus capitus anticus minor	Cervical plexus	Flexes neck backward.
Rectus lateralis	Cervical plexus	Moves head laterally.
Longus colli	Lower cervical	Flexes cervical spine.
Scalenus anticus	Lower cervical	Flexes neck laterally.
Scalenus medius	Lower cervical	Flexes neck laterally.
Scalenus posticus	Lower cervical	Flexes neck laterally.

Back.

NAME.	NERVE.	ACTION.
Trapezius	Spinal accessory and cervical plexus	Draws head backward and elevates shoulders.
Latissimus dorsi	Subscapular	Draws arm backward and downward.
Levator anguli scapulae	Third and fourth cervical	Elevates upper angle of scapula.
Rhomboideus minor	Fifth cervical	Retracts and elevates scapula.
Rhomboideus major	Fifth cervical	Elevates and retracts scapula.
Serratus posticus superior	Posterior branches of cervical	Raises ribs in inspiration.
Serratus posticus inferior	Posterior branches of dorsal	Depresses ribs in expiration.
Splenius capitus et colli	Posterior branches of cervical	Rotates head and holds it erect.
Splenius colli	Posterior branches of cervical	Rotates head and holds it erect.
Erector spine	Lumbar and dorsal	Holds spine erect.
Sacro-lumbalis	Branches of dorsal	Erects trunk and flexes it backward.
Musculus accessorius ad sacro-lumbalem	Branches of dorsal	Erects trunk and flexes it backward.
Longissimus dorsi	Branches of lumbar and dorsal	Erects trunk and flexes it backward.
Spinalis dorsi	Dorsal branches	Erects spinal column.
Cervicalis ascendens	Branches of cervical	Holds head erect and raises upper ribs.
Transversalis colli	Branches of cervical	Holds head erect.

Muscle	Nerve	Action
Trachelo-mastoid	Branches of cervical	Steadies head.
Complexus	Sub-occipital, great occipital, and branches of cervical	Retracts and rotates head.
Biventer cervicis	(The same as for complexus)	Retracts and rotates head.
Semispinalis dorsi	Branches of dorsal	Erects spinal column.
Semispinalis colli	Cervical branches	Erects spinal column.
Multifidus spinæ	Posterior spinal branches	Erects and rotates spinal column.
Rotatores spinæ	Dorsal branches of spine	Rotate spinal column.
Supraspinales	Posterior cervical	Approximate spinous processes.
Interspinales	Posterior cervical	Approximate spinous processes.
Extensor coccygis	Sacral branches	Extends coccyx.
Intertransversales	Posterior spinal nerves	Approximate transverse processes.
Rectus capitis posticus major	Sub. occipital	Rotates head.
Rectus capitis posticus minor	Sub. occipital	Draws head backward.
Obliquus capitis superior	Sub. occipital	Draws head backward.
Obliquus capitis inferior	Sub. and great occipital	Rotates head.

Abdomen.

Muscle	Nerve	Action
Obliquus externus	Intercostal, ilio-hypogastric, ilio-inguinal.	Compresses viscera and flexes thorax.
Obliquus internus	Intercostal, ilio-hypogastric, ilio-inguinal.	Compresses viscera and flexes thorax.
Transversalis	Intercostal, ilio-hypogastric, ilio-inguinal.	Compresses viscera and flexes thorax.
Rectus abdominis	Intercostal, ilio-hypogastric, ilio-inguinal.	Compresses viscera and flexes thorax.
Pyramidalis	Ilio-hypogastric	Renders linea alba tense.
Quadratus lumborum	Lumbar	Flexes thorax laterally.

Thorax.

Muscle	Nerve	Action
Intercostales externi	Intercostal	Depress ribs in expiration.
Intercostales interni	Intercostal	Raise ribs in inspiration.
Infracostales	Intercostal	Inspiration.
Triangularis sterni	Intercostal	Expiration.
Levatores costarum	Intercostal	Raise ribs.
Diaphragm	Phrenic	Inspiration.

Name.	Nerve.	Action.
Shoulder.		
Pectoralis major	Anterior thoracic	Draws arm down and forward.
Pectoralis minor	Anterior thoracic	Depresses point of shoulder.
Subclavius	Fifth and sixth cervical	Depresses shoulder.
Serratus magnus	Posterior thoracic	Raises shoulder and elevates ribs in inspiration.
Deltoid	Circumflex	Raises arm.
Subscapularis	Subscapular	Rotates humerus inward.
Supraspinatus	Suprascapular	Supports shoulder joint, raises arm.
Infraspinatus	Suprascapular	Rotates humerus outward.
Teres minor	Circumflex	Rotates humerus outward.
Teres major	Subscapular	Draws arm down and back.
Arm.		
Coraco-brachialis	Musculo-cutaneous	Draws arm forward and inward.
Biceps	Musculo-cutaneous	Flexes and supinates forearm.
Brachialis anticus	Musculo-cutaneous, musculo-spiral	Flexes forearm.
Triceps	Musculo-spiral	Extends forearm.
Subanconeus	Musculo-spiral	Tensor of posterior ligament of elbow.
Forearm.		
Pronator radii teres	Median	Pronates hand.
Flexor carpi radialis	Median	Flexes wrist.
Palmaris longus	Median	Tenses palmar fascia.
Flexor carpi ulnaris	Ulnar	Flexes wrist.
Flexor sublimus digitorum	Median	Flexes second phalanges.
Flexor profundus digitorum	Ulnar and anterior interosseus	Flexes the phalanges.
Flexor longus pollicis	Anterior interosseus	Flexes last phalanx of thumb.
Pronator quadratus	Anterior interosseus	Pronates hand.
Supinator longus	Musculo-spiral	Supinates hand.
Extensor carpi radialis longior	Musculo-spiral	Extends wrist.
Extensor carpi radialis brevier	Posterior interosseus	Extends wrist.
Extensor communis digitorum	Posterior interosseus	Extends fingers.

Extensor minimi digiti	Posterior interosseus	Extensor of little finger.
Extensor carpi ulnaris	Posterior interosseus	Extends wrist.
Anconeus	Musculo-spiral	Extends forearm.
Supinator brevis	Posterior interosseus	Supinates hand.
Extensor ossis metacarpi pollicis	Posterior interosseus	Extends thumb.
Extensor primi internodii pollicis	Posterior interosseus	Extends thumb.
Extensor secundi internodii pollicis	Posterior interosseus	Extends thumb.
Extensor indicis	Posterior interosseus	Extends index.
Abductor pollicis	Median	Draws thumb from median line.
Flexor ossis metacarpi pollicis (oppon).	Median	Flexes thumb.
Flexor brevis pollicis	Median and ulnar	Flexes thumb.
Hand.		
Adductor pollicis	Ulnar	Draws thumb to median line.
Palmaris brevis	Ulnar	Corrugates skin of palm.
Abductor minimi digiti	Ulnar	Abductor of little finger.
Flexor brevis minimi digiti	Ulnar	Flexes little finger.
Flexor minimi digiti (opponens)	Ulnar	Flexes little finger.
Lumbricales	Median and ulnar	Flex first phalanges and extend second and third.
Interossei palmaris	Ulnar	Adduct fingers.
Interossei dorsales	Ulnar	Abduct fingers, flex first phalanges, and extend second and third.
Lower extremity.		
Psoas magnus	Lumbar	Flexes and rotates thigh outward and flexes trunk on pelvis.
Psoas parvus	Lumbar	Tensor of iliac fascia.
Iliacus	Anterior crural	Flexes femur and rotates it outward.
Hip.		
Gluteus maximus	Small sciatic and sacral plexus	Extends and abducts thigh and rotates it outward.
Gluteus medius	Superior gluteal	Rotates outward and inward, abducts, extends, and flexes thigh.
Gluteus minimus	Superior gluteal	Rotates outward and inward, abducts, extends, and flexes thigh.

Name.	Nerve.	Action.
Pyriformis...............	Sacral	Rotates thigh outward, abducts it, and tilts pelvis forward.
Gemellus superior........	Sacral	Rotates thigh outward and abducts it.
Obturator internus......	Sacral	Rotates thigh outward and tilts pelvis forward.
Gemellus inferior........	Sacral	Rotates thigh outward and abducts it.
Obturator externus	Obturator....	Rotates thigh outward and tilts pelvis forward.
Quadratus femoris........	Sacral	Abducts thigh and rotates it outward.
Biceps.................	Great sciatic....	Flexes leg and rotates it outward.
Semitendinosus	Great sciatic....	Flexes leg on thigh and rotates it inward.
Semimembranosus	Great sciatic....	Flexes leg and rotates it inward.
Thigh.		
Tensor vaginæ femoris.....	Superior gluteal....	Tensor of fascia lata.
Sartorius.............	Anterior crural....	Flexes thigh and rotates it outward.
Rectus femoris...........	Anterior crural....	Extends leg.
Vastus externus.........	Anterior crural....	Extends leg.
Vastus internus.........	Anterior crural....	Extends leg.
Crureus................	Anterior crural....	Extends leg.
Quadriceps extensor (includes four preceding muscles).		
Subcrureus.............	Anterior crural....	Acts with crureus.
Gracilis................	Obturator........	Flexes and adducts thigh and rotates it inward.
Pectineus...............	Anterior crural, obturator	Flexes and adducts thigh and rotates it outward.
Adductor longus..........	Obturator........	Adducts and flexes thigh.
Adductor brevis.........	Obturator........	Adducts and flexes thigh.
Adductor magnus.........	Obturator and great sciatic....	Adducts thigh and rotates it outward.
Leg.		
Tibialis anticus.........	Anterior tibial.....	Flexes ankle and elevates inner border of foot.

Muscle	Nerve	Action
Extensor longus digitorum	Anterior tibial	Extends toes and flexes ankle.
Extensor proprius pollicis	Anterior tibial	Extends toes and flexes ankle.
Peroneus tertius	Anterior tibial	Flexes tarsus and raises outer border of foot.
Gastrocnemius	Internal popliteal	Extends foot.
Plantaris	Internal popliteal	Tenses plantar fascia.
Soleus	Internal popliteal	Extends foot.
Popliteus	Internal popliteal	Flexes leg and rotates it inward.
Flexor longus pollicis	Posterior tibial	Flexes great toe.
Flexor longus digitorum	Posterior tibial	Flexes phalanges and extends foot.
Tibialis posticus	Posterior tibial	Extends ankle and turns sole inward.
Peroneus longus	Musculo-cutaneous	Extends and everts foot.
Peroneus brevis	Musculo-cutaneous	Extends foot.

Foot.

Muscle	Nerve	Action
Extensor brevis digitorum	Anterior tibial	Extends toes.
Abductor pollicis	Internal plantar	Abducts great toe, flexes first phalanx, and extends second.
Flexor brevis digitorum	Internal plantar	Flexes lesser toes.
Abductor minimi digiti	External plantar	Abducts little toe.
Flexor accessorius	External plantar	Accessory flexor of toes.
Lumbricales	Internal and external plantar	Flex first phalanges and extend last two.
Flexor brevis pollicis	Internal plantar	Flexes first phalanx of great toe and extends second.
Adductor pollicis	External plantar	Adducts great toe and extends first and second phalanx.
Flexor brevis minimi digiti	External plantar	Flexes first phalanx of little toe and extends second.
Transversus pedis	External plantar	Adducts great toe.
Interossei dorsal	External plantar	Abduct toes.
Interossei	External plantar	Adduct toes.

The foregoing table has been arranged with much care, and with special reference to the needs of the student of massage. It is believed to be the most complete and correct resumé of the sort which has ever been published, embodying, as it does, the results of the very latest studies and authoritative statements relating to the nerve supply and actions of the various muscles of the body. The student of massage who desires to place himself in the front rank of his profession as a masseur, will find it not only profitable, but essential, to make a careful study of this table, and to become familiar with the facts which it very succinctly presents. The grouping of the muscles of the several regions of the body renders it convenient to study each section by itself, and by the aid of Plates V to X and XIII, it will not be found difficult to form a very correct idea of the precise location and outline of each particular muscle in the body, and of the origin and distribution of the nerve supply. Two hundred and seven different muscles or muscular groups are named in the table, by means of which one hundred and sixty-three different motor acts are performed. It may not be absolutely essential that every one of these should be held constantly in the memory, but those muscles, at least, which constitute the largest fleshy masses of the body, should be thoroughly studied and familiarized.

APPENDIX I.

Clinical Notes of Cases Treated by Massage.

In the following cases treated by myself and my colleagues at the Sanitarium at Battle Creek, Michigan, massage, manual Swedish movements, and gymnastics have been employed as the principal therapeutic means. Baths, and usually some electrical applications, together with other appropriate measures, have also been made use of, as in most cases treated in the institution; but these particular cases have been selected to illustrate the effects of massage, for the reason that in them more benefit was clearly attributable to this agent than to any other.

CASE I.

Obesity.—Mrs. W., aged fifty-three, was received for treatment in February, 1893. She had always been inclined to obesity, but had recently found herself increasing in weight so rapidly that life had come to be almost a burden. This patient remained under treatment six weeks, during which time, under vigorous massage administered daily, she lost in weight at the rate of nearly one pound a day. Baths and a systematic dietary were also used.

CASE II.

Mrs. A., aged twenty-five, was treated for obesity for two weeks. At the end of two weeks she weighed fourteen pounds less than at the beginning.of treatment.

CASE III.

Col. X., aged fifty-three, weighed at the beginning of treatment 334 pounds. He was naturally a very large man, but his weight had been gradually increasing for more than twenty years; and when received, he weighed fully one hundred pounds more than in health. As the result of treatment during eight weeks, the patient's weight was reduced seventy-five pounds. He was then obliged, by business engagements, to return home. He came back the following year, when he was found to have regained in part his former excess of weight; but a second course of treatment secured a still further reduction of the enormous accumulation of flesh about the trunk, which had given the patient's body most unwieldy proportions.

CASE IV.

Emaciation.— Miss B., aged thirty-two, had suffered from tuberculosis. A year in Colorado had effected a cure of the tuberculosis, but had left a large cavity in the upper lobe of the left lung. The patient had never recovered her normal weight or strength since this illness, and within two or three years had been still further reduced by uterine hemorrhages, until her condition had become very grave. Her physician sent her to the Sanitarium with the hope that the hemorrhages might be arrested and her general condition improved. She weighed less than one hundred pounds, was extremely anæmic, and was so weak that it was necessary to confine her strictly to bed for several weeks. At the end of six months this patient had improved to such a degree that she was enjoying better health than ever before in her life. Her weight had increased forty pounds, and her strength had improved proportionately. Digestion and all the other bodily functions were perfectly performed. The patient returned to her home enjoying excellent health, and has remained well to the present time, with the exception of an attack of la grippe.

CASE V.

Prof. W., aged sixty years, had been a dyspeptic since he was twenty years of age, and had for many years been greatly emaciated. He declared that his stomach was a "swill-barrel." Had been confined to his bed for six months before coming to the Sanitarium for treatment ; and was then barely able to stand upon his feet. He could take a few steps with assistance, but was obliged to use a wheel-chair in going to meals. During the first four weeks of treatment, this patient gained on an average one pound each day, and at the end of six weeks was so greatly improved that he walked a mile to the depot to meet a brother whom he had not seen for several months, and who, as he afterward stated, had difficulty in recognizing him, so greatly was his appearance changed for the better.

Many other similar cases might be cited. It is the author's custom to weigh each patient at the beginning of treatment, and regularly every week thereafter; and it is not an uncommon thing to find a patient who has gained three to five pounds in a single week. From twelve to twenty pounds is very frequently gained in the course of two or three weeks' treatment. Under the system advocated in this work, the patient gains not merely in flesh, but also in strength. A test of the strength is made at the beginning of treatment, and each month while the patient remains under observation. A gain of five hundred to six hundred pounds in strength capacity within four weeks is very common, and sometimes double this amount is gained within a month.

CASE VI.

Rheumatism.—Mrs. T., aged sixty, was received for treatment in September, 1893. In addition to general debility, anæmia, neurasthenia, dyspepsia, and disordered hepatic and renal functions, this patient was suffering from rheumatism and with much stiffness of the left shoulder. General tonic treatment, with general and local massage, especially directed to the shoulders, entirely relieved the rheumatic affection in six weeks.

CASE VII.

Mrs. C., aged seventy, was received for treatment in April, 1892. This patient had a fracture of the wrist which had been treated by means of a plaster bandage. The whole arm was useless; the fingers were extended and could not be flexed; the arm could not be raised as high as the shoulder; only a very slight movement of the elbow joint was possible; the entire arm was practically useless. The application of massage for two months entirely restored the arm, so that it was stronger than the other, as shown by the dynamometer. The patient, when she left, was able to use the arm and fingers freely in combing her hair and for any other purpose.

CASE VIII.

Miss R., aged twenty-three, was received in March, 1891. She had suffered from lameness in the left arm for seven years, the elbow being stiff, and the muscles of the arm considerably wasted. For a year she had not been able to use her hand or arm at all, and all the joints were more or less stiffened. The patient was under treatment for five months, at the end of which time the restoration of the arm was nearly complete. The motion of some of the joints was still slightly limited, but she had good use of the arm, and suffered no pain.

Case IX.

Mrs. K., aged fifty-three, was received for treatment in August, 1894. She had for several years suffered from stiffness of the shoulder joints, the limitation of movement being accompanied by pain, which was doubtless due to rheumatism. The disability was so great that the patient had for several years been unable to dress herself without assistance. At the end of one month's treatment, she was able to use the affected arm nearly as well as the other; could move it freely in all directions, lifting it above the head and placing it behind her,—movements which had not been possible for more than ten years previous.

Case X.

Neuritis.—Mr. X., aged fifty years, a carpenter, had for several months suffered from severe pain in his left shoulder joint. The muscles of the arm had wasted considerably, and the arm was wholly useless; he could not even raise it from his side. He had evidently suffered from neuritis of the nerves of the shoulder joint, and from muscular atrophy, which usually accompanies this disease. Massage, with applications of fomentations and electricity, effected a complete cure in the course of a few months, and the patient has now for seven or eight years enjoyed the full use of the arm as before.

Case XI.

Writers' Cramp.—Mr. A., aged twenty-seven years, cashier in a bank, presented the most extreme and graphic picture of writers' cramp which the author has ever encountered. The disease affected not only the hand, but the entire arm and the muscles of the neck and face; and spasms were excited, not only by writing, but by any movement of the body. If the patient attempted to rise from a chair, his head was immediately drawn to the right side, the right side of the face was contorted by muscular contraction, and the muscles of the hand and arm became rigid. The patient's gait seemed to be also slightly affected. He had submitted to several surgical operations, in which some of the nerves of the neck had been divided, and the sterno-cleido-mastoid and other muscles had also been twice divided. Slight temporary relief had followed the operations, but the disease, when the patient came under my care, was worse than it had ever been at any previous time. Upon examination, I found that the patient was suffering from all the different phases of writers' cramp. Whenever he undertook to write, the whole arm became rigid, and the head was drawn around toward the right side until the face looked nearly toward the shoulder. Strange grimaces played upon the countenance in consequence of the contraction of the facial muscles. Examination of the neck showed here and there points of induration. Massage and gymnastics applied to the arm, and thorough local massage of the muscles of the neck, together with revulsive applications of various sorts, including dry cupping, hot and cold applications, and mild counter-irritation, effected a complete cure; and the patient has remained well until the present time, it being now some five years since he was under treatment. Apparently little or no benefit was derived from other measures of treatment, nor until special attention was given to massage of the affected parts and to the points of induration above referred to. Many other equally successful cases might be cited from my experience, in which not only local but general neuritis has yielded completely as the result of the persevering and skillful application of massage.

Case XII.

Asthma.—Mrs. B., aged forty-one years, was received for treatment in July, 1890, having suffered from nervous exhaustion and asthma for many years. On examination, she was found to have prolapse of the stomach and bowels, and extreme hyperæsthesia of the lumbar ganglia of the sympathetic nerve. The patient was scarcely able to walk about, and could not sleep on account of continued asthmatic paroxysms. During the first two weeks after being received, she was confined in bed by asthmatic attacks, which were extremely aggravated by the slightest exercise. Within five weeks, however, the patient returned home wonderfully improved. The asthmatic paroxysms were especially relieved by percussion of the chest. Spatting and hacking movements were found most effective.

Case XIII.

Sprain.—Mrs. B., aged forty-four, was received in August, 1893, for treatment for severe sprain of the ankle. Derivative massage was applied at first ; later, massage of the joint, including gentle flexion and extension. At the end of ten days the patient was able to visit the World's Fair. She had the misfortune, however, to sprain the ankle again, and was obliged to return for treatment. At the end of two weeks the ankle showed no trace of injury.

Case XIV.

Miss M., aged twenty-nine years, was received for treatment in August, 1893, being unable to walk in consequence of lameness of the left ankle, the result of a sprain received some months before. Massage was applied for several weeks, at the end of which time she was able to walk with ease. Hot and cold applications, heating compresses, local applications of electricity, and other means were also employed, but the chief benefit was evidently derived from massage. A great number of similar cases might be cited.

CASE XV.

The writer had a personal experience of the benefits to be derived from massage in cases of sprain, which affords very conclusive evidence of the value of this simple method of treatment when skillfully administered in traumatisms of this character. The sprain involved both the ankle and the metatarso-phalangeal joints, chiefly the latter. The pain was so severe that it was impossible to sustain the weight of the body upon the anterior portion of the foot. It was only possible to walk by stepping in such a way as to keep the weight of the body over the heel of the affected foot. Being much engaged, the sprain was neglected for a couple of days, it being possible to hobble about after applying a tight bandage about the foot, with the hope that nature would effect a cure ; but on the morning of the second day, it was found that the pain had become so great that the whole foot was involved, and it was impossible to step at all without very great pain. A masseur was accordingly sent for, and derivative massage was applied with gentle friction of the foot and careful joint movements of the ankle.

At the end of a couple of hours the pain had disappeared, and in going about his usual duties, which require much exercise upon the feet, the writer was greatly surprised to find that the sprain was practically cured. No pain whatever was noticeable, and it was, indeed, impossible to place the foot in any position by which pain could be induced.

By the next morning, the third day following the accident, the foot seemed perfectly well. It was possible to run and jump, and to hop upon the affected foot without pain. Several mishaps to the foot caused a return of lameness before it was cured, but relief was invariably found in the application of local and derivative massage.

If the ordinary method of absolute rest, without massage, had been adopted, the writer feels confident that he would have been a cripple for at least three or four weeks.

CASE XVI.

Spinal Curvature.— Miss R., aged fourteen years, was suffering from double lateral curvature of the spine, with rotation. The curvature had first been noticed two years before. After eight months' treatment, the curvature had so nearly disappeared that the patient was allowed to return home. Electricity, baths, and Swedish gymnastics were employed in connection with massage.

CASE XVII.

Miss N., aged thirty-three years, was received in February, 1891, for treatment of double lateral curvature of the spine,—the result of sitting in a bad position in a large easy chair, a habit which had been maintained for many years. The curvature was first noticed five years previous. After five months' treatment the patient returned home so greatly improved that the curvature was no longer a matter requiring consideration.

CASE XVIII.

Miss B., aged twenty years, was received for treatment in December, 1891, suffering from double curvature of the spine, with rotation,—the result of an injury nine months before. In jumping from a wagon, she had fallen upon frozen ground, dislocating one shoulder, and causing partial paralysis of the arm and side. She was treated for a year and a half, wearing a plaster jacket for six months; and, at the time she came under my care, had worn a steel apparatus for six months. She complained of constant pain in the side and shoulder. The patient's strength was so much improved as the result of a few months' treatment, and the muscles of the trunk were developed to such a degree, that she was finally able to dispense with mechanical support of any kind. The total strength capacity was increased more than one thousand pounds, as shown by the dynamometer.

CASE XIX.

Mr. K., aged thirty-five years, was received for treatment in March, 1885. This patient had an extremely pronounced lateral curvature of the spine, involving both the dorsal and the lumbar region ; rotation to the right also existed. The disease had begun about one year previous, the chief symptom being severe pain in the right side. The muscles were extremely contracted. By massage, exercise, suspension, local applications of electricity, fomentations, and other measures of treatment, the patient was, in the course of three months, entirely cured, so that he was able to return to his business. His height was found to have increased two inches, and no trace of the curvature remained. The most important measures of treatment employed were massage and gymnastics, although the

17

baths and other means employed were doubtless to some extent beneficial.

CASE XX.

Paralysis.—Mrs. K., aged forty years, had been confined to her bed for many months as the result of paralysis of one lower half of the body, resulting from a fall in which the back was injured. After the daily application of massage for a few months the patient was able to walk, and at the end of ten months' treatment was able to ride a bicycle. Electricity, baths, and other measures were employed in connection with massage.

Scores of similar cases might be cited as illustrations of the benefit to be derived from massage in cases of paralysis of different forms. It is certainly of value, although not radically curative, in most forms of paralysis. The writer has seen marked beneficial results from massage in numerous cases of locomotor ataxia, and in a still larger number of cases of spinal sclerosis, and other forms of paralysis arising from degenerative processes in the general nervous system.

CASE XXI.

Infantile Paralysis.— Miss N., aged fourteen, had paralysis of one leg and arm, as the result of an attack of poliomyelitis when an infant. After several months' treatment by massage, with electricity and baths, the patient was able to dance, skate, and make good use of both arm and leg, although some evidences of the disease still remained.

CASE XXII.

Miss D., aged twelve, had suffered since infancy from infantile paralysis affecting the left leg. When received for treatment, the muscles below the knee were atrophied almost to complete disappearance. No response could be obtained to the application of faradic electricity, and only a slight one to the application of the galvanic current. The patient had scarcely any use of the limb, and was able to make only very slight movements of the toes. Her limb was constantly cold and moist. After one year's treatment by massage, galvanism, and baths, the patient was able to run about freely and make good use of the limb, and a very considerable degree of muscular development had taken place.

CASE XXIII.

Sclerosis.— Miss Z., aged twenty-six, entered the Sanitarium as a patient in January, 1883. She complained of an inability to use the right leg, having been compelled to use crutches in walking for several years. On examination, the right leg was found to be in a remarkable condition. Almost the entire limb had undergone such structural changes that it had become as hard as wood. The tissues were considerably shrunken, the surface was smooth as polished marble, the temperature was below normal, so that the limb felt cold to the hand, and the ankle and all the joints of the foot were fixed so that movement was impossible, although some mobility still remained in the knee joint. Below the knee the limb could not have been more rigid, hard, and lifeless in appearance if it had actually been made of wood or celluloid. The case seemed an utterly hopeless one, but the patient was so importunate that something should be done for her that we received the case on trial for a few months.

At the end of three months the changes which had occurred were truly remarkable. Above the knee the tissues had become quite soft and pliable; below the knee the hardness was disappearing somewhat; all the tissues of the foot were still hard, but the ankle and other joints had loosened somewhat, so that slight movement was possible. Continuance of the treatment at intervals for two years restored the limb to such a degree that the patient was able to walk without crutches, and scarcely a trace of the former condition remained. The improvement continued for several years. No relapse has occurred, and the patient at present is in the enjoyment of excellent health, and the disability of the right limb is comparatively slight. Electricity and hydrotherapeutic applications of various sorts were employed in connection with massage, but the paramount utility of massage in this case was unquestionable.

Case XXIV.

Constipation.—Mrs. H., aged thirty, was admitted for treatment in April, 1887. She had been an invalid since confinement, five years before, suffering from an aggravated form of dyspepsia and migraine. No natural movement of the bowels had occurred for three years. The constipation was entirely relieved by the employment of abdominal massage, together with general tonic treatment and a correct regimen.

Case XXV.

Miss H., aged twenty-two, had suffered extremely for a number of years from constipation, a natural movement very rarely occurring. At the end of two months' treatment the action of the bowels had become normal and regular. The patient has been enjoying good health ever since

Case XXVI.

Mr. X., a man of sedentary habits, had suffered from constipation for many years. After two weeks' treatment a daily natural evacuation of the bowels was secured without artificial means of any kind other than massage, although a natural movement had not occurred for more than three years previous.

Case XXVII.

Mrs. W., aged forty-four years, was received for treatment in April, 1877, having suffered from extreme constipation for more than twenty years. No movement of the bowels had occurred during this time without the use of medicines. The lady's husband was entirely faithless of any improvement under treatment, but at the end of three weeks the patient's bowels were moving regularly, without tonic medicine of any kind.

Case XXVIII.

Neurasthenia; General Debility.—Mrs. H., aged twenty-eight years, was received for treatment in June, 1893, having been an invalid for eight years. The patient had suffered greatly from acid dyspepsia, flatulence, distention of the bowels, aortic palpitation, and extreme constipation, with great hyperæsthesia of the lumbar ganglia of the sympathetic. The lower border of the stomach was found three inches below the umbilicus, also a floating kidney on the right side, and both ovaries prolapsed. Indeed, the conditions were sufficiently grave to render a person thoroughly miserable. The patient remained under treatment five months, during which time she received daily applications of massage, especially to the bowels, and electricity. At the end of five months she left the Sanitarium enjoying very comfortable health.

Case XXIX.

Hæmaturia and Anæmia.—Mrs. L., aged thirty-eight, was received for treatment in June, 1892. The patient was extremely anæmic, as the result of several months' suffering from a very aggravated form of hæmaturia. Her face was without color; she was emaciated, and so weak as to be confined to her bed. She could only be moved upon a stretcher or wheel-chair, from which it was necessary to lift her to the bed. She was able to walk at the end of three weeks, and left at the end of two months, entirely cured. She had gained greatly in flesh, and the natural color had returned to her cheeks. The patient pronounced herself entirely well. The hæmaturia ceased within a week after the beginning of treatment.

Case XXX.

Anæmia.— Miss A., aged twenty, had suffered from a variety of troubles which had resulted in a very grave form of anæmia. The chief of her troubles were chronic inflammation and prolapse of the left ovary; movable right kidney; enteroptosis and gastroptosis, the lower border of the stomach falling one inch below the umbilicus; extreme hyperæsthesia of the lumbar ganglia of the sympathetic; menorrhagia; and frequent attacks of acute gastritis. Strong anæmic murmurs were found at the base of the heart.

At the first examination the patient's nutrition was found to be reduced to such a low point that the hæmoglobin present was only four per cent — less than one third of the normal amount. The number of blood corpuscles per cubic millimeter was 1,510,000, or one third of the normal. Poikilocytes and microcytes were exceedingly abundant, and there were a few macrocytes. This case, if not one of pernicious anæmia, certainly bordered very closely on that class of anæmics. Under rational treatment, by which massage, both manual and mechanical, was a leading feature, the amount of hæmoglobin increased in ten days to seven per cent, and the blood count to 2,340,000 per cubic millimeter. A few macrocytes and poikilocytes still remained, showing that normal hæmatogenesis was not yet restored, but that the process was becoming normal.

A marked feature in this case was the small number of leucocytes contained in the blood. At the first examination the proportion of leucocytes to normal was only eighteen one hundredths; at the end of ten days the proportion had increased to fifty-four one hundredths. At the end of a few weeks' treatment the blood count was 3,210,000 and the hæmoglobin eight per cent, as measured by Henocque's hæmatoscope. The patient's improvement remained permanent, and at the present writing she is still improving.

Case XXXI.

Mrs. Z., aged twenty-five, was received at the Sanitarium for treatment in October, 1894. She had suffered for two years from marked anæmia, as the result of an attack of intermittent fever. On arrival, the examination of the blood gave the following results: Blood count, 3,760,000; hæmoglobin, 10.5 per cent.

Four weeks later a second examination showed an increase of the blood count to 3,930,000. The percentage of hæmoglobin was the same as at the first examination.

At the end of two weeks' further treatment, during which the patient made rapid gain, the blood count was found to be 4,370,000, and the hæmoglobin twelve per cent. The patient went home much benefited, and with a prospect of continued improvement.

Case XXXII.

Melancholia.— Mrs. B., aged thirty-one, was received for treatment in July, 1893. The patient was in an extremely weak and emaciated condition, and had been insane for three and a half years, as the result of a fright caused by the explosion of a lamp in a sleeping-car. For six months, marked suicidal tendencies had existed. After six months' treatment the patient returned to her home perfectly sound in health, mentally and physically. She has remained well up to the present time.

Case XXXIII.

Prolapsed Liver.— Mrs. N., aged fifty, was received for treatment in July, 1891. The abdominal muscles were found greatly contracted; but after the administration of massage for two weeks, the muscles became relaxed sufficiently to allow a minute exploration of the condition of the viscera, when a mass was found in the right side which, on further investigation, proved to be a prolapsed liver. This organ was daily replaced, in connection with abdominal massage. At the end of three months the patient returned to her home enjoying good health, the abdominal muscles well developed, and the liver in its normal position.

Such encouraging results as these cannot be obtained in every case, although almost equally good success has been reached in a number of others which have come under the writer's care. In a recent case the abdominal muscles had been so overstretched by repeated pregnancy, and had become so relaxed and wasted by disuse, that little could be accomplished by means of massage. The pyloric end of the stomach was in this case found three inches below the umbilicus, the lower border of the liver falling an inch below the umbilicus. Finding it impossible to support the organs in position by abdominal bandages or supports of any kind, and despairing of relieving the patient in any other way, the following surgical procedure was adopted: It being necessary to perform an operation upon this patient for the relief of an irreducible direct inguinal hernia, in which a mass of omentum had become incarcerated, I determined to make an attempt at the same time to restore the prolapsed stomach and liver to position by surgical means. An incision was accordingly made from a point one inch below the ensiform cartilage of the sternum nearly to the umbilicus. Passing two fingers downward through this incision, it was just possible to reach the lower border of the liver, which was forced up into its position under the ribs. The pyloric end of the stomach was drawn up to nearly its normal position, and by means of four silkworm-gut sutures inserted along the line of the lesser curvature of the stomach (including, of course, only the perineal coat) near its pyloric end, the organ was attached to the abdominal wall. The sutures were passed through the inner margins of the wound at its upper part, so that when tied they not only attached the stomach to the abdominal wall, but also brought together the edges of the peritoneum and the divided fascia. The sutures were buried in the wound by the closing sutures, being cut off short to remain permanently. The position of the sutures was made such as to cause them to fall at the notch between the right and left lobes of the liver, and thus serve as a means of supporting it in its normal position. The patient had no febrile reaction whatever following the operation, and was greatly improved by it, the stomach and liver being held in nearly normal position. Three weeks after the operation she was able to eat heartily, and the lower border of the stomach was found an inch above the umbilicus, instead of three inches below it.

CASE XXXIV.

Prolapsed Stomach and Bowels.— Mrs. A., aged twenty-seven, was received for treatment in July, 1891. The patient was very weak, anæmic, and nervously exhausted. Digestion was almost totally suspended. Upon examination, the lower border of the stomach was found two inches below the umbilicus. Special applications of massage to the abdomen; replacement of the stomach; and the employment of general massage, electricity, and baths restored the patient to complete health. At the end of six months the abdominal muscles were found to be vigorous and well developed. The stomach was held in normal position. The patient has since remained in good health.

After a thorough application of the procedures described elsewhere in this work for replacement of the stomach and lifting of the abdominal contents, the writer has frequently been able to demonstrate the lower border of the stomach at a point from two to four inches above the point at which it was found at the beginning of the treatment.

CASE XXXV.

Pelvic Disease and Constipation.— Mrs. T., aged thirty-two, had suffered for a number of years from severe constipation, extreme tenderness of the ovaries, uterine prolapse, and a variety of nervous symptoms arising from these conditions. At the end of four months' treatment, the patient returned home cured of the constipation and of her pelvic disorders, and has remained in good health ever since.

A large number of cases similar to the above might be cited, illustrating the beneficial results following the use of massage, both general and local, in cases of chronic constipation in its different forms. It is needless to remark that in the treatment of this class of cases, manual Swedish movements, gymnastics, and a proper regulation of the dietary are always combined with massage. In some instances, also, the sinusoidal electric current is employed, the chief value of this agent in these cases being the rhythmical exercise secured by it for the abdominal and other voluntary muscles which come within the influence of the application.

Case XXXVI.

Mrs C., aged thirty-four, was received in February, 1890. The patient had been an invalid for ten years, her ailments dating from the birth of her first child. She was nearly bedridden, emaciated, sallow, depressed, extremely nervous, and a constant sufferer from severe pain in the abdomen and pelvis, the result of chronic peritonitis. The abdomen was so tender that at first scarcely the weight of the hand could be tolerated. After a few weeks the patient was able to endure vigorous manipulation of the abdomen, also pelvic massage. She remained under treatment eleven months, at the end of which time she returned to her home restored to good health. Vaginal douches, fomentations to the abdomen, and applications of electricity were also used in connection with the massage.

Case XXXVII.

Ovarian Disease.— There is no class of functional disorders more amenable to the intelligent application of massage than disease of the ovaries. A great number of cases — some scores — might be quoted in demonstration of the truth of this statement. A few typical ones only will be cited.

Miss W., aged twenty-four, was admitted as a patient in September, 1892. She had spent the greater part of her life in boarding school, where she had been subjected to the usual deteriorating influences of boarding-school life. Examination showed that, in addition to a very marked anæmia and a great variety of neurasthenic symptoms, there was also a posterior curvature of the spine at the middle dorsal region, resulting in extreme flatness of the chest and abnormal prominence of the abdomen, marked hyperæsthesia of the abdominal sympathetic and pneumogastric ; stomach and bowels sunken ; left ovary prolapsed, enlarged, and extremely tender ; severe dysmenorrhœa and menorrhagia, menstrual flow lasting a full week ; and constant backache. She had had two attacks of pelvic inflammation ; could take no exercise at all without inducing severe pelvic pain ; for the last year and a half had been receiving treatment of the eyes from an eye specialist, who labored under the belief that muscular asthenopia, or eye-strain, was the cause of all the symptoms. She grew steadily worse, however, instead of better, although several operations were performed upon the muscles of the eye. At the end of three months the patient declared she felt stronger and better than ever before in her life. The pelvic inflammation, ovarian congestion, and other local disorders have entirely disappeared. The curvatures of the spine, which were wholly due to unbalanced muscular action, were cured. The total gain in strength was 1029 pounds, the increase being from 1582 to 2611. The patient returned to her home with rosy cheeks and ruddy lips, giving no evidence, either objective or subjective, that she was enjoying other than perfect health.

Case XXXVIII.

Miss H., aged twenty, entered the Sanitarium Hospital as a patient with the expectation that the ovaries would have to be removed, as they had been a source of great pain and suffering. She had been bedridden most of the time for three years. There was extreme pain in the left leg, which seemed to proceed from the left ovary ; also in the left ovarian region ; the uterus was antiflexed and retroverted ; the patient generally feeble and anæmic. A scar in the median line below the umbilicus was evidence of the fact that she had had, some months previous, an abdominal section performed, the purpose of the operator having been to remove what he supposed to be a diseased left ovary. A disagreement between the two physicians who were in charge of the case at the time of the operation, as to whether or not the ovary was sufficiently diseased to require removal, led to a conclusion of the operation as an exploratory incision. I took care to restore the prolapsed ovary to position, and replaced the uterus, supporting it by means of a suitably adjusted pessary, and rendered the replacement permanent by shortening the round ligaments. Under the influence of massage and proper exercise, coupled with local applications of electricity, vaginal douches, etc., the patient made an excellent recovery, and escaped mutilation by the removal of the ovaries.

Case XXXIX.

Miss. S., aged twenty-five, arrived at the Sanitarium in a wheel-chair, pale, weak, thoroughly discouraged,— an invalid,— having been in bed for nearly three years, and for two years unable to sit up long enough to take a single meal. The patient was extremely neurasthenic, anæmic to a marked degree, emotional, hysterical, and had constant ovarian pain, which was very greatly increased at the menstrual periods; bowels were constipated; gastric and intestinal catarrh were present. The patient was so susceptible to cold air that she was constantly muffled up in warm blankets, and the slightest draught gave rise to extreme neuralgic pains in various parts of the body.

An examination of the stomach fluid showed hyperpepsia. Physical examination discovered no disorder of the heart or lungs, but extreme hyperæsthesia of the abdominal sympathetic; great pelvic congestion, which was indicated by the almost universal throbbing of the pelvic vessels, the uterus being enlarged to more than twice its normal size, and in a state of extreme retroversion; prolapsus and tenderness of the ovaries, each being twice the normal size; extreme tenderness and irritability of all the pelvic viscera, with general prolapse of the abdominal organs.

This patient had been under the care of physicians for many years. For the last two years she had been under the care of eminent metropolitan physicians, who had employed "rest-cure," and the various methods of treatment commonly adopted in such cases, but without benefit; in fact, the patient had steadily grown worse. She was brought to the Sanitarium from a hospital in Chicago, where she had spent some time, but without receiving help. Massage, manual Swedish movements, and exercise with a wheel-crutch were employed, together with replacement of the uterus and ovaries, and pelvic massage twice a week.

As the patient gained strength, she was required to take more vigorous exercises from day to day; and at the end of six weeks her wheel-chair was taken from her, and regular walking exercises, with the aid of the wheel-crutch, were instituted. At the end of two months the blood had become normal, the amount of hæmoglobin being fourteen per cent, as shown by Henocque's hæmatoscope. The right ovary was still enlarged and somewhat tender, and had a disposition to prolapse; the left ovary was not at all tender, and remained in place. Less than four months after the patient's arrival, the uterus was normal in size and position. Neither ovary could be felt. The patient still complained occasionally of pain in the right ovarian region, but had so far recovered that she was able to begin to ride the bicycle; and since that time has made steady improvement. Her total strength was 2558 pounds, a gain of more than one thousand pounds. The patient was able to exercise freely, and to go about on her feet all day like a well person, and could ride seven or eight miles on a bicycle without the slightest inconvenience. The general sagging of the viscera, although a very noticeable feature at the beginning of the treatment, had entirely disappeared. The bowels were well held up; the lower border of the stomach had risen two inches; and the patient was discharged as cured. She has remained well.

CASE XL.

Miss D., aged twenty-two, came to the Sanitarium a very frail, undeveloped woman, a victim of nervousness, spinal irritation, and a multitude of symptoms, one of the worst of which was so-called muscular rheumatism. She had never in her life enjoyed good health. Menstruation was irregular, accompanied by extreme pain; uterus anteflexed, in a state of retrocession; left ovary prolapsed and tender; profuse leucorrhœal discharge. At the end of six weeks the patient had increased in weight from eighty-six to ninety-six pounds, and had gained 500 pounds in strength. Her waist measure had increased one inch. Her countenance, formerly sallow, was now fresh and full of color; cheeks plump; and her appetite, which had been almost wholly absent, was now so excellent as to oblige her to leave the table hungry, to avoid overeating. The patient was no longer depressed, but wore a happy, cheerful face, being as "busy as a bee" all day long, working for the health and vigor which she already enjoyed in greater measure than ever before in her life. Pelvic massage was administered twice a week. The result was complete relief from ovarian tenderness and pain.

CASE XLI.

Miss K., aged twenty-one, had suffered from constant backache, and was very nervous; had been for some time a student, but had become so ill that her studies were seriously interfered with, and she was unable to endure any physical exertion. Examination showed extreme tenderness of the spine, retroversion of the uterus, prolapse and tenderness of the ovaries, and, as usual in such cases, prolapse of stomach and bowels. The patient was under treatment for several months, during which time she continued her studies, when her health became so greatly improved that she entered the employ of the Sanitarium as a nurse. She now enjoys better health than ever before in her life. Her waist, which had been compressed by tight bands and corsets, expanded several inches as the result of physical exercise, and the vigor of respiration increased to such an extent that the waist enlarged fully six inches in taking a deep breath. Her waist measurement has increased four inches. The ovarian tenderness has disappeared, and not the slightest uterine displacement remains. There is no longer any complaint of backache, and the patient enjoys almost perfect health.

CASE XLII.

Miss T., aged twenty-two, had suffered constantly from great distress in the head, mental confusion, extreme nervousness and lassitude, backache, and severe dysmenorrhœa. The patient had been so long a sufferer that she had lost all interest in life, — a fact which was clearly indicated by her dejected and hopeless countenance. On examination, I found the uterus and ovaries prolapsed, and the ovaries tender. The patient had worn a corset since fifteen years of age. The waist measure was 23.5 inches ; waist expansion, with clothing entirely loose, 1.3 inches. The abdomen was sagging, and general visceral prolapse existed. The patient was so feeble that her aggregate strength was but 832 pounds. At the end of two months' treatment, by the methods previously outlined, this patient's total strength was increased to 1600 pounds, or nearly doubled. There was an increase of one and one half inches in waist measurement, and general improvement in every particular. Ovarian irritation, which was very marked at the beginning of treatment, had entirely disappeared. The patient soon entered the Sanitarium Training School for Nurses, and has since done very efficient work as a nurse. She has now (1894) followed her profession for five years, and is enjoying excellent health. At the end of one year from the beginning of treatment, and several months after the treatment and training had been discontinued, her aggregated strength was found to be 3031 pounds. Her waist measure had increased to thirty inches. There was a marked gain in the lung capacity, and the patient's entire appearance had undergone so decided a change that she could scarcely be recognized as the same person. The sallow complexion had disappeared, and a fresh, ruddy countenance had taken its place. The air of lassitude and dejection previously worn was wholly gone, and an expression of energy, vigor, and cheerful content had taken its place. The increase of strength in the several regions of the body, in this case, was so interesting as to be worth noting. The total increase in strength of arms was from 257 to 855 pounds ; in the legs, from 251 to 1058 pounds ; in the trunk, from 161 to 712 pounds ; in the chest, from 164 to 406 pounds : by which it appears that the arms had increased in strength seventy per cent; the legs, seventy-six per cent ; the trunk, seventy-seven per cent; and the chest, or respiratory muscles, sixty per cent. The greatest gain was in the trunk muscles, which I have almost uniformly found to be the case, as this is the weakest point with women suffering from displacement of the abdominal and pelvic viscera. Figures 93 and 94, Plate XXXIV, show the change which took place in this young woman's figure as the result of her treatment.

Case XLIII.

Miss T., aged twenty-one years, had been a miserable invalid for a number of years, having suffered extreme pain at the menstrual period, and being subject to constant headache, a great number of neurasthenic symptoms, and extreme nervousness. Examination showed the following conditions: Prolapse of stomach and bowels; movable right kidney; great tenderness of the abdominal sympathetic, and especially of the renal plexus and lumbar ganglia; the uterus in an abnormal position, and the left ovary prolapsed and exceedingly sensitive; congestion of all the pelvic viscera. After a few months' treatment, in which massage and exercise were the most prominent agents, although electricity and other means were employed, the patient returned home enjoying perfect health. The ovaries were in position and not sensitive. The stomach and bowels were elevated to nearly their normal position. The right kidney remained in place so long as the patient maintained a correct posture. Her stomach, which had been exceedingly foul, was clean, and the patient was relieved of all her previous symptoms of ill health. Since that time, now some three years, she has been constantly engaged in ordinary household employments without injury. In this patient the total strength increased in three months from 1004 pounds to 2647 pounds. The waist measure increased two and one half inches.

Case XLIV.

Miss L., aged twenty-two years, had for a number of years been a student at a boarding school. At the time I first saw her, she had been for several years a confirmed invalid, had suffered extremely, and was very nervous. I think I have never met a patient who suffered more severely from menstrual pains and dysmenorrhœa. She was so reduced in flesh as to be scarcely able to walk; had been under the care of leading New York gynæcologists, but without benefit. At the end of twelve months, by the careful employment of massage and other measures, with physical training, she returned home the picture of health, free from pain, without ovarian tenderness, which had been extreme, and able to walk several miles without injury or discomfort. Two months later she resumed her studies in the advanced classical course of a well-known college.

Case XLV.

Miss A., aged twenty-six, had been a confirmed invalid for a number of years; had suffered from severe dysmenorrhœa, and the menstrual pain was increasing from month to month. She had become extremely nervous, hysterical, and generally hyperæsthetic. Examination showed tenderness of the spine the whole length, the slightest touch being extremely painful; and the same was practically true of all portions of the body. The uterus and both ovaries were prolapsed, and the latter were extremely sensitive. There was also prolapse of the stomach and bowels. In addition to the symptoms mentioned, the patient was subject to very severe headaches, a symptom which I have found very common in these cases. I believe these headaches to be due, however, not to the ovarian disease, but to the accompanying stomach disorder, for the relief of which massage and careful regulation of the dietary are among the most efficient means of treatment. This patient was under treatment for four months, during which time physical culture, massage, Swedish movements, hydrotherapy, and electricity were employed, either in conjunction or consecutively, and with the result that at the end of the period named, I was able to send the patient home to her friends in excellent health. The menstrual suffering had entirely ceased. The patient's flesh and blood had increased so that she had become the picture of health. There was still slight ovarian tenderness, but it was disappearing so rapidly that there was every reason to believe it would be entirely gone in a very short time. Unfavorable conditions caused a partial relapse after the patient reached home, but a return to the same methods of treatment resulted ultimately in complete and permanent recovery.

Case XLVI.

Miss B., aged thirty-six years, entered the Sanitarium in February, 1893. She had never been well, and was so weak, anæmic, and emaciated that she was supposed to be suffering from serious lung trouble, for which she had been under treatment for some time. Diagnosis of some pulmonary disease was favored by a night cough. Examination showed the following conditions: Prolapse of the stomach; hyperæsthesia of the left lumbar ganglion and solar plexus; right kidney floating; both ovaries extremely sensitive. Examination of the stomach fluid showed hyperpepsia, with fermentation. After less than two months' application of massage and other treatment appropriate to the case, the patient went home improved in every particular; in fact, was so greatly changed for the better that she considered herself in excellent health.

Case XLVII.

Miss E., aged twenty-four, entered the Sanitarium in August, 1892. She had been a chronic invalid for many years, and had despaired of recovery. Her principal symptoms were general nervousness, exhaustion, and severe pelvic pains. Local examination showed left ovary to be extremely sensitive and prolapsed. The patient remained under treatment a little less than three months, at the end of which time she returned home with no trace of pelvic disease, and enjoying excellent health. This patient nearly doubled her muscular strength while under treatment, the aggregate lifting capacity of the muscles being increased from 1365 to 2350 pounds. In this case, as in a great majority of those of this kind, the greatest proportion of gain was in the muscles of the trunk. The gain in strength for the several parts of the body was as follows: Arms, from 414 to 571 pounds; legs, from 674 to 1168 pounds; trunk, from 197 to 451 pounds; chest, from 80 to 160 pounds. Massage of the muscles of the trunk and abdomen plays a very important part in a systematic course of treatment for the development of this part of the body, the weakness of which is one of the principal causes of disease in women.

Case XLVIII.

Miss B., aged twenty-five, entered the Sanitarium as a patient in July, 1891. She had been more or less an invalid ever since her twelfth year, having suffered from pelvic inflammation at various times, and from the beginning of menstruation at the age of twelve, from severe menstrual pain. Examination showed retrocession of the uterus; ovarian sensitiveness and congestion; prolapsed stomach and bowels; and floating right kidney. By the employment of abdominal massage, manual and mechanical Swedish movements, and a carefully conducted course of physical training, together with other appropriate treatment, the patient was, at the end of four and a half months, able to leave the Sanitarium in the enjoyment of very good health. The menstrual pain had ceased; ovarian irritation had disappeared; the stomach and bowels were well held in position, and there had been a gain in strength of from 1600 pounds to 3000 pounds. The gain in symmetry was even more remarkable than the gain in physical strength, as is well shown by the physical chart obtained in this case (Chart I). The radical improvement made in this patient's health has been permanent.

Case XLIX.

Miss. T., aged thirty-three, entered the Sanitarium as a patient in September, 1892. She had been an invalid for a long time ; had suffered greatly from ovarian pain and the usual accompanying symptoms,—general neurasthenia, hyperæsthesia of the spine, and hysteria. The patient was in an extremely wretched and helpless condition. In two months she returned to her home, having been absolutely free from pain for several weeks, and with entire relief from pelvic symptoms.

CASE L.

Miss X., aged forty-three, was received at the Sanitarium as a patient in July, 1893. She had been an invalid since her sixteenth year; had suffered from menstrual pain and leucorrhœal discharge ; right kidney palpable and sensitive; stomach prolapsed; uterus in retrocession; right ovary prolapsed and tender; left ovary prolapsed and very sensitive, and more than double the normal size. The slightest attempt to replace the uterus and ovaries gave extreme pain. At the end of six weeks, the patient had gained several hundred pounds in strength. The pelvic pains had disappeared. The digestion, which had formerly been very much disturbed, was greatly improved, and the patient had begun to enjoy good health. Pelvic and abdominal massage played the most important part in the cure of this case.

CASE LI.

Miss M., thirty-two years of age, became a patient in the institution in July, 1893. She had suffered for years from a great variety of nervous disturbances, which were mostly neurasthenic in character. Some of the most troublesome symptoms were a severe burning sensation of the spine, a constant ringing sound in the head, and great distress at the base of the brain. She had suffered also from severe dysmenorrhœa. On examination, I found the stomach prolapsed; extreme sensitiveness of the left lumbar ganglion of the sympathetic; right kidney movable; left ovary large, prolapsed, and tender. Examination of the stomach fluid showed that the patient was suffering from hyperpepsia, with fermentation. General and local massage, abdominal massage, Swedish gymnastics, apparatus work in the gymnasium, also general and local baths, applications of galvanic, faradic, and the sinusoidal electrical currents, together with the establishment of a suitable dietary, resulted in the restoration of this patient to good health in the course of a few months.

CASE LII.

Miss H., aged seventeen, came to the Sanitarium in December, 1893. This patient was sent from a distant State by her physician, for the removal of the ovaries, as she had suffered from severe dysmenorrhœa from the very beginning of menstruation, which first appeared two years previous, at the age of fifteen. The periods were irregular, the flow profuse; and pain, which was excruciating during the menstrual period, was constantly present between the periods to such an extent that the patient was practically disabled. The patient complained of a dragging sensation in the pelvis, and four weeks previous had suffered from what her family physician believed to be an abscess of the left ovary. Examination showed anteflexion of the uterus, with extreme sensitiveness of both ovaries. The patient also suffered from indigestion, was extremely anæmic and weak; and she, as well as her parents, was very desirous that the operation of ovariotomy should be performed without delay. Indeed, the patient seemed very much disappointed when I informed her that I thought ovariotomy not necessary in her case, but that she could probably be cured without the adoption of any such radical measures. Curettement relieved the profuse flow. The patient was gradually gotten upon her feet, and trained to active exercise in the gymnasium, taking daily breathing exercises, Swedish gymnastics, apparatus work, and mechanical Swedish movements, in addition to massage, baths, and electrical applications. Especial attention was given to pelvic massage, which was certainly a very important agent in securing a rapid disappearance of painful symptoms. In fact, the patient improved so rapidly that within a month all thought of a serious surgical operation was abandoned.

A little more than five months after her arrival, the patient was dismissed. She no longer suffered from pain at her menstrual periods, or at any time; had gained twenty pounds in flesh; and gave every indication of the enjoyment of absolutely perfect health, which condition continues to the present time.

CASE LIII.

Miss S., aged twenty-nine, was received in June, 1894. For the last eight months she had suffered extremely from constant pelvic pain. The spine was extremely sensitive; all the pelvic viscera were congested; the patient complained of a bearing-down pain, constant and severe headache, neuralgia, and a great variety of nervous symptoms. She was extremely anæmic and very weak, having been confined to the bed for nearly six months; had also severe dysmenorrhœa and menorrhagia. She had suffered several attacks of severe pelvic inflammation, and had steadily grown worse for months, until recovery was almost despaired of. Examination of the urine showed renal insufficiency, the amount of urea eliminated being but 5.86 grams, while the total solids were 18.63, indicating tissue waste and deficient elimination. Digestion was very greatly disturbed; there was no appetite. The patient was much emaciated. The same measures employed in the preceding case were adopted in this case also, and with equal success, although the progress was not quite so rapid. Especial attention was given to

18

abdominal and pelvic massage. The stomach symptoms were relieved by a diet of kumyss (New Era Kumyss). The following notes were made of the case two months after the patient was received for treatment:—

"Her appetite is good; she is able to take ordinary food, has gained in flesh; the menorrhagia has disappeared, also the neuralgia and general neurasthenic symptoms; the patient is well established on her feet, and no longer suffers from ovarian pain either at the menstrual period or at other times, and expects to return in a short time to her field of labor as a foreign missionary." The patient has since remained well.

CASE LIV.

Miss C., aged thirty, was first examined in June, 1892. The patient's general health was fair, but she had suffered for many years from severe dysmenorrhœa and constant ovarian pain, which had in part disabled her, so that she was not able to do ordinary housework, which had been her occupation. The patient did not at that time come under the writer's care for treatment, but fell into the hands of other physicians. In June, 1894, she was sent to me by her physician for the performance of the operation of ovariotomy, constant treatment having failed to cure her, or to prevent a steady decline. On examination, I found she was in every respect worse, having been for a year completely disabled. The ovaries were much enlarged, prolapsed, and sensitive. All the tissues about the uterus were in a hypersensitive condition, and the pelvic vessels throbbing. The patient was placed under treatment similar to that employed in other like cases, special prominence being given, however, to pelvic massage, which was employed every other day. After the third treatment the patient was relieved to a very marked degree, and after three weeks' treatment she was able to engage in vigorous work in a laundry, doing both washing and ironing, which she had not been able to do for more than two years. The menorrhagia and dysmenorrhœa, which had been very severe, had entirely disappeared. She was not obliged to stop work even during the menstrual period, although previously for several years she had been obliged to call a physician, and had habitually taken morphia at that time to relieve the severe menstrual pain. The patient's improved health has continued to the present time (April, 1895), and she pronounces herself in perfect health.

When medical men come to appreciate the fact that *patients*, not simply *maladies*, are to be treated ; that the woman suffering from functional ovarian disease needs, not simply the treatment of her diseased ovaries, but to be made a better "animal,"— a more vigorous, less sensitive, and more highly vitalized woman,—a vast number of women who now languish on beds of suffering, or drag out lives made miserable by chronic invalidism and perpetual local treatment, will be restored to health and usefulness; and a very large number of young women who are now subjected to the operation of ovariotomy, will escape the surgeon's knife, and become happy wives and mothers. Massage, manual Swedish movements, and gymnastics will be found to contribute more to the cure of these cases than any other one class of therapeutic means.

Case LV.

Fractures.— Mrs. P——, a lady about forty years of age, in attempting to enter a street-car, slipped and fell upon the ice, breaking the tibia and fibula just above the right ankle joint. The displacement was very great, and the ligaments were torn to such an extent that it was impossible to restore and maintain perfect symmetry of the limb, although this was accomplished as perfectly as possible by means of a properly adjusted splint. Fomentations were applied for an hour or two before the application of the splint A snug bandage was then applied to the limb, and the splint adjusted. After the fourth day the splint was removed daily, fomentations or hot and cold applications were made, and massage was carefully administered (for method see page 51 and paragraph 385). The case looked to be a very unpromising one, but an excellent recovery occurred. In a few weeks the patient was on her feet, and after a few months, during which time massage was quite persistently employed, the function of the joint was perfectly restored. The ankle joint was not at any time allowed to become stiffened by disuse.

Case LVI.

Ununited Fractures.— Mr. A——, a young man aged thirty years, from Idaho, presented an ununited fracture of the humerus, the result of a gunshot wound. About two inches of bone had been lost, shortening the humerus to that extent. Three operations had been performed, two of them by distinguished surgeons, but the fracture was still ununited. The muscles had wasted away, and the arm was practically useless. The elbow joint was completely stiffened as the result of long immobilization, to which the arm had been subjected. The patient was apparently in fair general health, but he was nevertheless subjected to a course of vigorous tonic baths, special attention being given to the improvement of the nutrition of the arm by means of fomentations, the hot and cold douche, and especially by the application of massage. After a few

weeks an incision was made, and it was found that there had been
no attempt whatever at union, though the ends of the bone had
apparently been nicely adjusted and secured together. The ends
of the bone were irritated by erosion, and another wire was introduced at right angles to the first. The wound was closed, and
motion was restored to the stiffened elbow by forcible flexion and
extension. The wound healed by immediate union, and at the end
of a week the baths and massage were resumed with the result
that solid union was obtained, and the patient sent home with a
useful arm.

CASE LVII.

Mr. H——, aged twenty-six years, sustained a severe compound
fracture of the left humerus as a result of a railroad accident. He
was received into a hospital in the Eastern city where the accident
occurred. After a few weeks he was discharged, but upon subse-
quent examination it was found that no union had taken place. The
patient urged an operation, but instead was encouraged to believe
that union might be secured by means of massage, which was applied daily, and with the result that at the end of three months
solid union had been obtained, and a few months later the patient
pronounced his arm as good as ever. The arm was not immobilized,
but care was taken to give it some support by means of a sling, so
that an excessive amount of motion might not occur at the point of
fracture.

The philosophy of this method of treating fractures is that it
improves the nutrition, encourages the circulation, and stimulates all
the vital activities of the affected parts, and thus promotes a healthy
and efficient reparative action.

APPENDIX II.

The so-called Schott method of treatment, employed by the Schott brothers, of Nauheim, Germany, in connection with the effervescing chloride of calcium baths, has acquired a great reputation, not only in Germany, but in England, where it is now much in vogue, especially in hospitals and sanitariums.

While this method is as yet little employed in this country, and seems to have been practically unknown in Germany until introduced by the brothers Schott, it is but fair to state that it presents no features essentially different from the system of manual Swedish movements which has for more than fifty years been employed in Sweden, Norway, and Denmark, by the practitioners of the so-called Ling, or Swedish, system of curative gymnastics.

Although we have no definite knowledge upon the subject, we feel confident that careful inquiry into the origin of the "Nauheim treatment" would show it to have been derived from the Swedish system. Great credit is due to the Schott brothers for having so thoroughly systematized the method, and for having by persevering and successful effort brought it to the attention of the medical profession in so favorable a manner as to command attention and respect. Under this form, the writer has for the last twenty years employed gymnastics in the treatment of cardiac affections. The exact procedure, as the system is now in use at the Battle Creek Sanitarium, under the author's direction, may be thus briefly described : —

Exercise.— Each of the following movements is taken with resistance in both directions.

1. Arms forward stretch, sidewise moving, returning.

2. Arms downward stretch, forearm flexion and extension.

3. Arms downward stretch, forward upward moving, returning.

4. Fingers flexed, knuckles in contact at umbilicus, arms raising to vertex, returning.

5. Arms downward stretch, forward raising to upward stretch.

6. Trunk forward bending; resistance, (*a*) hands sternum and loins; (*b*) hand at upper spine.

7. Trunk rotating; resistance (*a*) left hand in front of patient's right shoulder, right hand behind patient's left shoulder; (*b*) reversed.

8. Lateral trunk flexion; resistance, attendant in front of patient, (*a*) right hand under patient's left arm, left hand on patient's right hip; (*b*) reverse.

9. Same as 1, except fist firmly clenched.

10. Same as 2, except palmar surface is turned out, and fist firmly closed during exercise.

11. Arm circumduction, one arm at a time.

12. Arms backward raising — trunk must not bend forward.

13. Knee raising, body balanced by support of opposite hand.

14. Leg forward and backward raising.

15. Leg backward flexing; hand support.

16. Leg outward raising.

17. Arms rotating, extreme degree.

18. Wrist flexion and extension.

19. Foot flexion and extension.

RULES PERTAINING TO EXERCISE.

1. Movements must be slow and uniform.

2. Follow each movement by an interval of rest.

3. Movements of the same limb or group of muscles should not be repeated twice in succession.

4. Movements should be immediately interrupted if any of the following symptoms appear, and the patient must be watched closely to avoid the development of these signs, which indicate exhaustion : —

(1) Accelerated breathing.

(2) Marked movements of the nares in breathing.

(3) Slight drawing of the corners of the mouth.

(4) Pallor or duskiness of the cheeks or lips.

(5) Palpitation of the heart.

(6) Sweating.

(7) Yawning.

If any of the above signs should appear in the midst of the movement, the exercise must be instantly suspended, the limbs being carefully placed in a state of rest.

5. The patient should not be allowed to hold the breath. To prevent this the patient should count in a whisper from 1 to 8 while the movement is being executed, or during each half of it.

6. Constriction of the limbs or any other portion of the body whereby the blood-vessels may be compressed, must be carefully avoided.

7. The force of the movement must be very carefully graduated to the strength of the patient. It is sometimes necessary to employ only the very gentlest resistance. Patients who are bedridden, and those who are very feeble cannot at first take all the movements, but must take only such as are adapted to their condition or strength.

8. Examination of the heart should be very carefully made in every case before beginning treatment. In cases of emphysema, asthma, and in obstruction of the aortic orifice, great care must be taken, especially with the arm-raising movement, to avoid producing syncope, on account of the obstruc-

tion of the pulmonary circulation. The same rule applies to
any condition in which the respiratory area is diminished, as in
pleurisy with effusion, consolidation of the lung, dropsy of the
chest, pyothorax, or pneumothorax.

9. In these cases the movements must be executed very
slowly, so as to give time for the distribution of the blood.
They may have to be taken while the patient is lying down.
The right side of the heart being overloaded in these cases, the
arm movement should not at first extend above the level of the
shoulders, unless the patient is reclining, as the extension of
the right heart would be increased by giving the blood the
down grade in the arteries.

10. Special attention should be given also to the patient's
regimen and diet by enforcing an aseptic dietary. Such exercise as graduated mountain climbing is too severe for patients
requiring this treatment. It is only adapted to cases which
have made considerable advancement toward a cure. The object of the method is not to strengthen the muscles, but to
regulate the circulation.

11. The patient may, to some extent, administer the exercise himself, by executing the various movements, producing
the resistance by hardening the muscle, as though working
against the resistant force.

Baths.—The purpose of the baths is to dilate the
peripheral and stimulate the arterial circulation.

The bath contains graduated quantities of chloride of sodium
and chloride of calcium, as follows : —

Chloride of sodium 1%, chloride of calcium 2%.

Chloride of sodium 2%, chloride of calcium 3%.

Chloride of sodium 3%, chloride of calcium 5%.

Effervescence in three grades is produced by adding sodium
bicarbonate and hydrochloric acid in varying quantities as follows: —

Sodium bicarbonate $\frac{1}{2}$lb., hydrochloric acid (25%) $\frac{3}{4}$lb.

Sodium bicarbonate 1lb., hydrochloric acid (25%) 1½lbs.

Sodium bicarbonate 2lbs., hydrochloric acid (25%) 3lbs.

If a copper tub is used, one-fourth extra amount of bicarbonate should be employed to protect the copper from corrosion.

In mixing the ingredients, first dissolve the bicarbonate of soda in water in the tub. Then, for slow effervescence place the bottle containing the acid, with stopper removed, at the bottom of the bath, laying it down upon the bottom, and moving it around from time to time. The bath will be ready in two or three hours. For rapid effervescence, invert the bottle without removing the stopper, place the mouth of the bottle just below the surface of the water, withdraw the stopper, and move the bottle about over the surface of the bath, so as to distribute a uniform layer of acid. By this means the bath is prepared in five minutes. The temperature of the bath should be 92° F.

Generally the bath should be taken only two or three days in succession, one day's respite being allowed. With stronger persons four or five successive baths may be given. The chloride of calcium and the chloride of sodium increase the skin excitation. The effect of the bath should be to slow the pulse, to lessen the area of cardiac dullness, and to increase the force of the pulse. Examination of the cardiac area should be made before the bath, and marked on the chart, a diagram being preserved in each case. Sphygmographic tracing of the pulse should also be made, the pulse pressure being determined with Oliver's sphygmo-dynamometer.

INDEX.

www.ingramcontent.com/pod-product-compliance
Lightning Source LLC
Chambersburg PA
CBHW030002290326
41934CB00005B/199